Psoriatic Arthritis and Psoriasis

Adewale Adebajo
Wolf-Henning Boehncke
Dafna D. Gladman • Philip J. Mease
Editors

Psoriatic Arthritis and Psoriasis

Pathology and Clinical Aspects

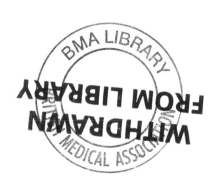

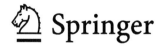

Springer

Editors
Adewale Adebajo
Faculty of Medicine
University of Sheffield
Sheffield
UK

Wolf-Henning Boehncke
Faculty of Medicine
University of Geneva
Geneva
Switzerland

Dafna D. Gladman
Toronto Western Hospital
Toronto, ON
Canada

Philip J. Mease
Seattle Rheumatology Associates
Seattle, WA
USA

ISBN 978-3-319-19529-2   ISBN 978-3-319-19530-8   (eBook)
DOI 10.1007/978-3-319-19530-8

Library of Congress Control Number: 2015960252

Springer Cham Heidelberg New York Dordrecht London

Printed on acid-free paper

Springer International Publishing AG Switzerland is part of Springer Science+Business Media (www.springer.com)

Preface

The last decade has seen a significant increase in our understanding of the burden of disease as well as the pathogenesis of both psoriasis and psoriatic arthritis. This has been paralleled by the development of new approaches to the assessment of, and novel therapies for these diseases.

Organizations such as the Group for Research and Assessment of Psoriasis and Psoriatic Arthritis (GRAPPA) have been at the forefront of education and research into these conditions, alongside other interested international and national organizations.

This new textbook addresses these advances and provides a state-of-the-art resource for psoriasis and psoriatic arthritis. Generalists and specialists, researchers and clinicians, together with other health care professionals who look after patients with these conditions will benefit from this textbook.

This comprehensive and authoritative textbook, written by experts in the field and supported by GRAPPA, is consequently an important resource in the assessment and management of psoriasis and psoriatic arthritis.

We particularly wish to acknowledge the various contributors to this textbook. In addition, however, we also want to thank the wider community of GRAPPA members and beyond. This textbook is a legacy to their commitment in advancing knowledge in the fields of psoriasis and psoriatic arthritis.

We also wish to thank the various members of staff of Springer who were involved in the production of this textbook.

Lastly, and most importantly, we wish to pay tribute to the many patients with these conditions who daily inspire us.

Sheffield, UK   Adewale Adebajo
Geneva, Switzerland   Wolf-Henning Boehncke
Toronto, ON, Canada   Dafna D. Gladman
Seattle, WA, USA   Philip J. Mease

Contents

Contributors

Ade Adebajo, FRCP, FACP, FAcMed Faculty of Medicine, Dentistry and Health, University of Sheffield, Sheffield, UK

Magaly Alva, MD Department of Rheumatology, H. Edgardo Rebagliati Martins, Lima, Peru

April W. Armstrong, MD, MPH Department of Dermatology, University of Colorado Denver, Aurora, CO, USA

Frank Behrens, MD Department of Rheumatology, University Hospital of Frankfurt, Frankfurt, Germany

Chiara Bertolazzi, MD Department of Rheumatology, Clinica Reumatologica, Università Politecnica delle Marche, Jesi, Ancona, Italy

Wolf-Henning Boehncke, MD, MA Service de Dermatologie et Vénéréologie, Hopitaux Universitaires de Genève, Geneve, Switzerland

Erica Bromberg, BA Department of Dermatology, Psoriasis Clinical Trials, University of Pittsburgh Medical Center, Pittsburgh, PA, USA

Laura Coates, MBChB, MCRP, PhD Leeds Institute of Rheumatic and Musculoskeletal Medicine, University of Leeds and Leeds Musculoskeletal Biomedical Research Unit, Leeds Teaching Hospitals NHS Trust, Leeds, UK

Kurt de Vlam, MD, PhD Department of Rheumatology, University Hospitals Leuven, Leuven, Belgium

Kristina Callis Duffin, MD Department of Dermatology, University of Utah, Salt Lake City, UT, USA

Lihi Eder, MD, PhD Department of Medicine, Centre for Prognosis Studies in the Rheumatic Diseases, Toronto Western Hospital, Toronto, ON, Canada

Luis R. Espinoza, MD Internal Medicine, Section of Rheumatology, LSU Health Sciences Center, New Orleans, LA, USA

María Laura Acosta Felquer, MD Rheumatology Unit, Internal Medical Service, Hospital Italiano de Buenos Aires, Capital Federal, Buenos Aires, Argentina

Bing-Jian Feng, PhD Department of Dermatology, University of Utah, Salt Lake City, UT, USA

Laura Korb Ferris, MD, PhD Department of Dermatology, University of Pittsburgh, Pittsburgh, PA, USA

Aleksandra Florek, MD Department of Dermatology, Northwestern University, Chicago, IL, USA

Dafna D. Gladman, MD, FRCPC Psoriatic Arthritis Program, Toronto Western Hospital, University Health Network, Toronto, ON, Cananda

Daniel Glinatsi, MD Center for Rheumatology and Spine Diseases, Rigshospitalet Glostrup, Copenhagen Center for Arthritis Research, Copenhagen, Denmark

Alice B. Gottlieb, MD, PhD Department of Dermatology, Tufts Medical Center, Boston, MA, USA

Marwin Gutierrez, MD Department of Rheumatology, Instituto Nacional de Rehabilitacion, Mexico City, Mexico

Nigil Haroon, MD, PhD Department of Medicine and Rheumatology, Toronto Western Hospital, University Health Network, University of Toronto, Toronto, ON, Canada

Jason E. Hawkes, MD Department of Dermatology, University of Utah, Salt Lake City, UT, USA

Philip H. Helliwell, MD, PhD Leeds Institute of Rheumatic and Musculoskeletal Medicine, University of Leeds, Leeds, UK

Deepak R. Jadon, MBBCh, MRCP Department of Rheumatology, Royal National Hospital for Rheumatic Diseases, Bath, UK

Bruce Kirkham, BA, MD, FRACP, FRCP Department of Rheumatology, Guy's & St Thomas' NHS Foundation Trust, Guy's Hospital, London, UK

Michaela Koehm, MD Department of Rheumatology, University Hospital of Frankfurt, Frankfurt, Germany

Rik J. Lories, MD, PhD Laboratory of Tissue Homeostasis and Disease, Skeletal Biology and Engineering Research Center, KU Leuven, Leuven, Belgium

Neil John McHugh, MBChB, MD, FRCP, FRCPath Pharmacy and Pharmacology, University of Bath, Bath, Bane, UK

Philip J. Mease, MD Department of Rheumatology, Swedish Medical Center, Seattle, WA, USA

Jacqueline Moreau, MD, MS Department of Internal Medicine, University of Pittsburgh Medical Center, Pittsburgh, PA, USA

Barbara Neerinckx, MD Laboratory of Tissue Homeostasis and Disease, Skeletal Biology and Engineering Research Center, KU Leuven, Leuven, Belgium

Darren D. O'Rielly, PhD, FCCMG Faculty of Medicine, Memorial University, St. John's, NL, Canada

Mikkel Østergaard, MD, PhD, DMSc Center for Rheumatology and Spine Diseases, Rigshospitalet Glostrup, Copenhagen Center for Arthritis Research, Copenhagen, Denmark

Rodolfo Perez-Alamino, MD Department of Rheumatology, Hospital Avellaneda, San Miguel De Tucuman, Argentina

Carlos Pineda, MD, MSc Research Department, Instituto Nacional de Rehabilitacion, Mexico City, Mexico

René Panduro Poggenborg, MD, PhD Center for Rheumatology and Spine Diseases, Rigshospitalet Glostrup, Copenhagen Center for Arthritis Research, Copenhagen, Denmark

Proton Rahman, MD, MSc Department of Medicine, Memorial University, St. John's, NL, Canada

Siba P. Raychaudhuri, MD Division of Rheumatology, Allergy & Clinical Immunology, School of Medicine, University of California Davis, Sacramento, CA, USA

Smriti K. Raychaudhuri, MD Division of Dermatology and Immunology, VA Sacramento Medical Center, Sacramento, CA, USA

Christopher Ritchlin, MD, MPH Immunology and Rheumatology Division, University of Rochester Medical Center, Rochester, NY, USA

Javier Rosa, MD Department of Rheumatology, Instituto Universitario Hospital Italiano de Buenos Aires, Buenos Aires, Argentina

Santiago Ruta, MD Rheumatology Unit, Hospital Italiano de Buenos Aires, La Plata, Buenos Aires, Argentina

Percival D. Sampaio-Barros, MD, PHD Division of Rheumatology, Faculdade de Medicina da Universidade de São Paulo, São Paulo, Brazil

Ami R. Saraiya, MD Department of Dermatology, Tufts Medical Center, Boston, MA, USA

Ankit Saxena, PhD Division of Immunology, Department of Pathology, Johns Hopkins University School of Medicine, Baltimore, MD, USA

Bahar Shafaeddin Schreve, MD Faculty of Medicine, University of Geneva, Geneva, Switzerland

Hisham Sharlala, MRCP (Rheumatology) Department of Rheumatology, Barnsley District General Hospital, Barnsley, South Yorkshire, UK

Enrique Roberto Soriano, MD, MSC Department of Rheumatology, Instituto Universitario Hospital Italiano de Buenos Aires, Buenos Aires, Argentina

William J. Taylor, MBChB, PhD, FAFRM, FRACP Department of Medicine, University of Otago Wellington, Wellington, New Zealand

William Tillett, MBChB, BSc, PhD, MRCP Department of Rheumatology, Royal National Hospital for Rheumatic Diseases, Bath, UK

William Tuong, MD Department of Dermatology, University of California Davis, Sacramento, CA, USA

Part I
Historical Aspects

Dafna D. Gladman

Historical Perspectives on Psoriatic Arthritis

Dafna D. Gladman

Abstract

Psoriatic arthritis is defined as an inflammatory musculoskeletal disease associated with psoriasis. First described in the nineteenth century, it was recognized as a unique entity in 1964, following detailed descriptions of the condition by Wright and Moll. Over that past several decades advances in the recognition, prognosis and outcome of psoriatic arthritis have been made, as well as therapeutic interventions which have improved the lives of individuals with this condition.

Keywords

Psoriasis • Psoriatic arthritis • Prognosis • Diagnosis • Pathogenesis

Concept of Psoriatic Arthritis as a Unique Entity

Although Luis Alibert is credited with the first description of psoriatic arthritis in 1818, Thomas Bateman actually reported on arthritis among psoriasis patients in 1813 [1, 2]. Subsequently, in 1860, Piere Bazin described "psoriasis arthritique". This was followed in 1888 by a report on "psoriasis et arthropathies" by Charles Bourdillon. Jeghers and Robinson described psoriatic arthritis as a unique entity in 1937, but in

1939 Walter Bauer found "little justification for considering these patients as suffering from a distinct disease entity". Vilanova and Pinol disagreed and described psoriatic arthritis as an entity in 1951 [3].

Despite this earlier recognition of psoriatic arthritis as a unique form of arthritis, it was the seminal papers of the late Professor Verna Wright of Leeds, England that psoriatic arthritis became widely recognized. Wright published on psoriasis and arthritis first in 1956 and re-evaluated the subject again in 1959, when he also performed a comparative study of rheumatoid arthritis, psoriasis and arthritis associated with psoriasis [4, 5]. A more detailed comparison of patients with rheumatoid arthritis and psoriatic arthritis followed [6]. Based on Wright's work the American Rheumatism Association (now known as the

D.D. Gladman, MD, FRCPC
Psoriatic Arthritis Program, Toronto Western Hospital, University Health Network,
399 Bathurst Street, Toronto, ON 1E-410B, Cananda
e-mail: dafna.gladman@utoronto.ca

© Springer International Publishing Switzerland 2016
A. Adebajo et al. (eds.), *Psoriatic Arthritis and Psoriasis: Pathology and Clinical Aspects*,
DOI 10.1007/978-3-319-19530-8_1

American College of Rheumatology) recognized psoriatic arthritis as a distinct entity in 1964 [7].

John Moll joined Verna Wright in Leeds and together they continued to make important contributions to the field of spondyloarthritis and psoriatic arthritis. Their review paper in 1973 outlined the evidence that supported the concept of psoriatic arthritis as a specific disease entity. They provided evidence from clinical, serological, radiological as well as epidemiological studies which confirmed the association between psoriasis and a specific form of arthritis [8].

Over 50 Years of Study of Psoriatic Arthritis

The initial description of psoriatic arthritis depicted the disease as a mild disease. However, studies performed over the past several decades have demonstrated that the disease is much more severe that previously thought. Moll and Wright described the majority of patients with psoriatic arthritis presenting with oligoarthritis. Although Wright described a mutilating form of arthritis, it was thought to occur in only 5 % of the cases, and the majority of patients presented with oligoarthritis. However, subsequent studies have shown that the majority of patients with psoriatic arthritis have polyarticular involvement. Helliewll et al actually developed a mathematical model demonstrating that the more joints are involved the more likely symmetric the disease might be [9]. It was first noted in 1987 that psoriatic arthritis is a severe disease [10]. Of the first 220 patients registered in the Toronto longitudinal observational cohort 67 % had at least one erosion, and 20 % developed clinical deformities and marked radiological damage resulting in functional disability. Over a 10-year follow up it was noted that 55 % of the patients developed ≥5 deformities [11]. Progression of erosions was also noted over a 5-year period by McHugh et al. [12]. A study of psoriatic arthritis patients presenting within 10 months of onset of symptoms revealed that 27 % of the patients already had at least one erosion, and by 2 years of follow-up 47 % of the patients developed erosive disease [13].

Indeed the severity of psoriatic arthritis was noted to be similar to that of rheumatoid arthritis, both in terms of radiographic damage and in terms of patient reported outcomes [14–16]. Helliwell has also demonstrated that polyarticular disease in psoriatic arthritis is more similar to oligoarticular psoriatic disease than to rheumatoid arthritis [17].

Polyarticular presentation was identified as a predictor for future deformities and erosions [18, 19]. Moreover, the number of actively inflamed joints at each visit, as well as elevated erythrocyte sedimentation rate, predict progression of clinical and radiological damage at subsequent visits [20, 21]. In addition, the number of damaged joints is an independent predictor of subsequent clinical and radiological damage. Digits with dactylitis are more likely to have erosive disease than digits without dactylitis [22]. Certain genetic markers are associated with disease progression, including HLA-B27 in the absence of DR7, HLA-B39 and HLA-DQw3 in the absence of DR7, while HLA-B22 is protective [23]. A variant of interleukin 4 (IL4-I50V) is associated with erosive disease in psoriatic arthritis [24].

Further evidence supporting the concept that psoriatic arthritis is a severe disease comes from studies demonstrating increased mortality among patients with psoriatic arthritis compared to the general population [25]. Although there appears to be a trend towards improved survival, the standardized mortality ratio is still elevated at 1.36 [26, 27]. Causes of death are primarily related to cardiovascular and respiratory problems as well as injuries/poisonings. Predictors for mortality are more active and severe disease at presentation [28].

Psoriatic arthritis impairs quality of life and function as measured by the Health Assessment Questionnaire (HAQ) and the Medical Outcome Survey Short Form 36 (SF-36) [29–31]. It was further demonstrated that the SF-36 is more sensitive to change than other instruments [32]. The HAQ varies over time in patients with psoriatic arthritis. Worsening HAQ scores are associated with female gender, longer disease duration and higher actively inflamed joint counts whereas improvement is related to shorter disease duration and lower number of joints involved at onset [33].

It has become clear that patients with psoriatic arthritis need to be identified and treated early in order to avoid these untoward outcomes. Patients seen in clinic within 2 years of diagnosis had less damage progression than those seen later in their course, and even a delay of 6 months in consultation led to more severe disease [34, 35]. There are a number of clinical features which can help identify patients with psoriasis destined to develop arthritis, including severity of psoriasis, certain sites such as scalp and intergluteal areas, and the presence of nail disease. In addition, there are genetic factors which have been identified, in particular HLA alleles [36, 37].

In recent years several studies have identified genes associated with psoriasis and psoriatic arthritis [38]. At the same time studies into environmental factors which may play a role in the etiology of psoriatic arthritis have also been performed, and suggest that infection and trauma play a role [39, 40]. Several studies have concentrated on elucidating the factors responsible for the pathogenesis of psoriatic arthritis [41, 42].

Major advances in the management of psoriatic arthritis have been achieved in the past 15 years. Understanding the pathogenesis of the disease, attention to outcome measures to be included in clinical trials, and the availability of a number of medications which work for both skin and joint manifestations of the disease have contributed to these. In addition, the development of international collaboration through the Group for Research and Assessment of Psoriasis and Psoriatic Arthritis (GRAPPA) have facilitated further work and provided evidence based recommendation for management of patients with psoriatic arthritis. The accomplishments of GRAPPA are reviewed in the next chapter.

References

1. O'Neill T, Silman AJ. Historical background and epidemiology. In: Wright V, Helliwell P, editors. Psoriatic arthritis in Baillière's clinical rheumatology. International Practice and Research. London: Baillière's Tindall; 1994. 8, p. 245–61.

2. Benedek TG. Psoriasis and psoriatic arthropathy, historical aspects: part I. J Clin Rheumatol. 2013;19: 193–8.

3. Vilanova X, Pinol J. Psoriasis arhtopathica. Rheumatism. 1951;7:197–208.

4. Wright V. Psoriasis and arthritis. Ann Rheum Dis. 1956;15:348–56.

5. Wright V. Rheumatism and psoriasis a re-evaluation. Am J Med. 1959;27:454–62.

6. Wright V. Psoriatic arhtirtis: a caomparative study of rheumatoid arthritis, psoriasis and arthritis associated with psoriasis. AMA Arch Derm. 1959;80:27–35.

7. Blumberg BS, Bunim JJ, Calkins E, Pirani CL, Zvaifler NJ. ARA nomenclature and classification of arthritis and rheumatism (tentative). Arhtritis Rheum. 1964;7:93–7.

8. Moll JMH, Wright V. Psoriatic arthritis. Semin Arthritis Rheum. 1973;3:55–78.

9. Helliwell PS, Hetthen J, Sokoll K, Green M, Marchesoni A, Lubrano E, et al. Joint symmetry in early and late rheumatoid and psoriatic arthritis: comparison with a mathematical model. Arthritis Rheum. 2000;43:865–71.

10. Gladman DD, Shuckett R, Russell ML, Thorne JC, Schachter RK. Psoriatic arthritis – clinical and laboratory analysis of 220 patients. Quart J Med. 1987;62: 127–41.

11. Gladman DD. The natural history of psoriatic arthritis. In: Wright V, Helliwell PS, editors. Psoriatic arthritis in Baillière's clinical rheumatology. International Practice and Research. London: Baillière's Tindall; 1994. p. 379–94.

12. McHugh NJ, Balachrishnan C, Jones SM. Progression of peripheral joint disease in psoriatic arthritis: a 5-yr prospective study. Rheumatology (Oxford). 2003;42: 778–83.

13. Kane D, Stafford L, Bresniham B, Fitzgerald O. A prospective, clinical and radiological study of early psoriatic arthritis: an early synovitis clinic experience. Rheumatology. 2003;42:1460–8.

14. Husted JA, Gladman DD, Farewell VT, Cook R. Health-related quality of life of patients with psoriatic arthritis: a comparison with patients with rheumatoid arthritis. Arthritis Care Res. 2001;45: 151–8.

15. Rahman P, Nguyen E, Cheung C, Schentag C, Gladman DD. Comparison of radiological severity in psoriatic arthritis and rheumatoid arthritis. J Rheumatol. 2001;28:1041–4.

16. Sokoll KB, Helliwell PS. Comparison of disability and quality of life in rheumatoid and psoriatic arthritis. J Rheumatol. 2001;28:1842–6.

17. Helliwell PS, Porter G, Taylor WJ. Polyarticular psoriatic arthritis is more like oligoarticular psoriatic arthritis, than rheumatoid arthritis. Ann Rheum Dis. 2007;66:113–7.

18. Gladman DD, Farewell VT, Nadeau C. Clinical indicators of progression in psoriatic arthritis (PSA): multivariate relative risk model. J Rheumatol. 1995;22: 675–9.

19. Queiro-Silva R, Torre-Alonso JC, Tinture-Eguren T, et al. A polyarticular onset predicts erosive and deforming disease in psoriatic arthritis. Ann Rheum Dis. 2003;62:68–70.

20. Gladman DD, Farewell VT. Progression in psoriatic arthritis: role of time varying clinical indicators. J Rheumatol. 1999;26:2409–13.

21. Bond SJ, Farewell VT, Schentag CT, Gladman DD. Predictors for radiological damage in psoriatic arthritis. Results from a single centre. Ann Rheum Dis. 2007;66:370–6.

22. Brockbank J, Stein M, Schentag CT, Gladman DD. Dactylitis in psoriatic arthritis (PsA): a marker for disease severity? Ann Rheum Dis. 2005;62:188–90.

23. Gladman DD, Farewell VT, Kopciuk K, Cook RJ. HLA markers and progression in psoriatic arthritis. J Rheumatol. 1998;25:730–3.

24. Rahman P, Snelgrove T, Peddle L, Siannis F, Farewell V, Schentag C, et al. A variant of the IL4 I50V single-nucleotide polymorphism is associated with erosive joint disease in psoriatic arthritis. Arthritis Rheum. 2008;58:2207–8.

25. Wong K, Gladman DD, Husted J, Long J, Farewell VT. Mortality studies in psoriatic arthritis. Results from a single centre. I. Risk and causes of death. Arthritis Rheum. 1997;40:1868–72.

26. Ali Y, Tom BDM, Schentag CT, Farewell VT, Gladman DD. Improved survival in psoriatic arthritis (PsA) with calendar time. Arthritis Rheum. 2007;56:2708–14.

27. Buckley C, Cavill C, Taylor G, Kay H, Waldron N, Korendowych E, et al. Mortality in psoriatic arthritis – a single-center study from the UK. J Rheumatol. 2010;37:2141–4.

28. Gladman DD, Farewell VT, Husted J, Wong K. Mortality studies in psoriatic arthritis. Results from a single centre. II. Prognostic indicators for mortality. Arthritis Rheum. 1998;41:1103–10.

29. Blackmore M, Gladman DD, Husted J, Long J, Farewell VT. Measuring health status in psoriatic arthritis: the health assessment questionnaire and its modification. J Rheumatol. 1995;22:886–93.

30. Husted J, Gladman DD, Farewell V, Long J. A modified version of the Health Assessment Questionnaire (HAQ) for psoriatic arthritis. Clin Exp Rheumatol. 1995;13:439–44.

31. Husted J, Gladman DD, Long JA, Farewell VT, Cook R. Validating the SF-36 health questionnaire in patients with psoriatic arthritis. J Rheumatol. 1997;24:511–7.

32. Husted JA, Gladman DD, Cook RJ, Farewell VJ. Responsiveness of health status instruments to changes in articular status and perceived health in patients with psoriatic arthritis (PsA). J Rheumatol. 1998;25:2146–55.

33. Husted JA, Brian T, Farewell VT, Schentag CT, Gladman DD. Description and prediction of physical functional disability in Psoriatic Arthritis (PsA): a longitudinal analysis using a Markov model approach. Arthritis Rheum. 2005;53:404–9.

34. Gladman DD, Thavaneswaran A, Chandran V, Cook RJ. Do patients with psoriatic arthritis who present early fare better than those presenting later in the disease? Ann Rheum Dis. 2011;70:2152–4.

35. Haroon M, Gallagher P, Fitzgerald O. Diagnostic delay of more than 6 months contributes to poor radiographic and functional outcome in psoriatic arthritis. Ann Rheum Dis. 2015;74:1045–50.

36. Eder L, Chandran V, Pellet F, Shanmugarajah S, Rosen CF, Bull SB, Gladman DD. Human leukocyte antigen risk alleles for psoriatic arthritis among psoriasis patients. Ann Rheum Dis. 2012;71:50–5.

37. Winchester R, Minevich G, Steshenko V, Kirby B, Kane D, Greenberg DA, et al. HLA associations reveal genetic heterogeneity in psoriatic arthritis and in the psoriasis phenotype. Arthritis Rheum. 2012;64:1134–44.

38. Ellinghaus E, Stuart PE, Ellinghaus D, Nair RP, Debrus S, Raelson JV, et al. Genome-wide meta-analysis of psoriatic arthritis identifies susceptibility locus at REL. J Invest Dermatol. 2012;132:1133–40.

39. Pattison E, Harrison BJ, Griffiths CE, et al. Environmental risk factors for the development of psoriatic arthritis: results from a case–control study. Ann Rheum Dis. 2008;67:672–6.

40. Eder L, Law T, Chandran V, Kalman-Lamb G, Shanmugarajah S, Shen H, et al. The association between environmental factors and onset of psoriatic arthritis in patients with psoriasis. Arthritis Care Res. 2011;63:1091–7.

41. Raychaudhuri SP. A cutting edge overview: psoriatic disease. Clin Rev Allergy Immunol. 2013;44:109–13.

42. Haroon M, Fitzgerald O. Pathogenetic overview of psoriatic disease. J Rheumatol Suppl. 2012;89:7–10.

GRAPPA Historical Perspective

Dafna D. Gladman, Philip J. Mease,
and Philip H. Helliwell

Abstract

The Group for Research and Assessment of Psoriasis and Psoriatic Arthritis (GRAPPA) was established in 2003 as an international collaborative group focused on psoriatic disease. GRAPPA has matured and become the foremost research and education society for psoriasis and psoriatic arthritis in the world, involving dermatologists and rheumatologists from many countries. GRAPPA collaborates with other societies including the ACR, EULAR, SPARTAN, ASAS, and OMERACT in fostering its goals. As an investment in the future, GRAPPA nurtures young researchers and clinicians interested in psoriasis and PsA in order to develop the next generation of leaders in these fields of medicine.

Keywords

Psoriasis • Psoriatic arthritis • GRAPPA • Treatment recommendations
Research • Education

D.D. Gladman, MD, FRCPC (✉)
Psoriatic Arthritis Program,
University Health Network, Toronto Western Hospital, 399 Bathurst Street,
Toronto, ON 1E-410B, Canada
e-mail: dafna.gladman@utoronto.ca

P.J. Mease, MD
Department of Rheumatology,
Swedish Medical Center,
Seattle, WA, USA

P.H. Helliwell, MD, PhD
Leeds Institute of Rheumatic and Musculoskeletal Medicine, University of Leeds, Leeds, UK

GRAPPA is not just a digestive taken after dinner. It is the Group for Research and Assessment of Psoriasis and Psoriatic Arthritis, an international group of clinicians and other stakeholders with a special interest in psoriasis and psoriatic arthritis (PsA), which was established in 2003. The following is a description of the development and launching of GRAPPA, as well as some of its accomplishments in the past 12 years.

GRAPPA was developed following the establishment of the Classification of Psoriatic Arthritis (CASPAR) study group. Initially only several European investigators were included in the study that was initiated by Philip Helliwell to

© Springer International Publishing Switzerland 2016
A. Adebajo et al. (eds.), *Psoriatic Arthritis and Psoriasis: Pathology and Clinical Aspects*,
DOI 10.1007/978-3-319-19530-8_2

develop classification criteria for psoriatic arthritis (PsA). However, at the same time several Italian rheumatologists approached Gladman to develop classification criteria for PsA. Gladman then approached Hermann Mielants, who was European League Against Rheumatism (EULAR) president at the time, who revealed that Philip Helliwell had already set up such a study. Helliwell was approached to increase his study group and the Italians and Gladman were included. Gladman also recommended that several North American centres be included such as Philip Mease and Luis Espinoza. A larger group of investigators was thus assembled and named CASPAR. EULAR provided financial support.

At a meeting of the CASPAR investigators during the International League Against Rheumatism (ILAR) in Edmonton in 2001, the idea of a broader approach to study PsA was brought forth by Philip Mease, who had run an independent investigator trial of etanercept in PsA. Mease was impressed by the way the Ankylosing Spondylitis ASsessment (ASAS) group had developed to further research on anky-losing spondylitis, and suggested that it would be appropriate to broaden the efforts of the CASPAR group to collaboratively advance research on PsA and psoriasis, and work more closely with indus-try to set up a group where people could get to know each other and share research ideas. This was enhanced by an additional meeting with Arthur Kavanaugh and Christian Antoni who were conducting the infliximab trials in PsA. Mease met with Desiree van der Heijde dur-ing the spondyloarthritis congress in Gent in 2002 to discuss whether to incorporate PsA work within ASAS or, because the goal was to have equal involvement with dermatologists, to estab-lish a separate organization. The latter was decided upon and over the course of 2003, numerous thought leaders involved in psoriasis and PsA research and education around the world, including rheumatologists, dermatolo-gists, representatives of patient service leagues and the pharmaceutical industry teleconferenced and emailed about establishing a society that could meet, exchange knowledge and ideas, and conduct collaborative research.

Robin Shapiro, who headed a company called Health Advocacy Strategies, was recruited to help organize the inaugural meeting. A number of people helped develop this group including rheumatologists Philip Mease (USA), Dafna Gladman (Canada), Desiree van der Heijde (The Netherlands), Robert Landewé (the Netherlands), Philip Helliwell (United Kingdom), Herman Mielants (Belgium), Annelies Boonen (The Netherlands), Peter Nash (Australia), Christopher Ritchlin (USA), Christian Antoni (Germany), Artie Kavanaugh (USA), Josef Smolen (Austria), Joachim Kalden (Germany), and dermatologists Mark Lebwohl (USA), Jerry Krueger (USA), Alice Gottlieb (USA), Steve Feldman (USA), Allan Menter (USA), Christopher Griffiths (UK), and the heads of various countries patient service leagues.

The first meeting of the "PsA Working Group" was scheduled to take place in New York City August 15–17, 2003. As it turned out, the day the meeting was to start was the beginning of the largest electrical blackout to affect the Eastern Seaboard of North America. The city was dark-ened, flights were canceled, local transportation precarious but nonetheless 40 intrepid people made it to the meeting hotel. Shortly after the first delegates arrived at the Marriott Hotel Downtown the city went into darkness, putting the plans in jeopardy. There was nothing to be done that eve-ning except climb 30 flights to one's room in the hotel. The next morning, Robin Shapiro who had organized the meeting, walked up Manhattan until she saw lights. She found the Warwick Hotel open and able to accommodate our meet-ing. Forty people were able to make it to the meeting, which turned out a great success. One of the first items on the agenda was to identify a name for the group. Philip Helliwell came up with the acronym GRAPPA - Group for Research and Assessment of Psoriasis and Psoriatic Arthritis, which was immediately adopted by the delegates, and GRAPPA was established.

The mission of GRAPPA was set to include: increasing awareness and early diagnosis of psoriasis and PsA; development and validation of research assessment tools to measure clinical status and disease outcome; evaluation of treatment modalities; supporting and conducting basic research on disease pathophysiology; fostering communication between rheumatologists, dermatologists, representatives of patient advocacy organisations, biopharmaceutical companies, regulatory agencies, and others who are interested in the advancement of care of psoriasis and PsA.

The goals of GRAPPA were set up at its first meeting:

1. Provide a forum for acquaintance, networking, and communication between international researchers in rheumatology and dermatology, industry, patient advocacy organisations, and regulatory agencies.
2. Develop and conduct collaborative research, education and other projects, and provide the opportunity for in-person meetings and intranet communication to share knowledge and research findings with others.
3. Develop and validate a criteria set for the definition of PsA.
4. Prioritise domains of enquiry within PsA and psoriasis for research.
5. Review, develop, and validate effective and feasible outcome measures for the assessment of PsA and psoriasis.
6. Promote the development of national and international collaborative registries of PsA and psoriasis patients to standardise the data being obtained and learn more about the natural history of the disease as well as its genetic underpinnings.

7. Work closely with representatives of patient advocacy organisations to promote public education and awareness of PsA and psoriasis and improve our understanding of patient needs.
8. Work closely with representatives of biopharmaceutical companies to promote and conduct research on effective therapies for PsA and psoriasis.
9. Work closely with representatives of regulatory agencies to establish appropriate guidelines for regulatory approval of new therapies.
10. Work with other professional bodies, such as the American College of Rheumatology, American Academy of Dermatology, OMERACT, etc. to promote knowledge of and research about PsA and psoriasis within the context of those disciplines.
11. Develop treatment guidelines for governmental and other interested parties.

The topics discussed at the first meeting are all summarized in a supplement published in the Annals of the Rheumatic diseases [1].

How has GRAPPA fared in achieving these goals and developing new ones?

Over the past 12 years, GRAPPA has grown and now includes 567 members (Table 2.1). GRAPPA has developed a website (http://grappanetwork.org) which provides information on the purpose of the organization, meetings, resources, publications and other information available to its members. GRAPPA is supported

Table 2.1 GRAPPA membership

Participant type	Non-north American	North American	Total
Dermatologist	91	80	171 (30%)
Geneticist	1	5	6 (1%)
Methodologist	8	3	11 (2%)
Patient group/Gov.	12	9	21 (4%)
Radiologist	4	3	7 (1%)
Rheumatologist	235	101	336 (59%)
Not filed	0	1	1 (0%)
Other	9	5	14 (3%)
(SubTotal)	360	207	567 (100 %)
Sponsors	66	88	154 (100 %)

Table 2.2 GRAPPA annual meetings

Date	Site	Type	Comment
August 13–15, 2003	New York, USA	Inaugural meeting	
May 31, 2006	Stockholm, Sweden	Annual meeting	Adjacent to 1st World Congress Psoriatic Disease
September 7–9, 2007	Boston, USA	Annual meeting	
September 5–7, 2008	Leeds, UK	Annual meeting	
June 23–24, 2009	Stockholm, Sweden	Annual meeting	Adjacent to 2nd World Congress Psoriatic Disease
December 9–11,2010	Miami, USA	Annual meeting	
July 7–9, 2011	Naples, Italy	Annual meeting	
June 25–27, 2012	Stockholm, Sweden	Annual meeting	Adjacent to 3rd World Congress Psoriatic Disease
July 11–14, 2013	Toronto, Canada	Annual meeting	GRAPPA 10th anniversary
July 9–11, 2014	New York, USA	Annual meeting	Joint meeting with SPARTAN
July 7, 2015	Stockholm, Sweden	Annual meeting	Adjacent to 4th World Congress Psoriatic Disease

by an administrative team currently led by Pam Love. It is incorporated as a non-profit organization with bylaws and a leadership structure which includes an executive and steering committee. GRAPPA is financially supported by unrestricted grants from a number of pharmaceutical companies which are stakeholders in psoriasis and PsA, including Amgen, BMS, Celgene, Janssen, Lilly, Novartis, Pfizer, and UCB.

To achieve the first 2 goals listed above GRAPPA has annual meetings at which its members are able to network and communicate and which have provided an opportunity to carry out many of its research activities (Table 2.2). These have included stand alone meetings, which rheumatologists and dermatologists attend, as well as meetings associated with the American College of Rheumatology (ACR) and EULAR, which are attended primarily by rheumatologists, and meeting associated with the American Academy of Dermatology (AAD) and the European Academy of Dermatology and Venereology (EADV) which are attended primarily by dermatologists. The annual meeting, spanning 2 days, is primarily devoted to plenary and small group discussions regarding a wide array of research and education projects being undertaken by GRAPPA, as well as business matters. In addition, a significant portion of the program is devoted to presentations by rheumatology and dermatology trainees, mentored by GRAPPA members, providing the next generation of researchers and clinicians the

opportunity to become engaged with GRAPPA activities. These meetings result in meeting reports which describe the deliberations that took place about various subjects related to the GRAPPA goals.

Numerous education projects have been and are being conducted. Since 2012, GRAPPA has collaborated with SPARTAN (Spondyloarthritis Research and Therapy Network) in the United States of America (USA) to conduct over 25 continuing medical education (CME) programs to educate rheumatologists and trainees about psoriatic arthritis and spondyloarthritis in cities around the USA. More recently, GRAPPA, SPARTAN, and ASAS (Ankylosing Spondylitis Assessment international Society) have collaborated on educational programs at the ACR meeting. Utilizing unrestricted pharmaceutical support, GRAPPA has conducted combined rheumatology-dermatology educational symposia in many countries around the world including Brazil, Argentina, Mexico, Japan, Korea, China, India, UK, Spain, Norway, Netherlands, Saudi Arabia, and in Africa. A comprehensive educational slide deck about all aspects of PsA and its care has been developed for use by GRAPPA educators.

Goal 3, to develop and validate criteria for PsA, was met earlier on as the CASPAR group had already collected the data for the CASPAR criteria which were published in 2006 [2]. That study included 30 sites from 17 countries and clearly demonstrated the ability of the group to work together to achieve a common goal. Moreover, the criteria have since been validated by a number of studies demonstrating their usefulness in early arthritis clinics, early PsA and in various clinical settings [3–6].

Goal 4, to prioritize domains of inquiry in PsA and psoriasis, was achieved through a collaborative effort between GRAPPA and OMERACT. In early 2003 Gladman submitted a proposal to OMERACT to develop a workshop/module devoted to outcome measures in PsA. This was accepted as a workshop under the leadership of Dafna Gladman (Canada), Philip Mease (USA), and Peter Nash (Australia). Christian Antoni, Artie Kavanaugh and Vibeke Strand were added to the steering committee for the OMERACT workshop. In preparation for the OMERACT workshop a literature review was undertaken of all outcome measures used in clinical trials and other studies in PsA [7]. At the first GRAPPA meeting breakout groups were conducted during which the domains of inquiry in PsA were identified, and this work was subsequently presented at OMERACT in Asilomar in May 2004. Further work on the domains was done during the OMERACT meeting [8]. A module on PsA outcome measures at the 2006 OMERACT meeting in Malta finalized the domains of inquiry and also identified some of the outcome measures to be used in clinical trials and observational studies of PsA [9]. A research agenda was set as well. GRAPPA participated in subsequent OMERACT meetings, and at the last meeting a PsA workshop was conducted with enhanced patient involvement. As OMERACT has established an enhanced mechanism for reporting on patient outcomes, GRAPPA will be the first disease group to modify the domains and instruments to accommodate filter two [10].

Subsequent studies of individual outcome measures were performed through the GRAPPA collaboration. A reliability study of clinical measures of musculoskeletal disease was carried out evaluating peripheral joint assessment, dactylitis and enthesitis, as well as spinal measurements. This study was carried out in collaboration with ASAS, and demonstrated that there was good agreement in assessing tender joints, but not as good an agreement for swollen joints. Dactylitis assessment also provided a moderately high agreement. Enthesitis point count was highly reliable while the specific enthesitis indices provided somewhat different results for axial PsA, where the SPARCC enthesitis tool and the Leeds Enthesitis index functioned better, whereas in AS the Berlin, MASES and San Francisco indices were somewhat better. Axial disease assessment was also reasonably reliable in both axial PsA and AS [11, 12]. Another study testing the reliability of rheumatologists and dermatologist to perform assessments of patients with PsA was carried out and demonstrated that dermatologists and rheumatologists agree on tender joint count although the agreement with regards to swollen joints is much lower. Dactylitis assessment was not reliable among dermatologists. On the other hand, assessment of skin disease using the PASI provided moderate agreement among rheumatologists and dermatologists, and the nail assessment was highly reliable among rheumatologists and dermatologists. It was noted that there was less agreement in PGA and body surface area scores among rheumatologists than dermatologist [13].

An evaluation of patient and physician global assessment was carried out through a GRAPPA collaborative study. The results recommended that the PGA include components on joints and skin separately as well as a joint question on psoriatic disease [14].

Goal 5, to develop composite outcome measures was achieved through a GRAPPA study directed by Philip Helliwell to develop composite indices (The GRACE study) resulted in the development of two indices, the Psoriatic Arthritis Disease Activity Score (PASDAS) and the GRACE instrument [15]. These two instruments are currently being validated in clinical trials.

Through the GRAPPA OMERACT collaboration, another effort is underway to develop outcome measures for psoriasis as well as other dermatology outcomes. Alice Gottlieb has spearheaded this project along with a number of other GRAPPA members including Kristina Callis-Duffin, April Armstrong, Amit Garg, and Joe Merola. The organization is known as IDEOM

(International Dermatology Outcome Measures). This group has successfully engaged a broad array of members including internationally representative dermatologists, patient research partners, and representatives of patient service organizations, the pharmaceutical industry, payers, and regulatory agencies. A number of meetings have already taken place both within and independent of GRAPPA meetings and the effort is well on its way to develop widely accepted outcome measures for skin and nail assessment [16].

Goal 6, to develop and promote international registries, has been addressed by the International Psoriasis and Arthritis Research Team (IPART), a network developed through funding from the Canadian Institute of Health Research (CIHR), and directed by Dafna Gladman. A web-based data base was developed which is currently being used by a number of GRAPPA members to record patients with psoriasis without arthritis as well as patients with psoriatic arthritis [17]. Through this initiative a number of genetic studies have been performed including patients with cutaneous psoriasis only and patients with psoriatic arthritis [18, 19]. Other GRAPPA members are currently developing registries including the same content, and have also performed genetic studies in PsA [20]. Examples of these registries include the CORRONA (Consortium of Rheumatology Researchers of North America) registry in the USA, The British Society of Rheumatology Biologics Registry (BSRBR), The Norwegian DMARD registry (NOR-DMARD), the Danish National Board of Health (DANBIO) registry, to name a few. Collaboration among these registries is expected in the future. More recently, a GRAPPA initiative to identify biomarkers for disease damage in PsA was established. A protocol has been prepared and funding is currently sought to support this effort [21]. The GRAPPA biomarker group is collaborating with several current pharmaceutical trials to collect pilot biomarker data for this initiative.

Goal 7, to work closely with representatives of patient advocacy organizations and develop educational module has also been addressed. Working with the National Psoriasis Foundation in the United States a program for training health professionals and patients has been developed, and a similar program has been developed in Europe. The European initiative has mirrored the efforts of GRAPPA and the NPF. Small meetings, with up to 50 attendees, preferably a mix of rheumatologist and dermatologists have met to promote knowledge about psoriatic disease and to facilitate inter-disciplinary working. A total of nine meetings are planned throughout Europe in 2015 and a full evaluation of the educational content will follow.

In addition, GRAPPA has developed video modules to train health professionals how to assess patients with psoriasis and psoriatic arthritis. The videos include sections on skin and nail assessment, evaluation of peripheral joints, axial disease, dactylitis and enthesitis. The videos have been used to train investigators in clinical trials [22].

Goal 8, to work closely with representatives of biopharmaceutical companies to promote and conduct research on effective therapies for PsA and psoriasis, has been met through participation in clinical trials. Many members of GRAPPA have not only participated in clinical trials of new medications for PsA, but have been members of steering committees, and have helped design the trials.

Goal 9, to work closely with representatives of regulatory agencies to establish appropriate guidelines for regulatory approval of new therapies, has been a challenge since in many jurisdictions it has been difficult to participate in this process. Nonetheless, members of GRAPPA have counseled the FDA and participated in deliberations of the National Institute for Health and Care Excellence (NICE) in the United Kingdom.

Goal 10, members of GRAPPA have worked with other professional bodies, such as the ACR, AAD, EULAR, EADV, and OMERACT to promote knowledge of and research about PsA and psoriasis within the context of those disciplines.

Goal 11, to develop treatment guidelines, has been achieved. Through the first few years of GRAPPA Artie Kavanaugh and Christopher Ritchlin spearheaded the GRAPPA treatment recommendations project. This resulted in a literature review covering the domains of PsA and psoriasis, which led to a publication on treatment recommendations [23–31]. Based on the literature review it was recommended that all aspects of psoriatic disease need to be treated. Each domain was defined in terms of severity levels and it was suggested that the treatment for the domain most severe in an individual patient should be provide [31]. The recommendations were aimed for practicing physicians, governmental and other interested parties.

In 2012 GRAPPA embarked on a revision of the treatment recommendations. Again a literature review process was carried out which resulted in updated publications for the various domains of PsA. This time comorbidities were included [32–39]. The full recommendations will be submitted for publication soon.

In summary, GRAPPA has matured and become the foremost research and education society for psoriasis and psoriatic arthritis in the world, involving dermatologists and rheumatologists from many countries. GRAPPA collaborates with other societies including the ACR, EULAR, SPARTAN, ASAS, and OMERACT in fostering its goals. As an investment in the future, GRAPPA nurtures young researchers and clinicians who are interested in psoriasis and PsA in order to develop the next generation of leaders in these fields of medicine. GRAPPA has matured and become the foremost research and education society for psoriasis and psoriatic arthritis in the world, involving dermatologists and rheumatologists from many countries. GRAPPA collaborates with other societies including the ACR, EULAR, SPARTAN, ASAS, and OMERACT in fostering its goals. As an investment in the future, GRAPPA nurtures young researchers and clinicians who are interested in psoriasis and PsA in order to develop the next generation of leaders in these fields of medicine.

References

1. Mease P, Gladman D, Krueger G, Antoni C. Psoriatic arthritis and psoriasis. Ann Rheum Dis. 2005;64(Suppl II):1–117.
2. Taylor WJ, Gladman DD, Helliwell PS, Marchesoni A, Mease P, Mielants H. Classification criteria for psoriatic arthritis: development of new criteria from a large international study. Arthritis Rheum. 2006;54: 2665–73.
3. Chandran V, Schentag CT, Gladman DD. Sensitivity of the Classification of psoriatic arthritis (CASPAR) Criteria in early psoriatic arthritis. Arthritis Rheum (Arthritis Care & Research). 2007;57:1560–3.
4. D'Angelo S, Mennillo GA, Cutro MS, Leccese P, Nigro A, Padula A, Olivieri I. Sensitivity of the classification of psoriatic arthritis criteria in early psoriatic arthritis. J Rheumatol. 2009;36:368–70.
5. Coates L, Conaghan PG, Emery P, Green MJ, Ibrahim G, MacIver H, Helliwell PS. Sensitivity and specificity of the classification of psoriatic arthritis criteria in early psoriatic arthritis. Arthritis Rheum. 2012;64: 3150–5.
6. Chandran V, Schentag CT, Gladman DD. Sensitivity and specificity of the CASPAR criteria for psoriatic arthritis when applied to patients attending a family medicine clinic. J Rheumatol. 2008;35:2069–70.
7. Gladman DD, Helliwell P, Mease PJ, Nash P, Ritchlin C, Taylor W. Assessment of patients with psoriatic arthritis. A review of currently available measures. Arthritis Rheum. 2004;50:24–35.
8. Gladman DD, Mease P, Krueger G, van der Heijde D, Antoni C, Helliwell P, et al. Outcome measures in psoriatic arthritis (PsA): OMERACT VII Psoriatic Arthritis Workshop. J Rheumatol. 2005;32: 2262–9.
9. Gladman DD, Mease PJ, Strand V, Healy P, Helliwell PS, FitzGerald O, et al. Consensus on a core set of domains for psoriatic arthritis. OMERACT 8 PsA Module Report. J Rheumatol. 2007;34:1167–70.
10. Tillett W, Eder L, De Wit M, Gladman D, FitzGerald O, Goel N, et al. Enhanced patient involvement and the need to revise the core set- report from the Psoriatic Arthritis workshop at OMERACT 2014. J Rheumatol. 2015;42:2198–203.
11. Gladman DD, Inman R, Cook R, Maksymowych W, Braun J, Davis JC, et al. International spondyloarthritis inter-observer reliability exercise – the INSPIRE study: I. Assessment of spinal measures. J Rheumatol. 2007;34:1733–9.
12. Gladman DD, Inman R, Cook R, Maksymowych W, Braun J, Davis JC, et al. International spondyloarthritis inter-observer reliability exercise – the INSPIRE study: II. Assessment of peripheral joints, enthesitis and dactylitis. J Rheumatol. 2007;34: 1740–5.
13. Chandran V, Gottlieb AB, Cook RJ, Callis Duffin K, Garg A, Helliwell PS, et al. International Multi-centre Psoriasis and Psoriatic Arthritis Reliability Trial (GRAPPA-IMPART): assessment of skin, joints, nails and dactylitis. Arthritis Rheum (Arthritis Care & Res). 2009;61:1235–42.
14. Cauli C, Gladman D, Mathieu A, Olivieri I, Porru G, Tak PP, GRAPPA 3PPsA Study Group. Patient global assessment in psoriatic arthritis (PsA). A multicentre GRAPPA and OMERACT study. J Rheumatol. 2011;38:898–903.

15. Helliwell PS, FitzGerald O, Fransen J, Gladman DD, Kreuger GG, Callis-Duffin K, et al. The development of candidate composite disease activity and responder indices for psoriatic arthritis (GRACE project). Ann Rheum Dis. 2013;72:986–91.

16. Gottlieb AB, Armstrong AW, Christensen R, Garg A, Duffin KC, Boehncke WH, et al. The international dermatology outcome measures initiative as applied to psoriatic disease outcomes: a report from the GRAPPA 2013 meeting. J Rheumatol. 2014;41: 1227–9.

17. Gladman DD, Chandran V. Review of clinical registries of psoriatic arthritis: lessons learned? Value for the future? Curr Rheumatol Rep. 2011;13:346–52.

18. Nair RP, Duffin KC, Helms C, Ding J, Stuart PE, Goldgar D, et al. The Collaborative Association Study of Psoriasis. Genome-wide scan reveals association of psoriasis with IL-23 and NF-κB pathways. Nat Genet. 2009;41:199–204.

19. Tsoi LC, Spain SL, Knight J, Ellinghaus E, Stuart PE, Capon F, et al. Identification of 15 new psoriasis susceptibility loci highlights the role of innate immunity. Nat Genet. 2012;44:1341–8.

20. Bowes J, Budu-Aggrey A, Huffmeier U, Uebe S, Steel K, Hebert HL, et al. Dense genotyping of immune-related susceptibility loci reveals new insights into the genetics of psoriatic arthritis. Nat Commun. 2015;6:6046.

21. FitzGerald O, Chandran V. Update on biomarkers in psoriatic arthritis: a report from the GRAPPA 2010 annual meeting. J Rheumatol. 2012;39:427–30.

22. Callis DK, Armstrong AW, Mease PJ. Psoriasis and psoriatic arthritis video project: an update from the 2012 GRAPPA annual meeting. J Rheumatol. 2013;40:1455–6.

23. Gladman DD, Mease PJ. Towards international guidelines for the management of psoriatic arthritis. J Rheumatol. 2006;33:1228–30.

24. Soriano ER, McHugh NJ. Therapies for peripheral joint disease in psoriatic arthritis. A systematic review. J Rheumatol. 2006;33:1422–30.

25. Nash P. Therapies for axial disease in psoriatic arthritis. A systematic review. J Rheumatol. 2006;33: 1431–4.

26. Ritchlin CT. Therapies for psoriatic enthesopathy. A systematic review. J Rheumatol. 2006;33:1435–8.

27. Helliwell PS. Therapies for dactylitis in psoriatic arthritis. A systematic review. J Rheumatol. 2006;33: 1439–41.

28. Cassell S, Kavanaugh AF. Therapies for psoriatic nail disease. A systematic review. J Rheumatol. 2006;33: 1452–6.

29. Boehncke WH, Prinz J, Gottlieb AB. Biologic therapies for psoriasis. A systematic review. J Rheumatol. 2006;33:1447–51.

30. Strober BE, Siu K, Menon K. Conventional systemic agents for psoriasis. A systematic review. J Rheumatol. 2006;33:1442–6.

31. Ritchlin CT, Kavanaugh A, Gladman DD, Mease PJ, Boehncke WH, de Vlam K, et al. Treatment recommendations for psoriatic arthritis. Ann Rheum Dis. 2009;68:1387–94.

32. Coates LC, Kavanaugh A, Ritchlin CT, GRAPPA Treatment Guideline Committee. Systemic review of treatments for psoriatic arthritis: 2014 update for GRAPPA. J Rheumatol. 2014;41:2273–6.

33. Acosta Felquer ML, Coates LC, Soriano ER, Ranza R, Espinoza LR, Helliwell PS, et al. Drug therapies for peripheral joint disease in psoriatic arthritis: a systematic review. J Rheumatol. 2014;41: 2277–85.

34. Nash P, Lubrano E, Cauli A, Taylor W, Gladman DD, Chandran V. Updated guidelines for the management of axial disease in psoriatic arthritis. J Rheumatol. 2014;41:2286–9.

35. Orbai AM, Weitz J, Siegel EL, Siebert S, Savage LJ, Aydin SZ, et al. Systematic review of treatment effectiveness and outcome measures for enthesitis in psoriatic arthritis. J Rheumatol. 2014;41:2290–4.

36. Rose S, Toloza S, Bautista-Molano W, Helliwell PS, GRAPPA Dactylitis Study Group. Comprehensive treatment of dactylitis in psoriatic arthritis. J Rheumatol. 2014;41:2295–3000.

37. Wolf-Henning Boehncke WH, David Alvarez Martinez D, James A, Solomon JA, Gottlieb AB. Safety and efficacy of therapies for skin symptoms of psoriasis in patients with psoriatic arthritis: a systematic review. J Rheumatol. 2014;41:2301–5.

38. Armstrong AW, Tuong W, Love TJ, Carneiro S, Grynszpan R, Lee SS, Kavanaugh A. Treatments for nail psoriasis: a systematic review by the GRAPPA nail psoriasis work group. J Rheumatol. 2014;41: 2306–14.

39. Ogdie A, Schwartzman S, Coates L, Eder L, Maharaj A, Zisman D, et al. Comprehensive treatment of psoriatic arthritis: managing comorbidities and extra-articular manifestations. J Rheumatol. 2014;41:2315–22.

Part II

Epidemiological Aspects

Philip H. Helliwell

Classification Criteria for Psoriasis and Psoriatic Arthritis

3

William J. Taylor

Abstract

Classification criteria are primarily for assembling meaningfully homogenous groups of patients for the purpose of clinical research. They are not for diagnosis in clinical interactions between physicians and patients. The classification criteria most commonly used for psoriatic arthritis currently are the CASPAR criteria, which demonstrate high levels of accuracy in a variety of contexts. Classification criteria do not resolve challenges to disease concept but simply reflect current understanding and may evolve with greater knowledge of the pathophysiological basis of psoriatic arthritis. Recent classification criteria for spondyloarthritis, among which psoriatic arthritis is included, has identified additional challenges for disease concept.

Keywords

Psoriatic arthritis • Psoriasis • Classification criteria • CASPAR

The Nature of Classification Criteria

It is important to distinguish between diagnostic criteria and classification criteria. Diagnosis is what clinicians do in the clinic when they want to be able to name the pathological process that is affecting the patient in order to come to an effective treatment plan and provide accurate advice to the patient about what is wrong and what is likely to happen in the future. The diagnostic process brings to bear all available pieces of evidence in order to assign or not assign a particular diagnostic label. Such labels can vary in the level of detail or precision but the process is the same, so that the process of making a diagnosis of 'heart failure' is the same as the process of making a diagnosis of 'alcoholic cardiomyopathy' even though one condition subsumes another and requires a different set of information. Since physicians differ in the informational

W.J. Taylor, MBChB, PhD, FAFRM, FRACP
Department of Medicine, University of Otago
Wellington, Wellington, PO Box 7343 6242,
New Zealand
e-mail: william.taylor@otago.ac.nz

© Springer International Publishing Switzerland 2016
A. Adebajo et al. (eds.), *Psoriatic Arthritis and Psoriasis: Pathology and Clinical Aspects*,
DOI 10.1007/978-3-319-19530-8_3

data-base available to them or how the same pieces of data are weighed and yet are still able to make the same diagnoses, standardization in diagnosis is not feasible unless the diagnosis is of a very precise nature. There may be some conditions where a diagnosis is not possible without a very particular piece of information being present. In such cases, diagnostic criteria could be imaged; for example diabetes mellitus could not be diagnosed without hyperglycemia. In rheumatology, such well-identified pathological markers are seldom known, so that diagnostic criteria are very rare for rheumatic diseases. The term 'gold-standard' is sometimes used for diagnostic criteria, and is an essentially equivalent term.

In rheumatology, the 'gold standard' of diagnosis is usually expert opinion. For clinical research, expert opinion may not always be obtainable. Furthermore, expert opinion is not only fallible, it is un-measurably fallible. That is, diagnostic errors are probably made from time to time but the extent of the error is unknown. For clinical research purposes, such a process is not adequate.

In contrast, classification is the process of defining case-ness for the purpose of studying the condition, that is, for research. In such a setting, standardization is very important since it is necessary for the same condition to be studied to make sense of all the research that considers this condition. The process of standardization inevitably means that only a limited part of the informational database is used to define whether the patient has the disease or not, but the critical issue is that same segment of information is used in the same way in every research study to ensure homogeneity of the population under study. In addition, it is inevitable that the criteria will not agree with the 'gold standard' of diagnosis, but in this case it is possible to quantify the degree of disagreement: the false positive rate and the false negative rate.

Classification therefore resolves to a problem of finding the smallest informational database that leads to the smallest false positive rate and false negative rate.

Classification Criteria for Psoriasis

Classification criteria for psoriasis do not exist. Typically, patients with psoriasis are easily identified on the basis of their characteristic skin lesions. Disease entry criteria for clinical trials of treatment for psoriasis are generally of this form: "patients were 18 years of age or older with moderate-to-severe plaque psoriasis that had been diagnosed at least 6 months before randomization" [1]. The protocol for the quoted secukinumab study does not specify how the condition was diagnosed, or whether a specific kind of physician (eg dermatologist) was needed to make the diagnosis. Since plaque psoriasis cannot be diagnosed without the clinical sign of plaque psoriasis, diagnosis and classification come to the same thing and formalized classification criteria are not necessary.

Classification Criteria Prior to CASPAR

In contrast, there are a plethora of classification criteria for PsA. There has been a virtually linear evolution of proposed classification criteria for PsA since the earliest concept of the disease proposed by Moll and Wright (Fig. 3.1).

The key features of the criteria prior to CASPAR are shown in Table 3.1. The original criteria of Moll and Wright are the simplest and the most frequently used in studies prior to 2006. These criteria were designed to be sensitive without being too specific but it is possible that Moll and Wright were using other (non-explicit) features of the disease to make their diagnosis. As a consequence of omitting from the criteria what would now be regarded as characteristic features of psoriatic arthritis (such as enthesitis, spondylitis, dactylitis, nail disease) it is possible that many of the patients included in later studies had seronegative rheumatoid arthritis with co-incidental psoriasis.

The issue with using RF as an exclusion criterion was highlighted by Gladman, who found that 12 % of her cohort with PsA had a positive RF. The criteria that she used to define PsA in the

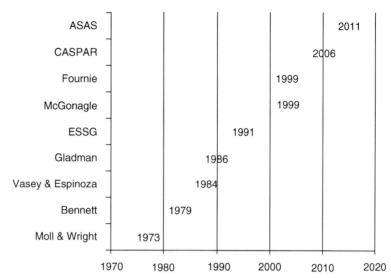

Fig. 3.1 Time-line for the evolution of PsA classification criteria

Toronto cohort was therefore less rigid concerning RF positivity, but still excluded patients with rheumatoid nodules or other kinds of inflammatory arthritis [2].

Other proposed classification criteria have not been widely adopted. They are of interest mainly in terms of the selection of features included, which highlight salient features of PsA. Bennett's criteria combined the clinical features unique to psoriatic arthritis together with characteristic radiologic features [3]. In addition two pathological criteria, one based on synovial fluid analysis and the other based on synovial histology, were included. Vasey and Espinoza simplified the Bennett criteria recognizing that there are two principle manifestations of psoriatic arthritis; only two criteria are required – psoriasis and one manifestation of either peripheral joint disease or spinal disease [4]. Although the European Spondyloarthropathy Study Group (ESSG) developed criteria for the diagnostic classification of the spondyloarthropathy (SpA) group as a whole, particular types of SpA can be identified from the published classification criteria, including psoriatic arthritis [5]. These criteria meant for the first time that it was possible for PsA to be classified in the absence of psoriasis, if a family history of psoriasis was present. McGonagle et al. proposed a definition of psoriatic arthritis based on enthesopathy [6]. As the first proper

attempt to define and validate criteria from actual patient data, the study by Fournié (23) represented an important step. In this study, the criteria items and weighting were selected using discriminant function and logistic regression analysis. The data were derived from a population of patients diagnosed by rheumatologists from a single clinic as having PsA, ankylosing spondylitis or rheumatoid arthritis. A score of 11 points is required for the diagnosis of PsA (sensitivity 95 %, specificity 98 %, LR +47.5) and, although the criteria include HLA data, it is possible to attain this threshold on clinical data alone.

There have been a few studies that have sought to identify the best performing classification criteria. A retrospective study using data from clinical records and existing radiographs in 343 patients with PsA and 156 with RA found that the criteria of Vasey & Espinoza had the best combination of specificity, sensitivity and feasibility, although there wasn't a statistically significant difference between Vasey, Gladman and McGonagle [7]. The CASPAR study also found that the criteria of Vasey & Espinoza performed the best of all the pre-CASPAR classification criteria [8]. Another small study of patients with PsA found that the CASPAR criteria had the best sensitivity compared to Bennett's criteria, Moll & Wright, ESSG, Vasey & Espinoza, Fournié with the proportion of those patients who did not fulfil

Table 3.1 Classification criteria prior to CASPAR

Criteria name (year)	Main features	Number of citations to 2014[a, b]
Moll & Wright (1973)	An inflammatory arthritis (peripheral arthritis and/or sacroiliitis or spondylitis) The presence of psoriasis The (usual) absence of serological tests for rheumatoid factor (RF)	777

Bennett (1979)	Mandatory:
	  Clinically apparent psoriasis (skin or nails)
	  Pain and soft-tissue swelling and/or limitation of motion in at least one joint observed by a physician for 6 weeks or longer
	Supportive:
	  Pain and soft-tissue swelling and/or limitation of motion in one or more other joints observed by a physician
	  Presence of an inflammatory arthritis in distal inter-phalangeal joint. Specific exclusions: Bouchards or Heberden's node
	  Presence of 'sausage' fingers or toes
	  An asymmetrical distribution of arthritis in the hands and feet
	  Absence of subcutaneous nodules
	  A negative test for rheumatoid factor in the serum
	  An inflammatory synovial fluid with a normal or increased C3 or C4 level and an absence of infection (including acid fast bacilli) and crystals of monosodium urate or pyrophosphate
	  A synovial biopsy showing hypertrophy of the synovial lining with a predominant mononuclear cell infiltration and an absence of granuloma or tumour
	  Peripheral radiographs showing erosive arthritis of small joints with a relative lack of osteoporosis. Specific exclusion: erosive osteoarthritis
	  Axial radiographs showing any of the following: sacroiliitis, syndesmophytes, paravertebral ossification
	Definite PsA: mandatory plus 6 supportive
	Probable PsA: mandatory plus 4 supportive
	Possible PsA: mandatory plus 2 supportive
		184

Vasey & Espinoza (1984)	Criteria I plus one from either Criteria II or III
	Criteria I: Psoriatic skin or nail involvement
	Criteria II: Peripheral pattern
	  Pain and soft tissue swelling with or without limitation of movement of the distal interphalangeal joint for over 4 weeks
	  Pain and soft-tissue swelling with or without limitation of motion of the peripheral joints involved in an asymmetric peripheral pattern for over 4 weeks. This includes a sausage digit
	  Symmetric peripheral arthritis for over 4 weeks, in the absence of rheumatoid factor or subcutaneous nodules
	  Pencil-in-cup deformity, whittling of terminal phalanges, fluffy periostitis and bony ankylosis
	Criteria III: Central pattern
	  Spinal pain and stiffness with the restriction of motion present for over 4 weeks
	  Grade 2 symmetric sacroiliitis according to the New York criteria
	  Grade 3 or 4 unilateral sacroiliitis
		151

Gladman (1987)	Inflammatory arthritis Presence of psoriasis No other cause of inflammatory arthritis (rheumatoid arthritis, crystal arthritis, severe osteoarthritis, reactive arthritis, inflammatory bowel disease arthritis)	441

ESSG (1991)	Inflammatory spinal pain
	OR
	Synovitis (either asymmetric or predominantly lower limb)
	AND
	One or more of the following:
	  Positive family history of psoriasis
	  Psoriasis
		1551

McGonagle (1999)	Psoriasis or family history of psoriasis
	Plus any one of:
	  Clinical inflammatory enthesitis
	  Radiographic enthesitis (replaces MRI evidence of enthesitis)
	  DIP disease
	  Sacroiliitis/spinal inflammation
	  Uncommon arthropathies (SAPHO, spondylodiscitis, arthritis mutilans, onchyo-pachydermo-periostitis, chronic multifocal recurrent osteomyelitis)
	  Dactylitis
	  Monoarthritis
	  Oligoarthritis (four or less swollen joints)
		225

Fournié (1999)	Psoriasis antedating or concomitant with joint symptom onset – 6 points Family history of psoriasis (if criterion one negative) or psoriasis postdating joint symptom onset – 3 points Arthritis of a DIP – 3 points Inflammatory involvement of cervical and thoracic spine – 3 points Asymmetric monarthritis or oligoarthritis – 1 point Buttock pain, heel pain, spontaneous anterior chest wall pain, or diffuse inflammatory pain in the entheses – 2 points Radiological criterion (any one present): Erosion DIP, Osteolysis, Ankylosis, Juxtaarticular periostitis, Phalangeal tuft resorption – 5 points HLA B16 (38,39) or B17 – 6 points Negative RF – 4 points Psoriatic arthritis ≥11 points	86

[a]Using Scopus for journal articles or Google scholar for chapters in text books
[b]In comparison, the CASPAR criteria article has been cited 825 times

all six criteria fulfilling each criteria being 90 %, 10 %, 31 %, 44 %, 46 %, and 79 % respectively [9]. In Han Chinese patients with inflammatory arthritis, the performance (sensitivity, specificity) of Moll & Wright, ESSG, Vasey & Espinoza and CASPAR criteria were 85/100, 81/99, 98/100, 98/100 respectively [10]. In another study, the performance (sensitivity, specificity) of CASPAR, Moll and Wright and ESSG criteria was 92/99, 86/100, 63/94 respectively [11].

The CASPAR Criteria

The Classification of Psoriatic Arthritis (CASPAR) criteria, published in 2006, arose from an international collaboration of interested rheumatologists, motivated by the multiplicity of classification criteria for PsA and the clear need to have internationally agreed criteria that were data-driven and validated [8]. The project was essentially unfunded, although some central coordinating costs were covered by a grant from the European League Against Rheumatism (EULAR). This study was conducted across 13 countries and involved over 1000 patients consecutively recruited from rheumatology clinics.

Patients with other inflammatory arthritis were controls – these included RA (70 % of controls), ankylosing spondylitis, undifferentiated arthritis and a smaller number of other diseases. Using items derived from two different statistical techniques (classification and regression tree, logistic regression), new criteria were derived that had very high specificity but slightly less sensitivity than the Vasey & Espinoza criteria. The criteria are shown in Table 3.2.

The performance of these criteria has been subsequently examined in a number of settings (summarized in Table 3.3) and generally the criteria retain high sensitivity and specificity.

The CASPAR criteria have also been used to identify patients with PsA from dermatology clinic patients with psoriasis, although the criteria were not specifically designed with that purpose in mind. For example, Hernán et al. [17] showed that 17 % of patients attending a psoriasis clinic met CASPAR criteria. The criteria have also been used as the reference standard to test the performance of screening questionnaires to identify patients with PsA amongst patients with psoriasis [18].

One of the difficulties with using CASPAR as a diagnostic or screening tool for dermatologists to

Table 3.2 The CASPAR criteria

Inflammatory articular disease (joint, spine, or entheseal)		
With three or more points from the following:		
1. Evidence of psoriasis (one of a, b, c)	(a) Current psoriasis[a]	Psoriatic skin or scalp disease present today as judged by a rheumatologist or dermatologist
	(b) Personal history of psoriasis	A history of psoriasis that may be obtained from patient, family doctor, dermatologist, rheumatologist or other qualified health-care provider
	(c) Family history of psoriasis	A history of psoriasis in a first or second degree relative according to patient report
2. Psoriatic nail dystrophy		Typical psoriatic nail dystrophy including onycholysis, pitting and hyperkeratosis observed on current physical examination
3. A negative test for rheumatoid factor		By any method except latex but preferably by ELISA or nephelometry, according to the local laboratory reference range
4. Dactylitis (one of a, b)	(a) Current	Swelling of an entire digit
	(b) History	A history of dactylitis recorded by a rheumatologist
5. Radiological evidence of juxta-articular new bone formation		Ill-defined ossification near joint margins (but excluding osteophyte formation) on plain xrays of hand or foot

Reprinted from Taylor et al. [8]. With permission from John Wiley & Sons
Specificity 0.987, sensitivity 0.914
[a]Current psoriasis scores 2 whereas all other items score 1

Table 3.3 Performance of the CASPAR criteria

First author (year)	Sensitivity	Specificity	Comment
Zlatkovic-Svenda (2013) [11]	0.917	0.992, 0.991	Rheumatology centre patients. Specificity calculated in patients with RA and non-inflammatory musculoskeletal disease separately
Coates (2012) [12]	0.874	0.991	In patients with early inflammatory arthritis (median disease duration 5–8 months)
Tillett (2012) [13]	0.997	0.991	Data retrospectively ascertained from medical records of a rheumatology clinic
Congi (2010) [9]	0.933	NA	Only applied to PsA patients
Leung (2010) [10]	0.982	0.995	In Chinese patients with inflammatory arthritis
D'Angelo (2009) [14]	0.773	NA	In patients with very early PsA (mean disease duration 16 weeks)
Chandran (2008) [15]	1.00	0.988	In a family medicine clinic (only two patients with PsA)
Chandran (2007) [16]	0.991, 0.972	NA	In patients with early and established PsA (mean disease duration 1.1 and 11 years)

identify PsA in people with psoriasis is the undefined nature of the entry criteria: inflammatory musculoskeletal disease. Since this entity is confidently identified by rheumatologists but not, in the absence of clearer definitions, other physicians, it has been proposed that the CASPAR criteria be modified to make this entry criteria more defined. This will be discussed in more detail below.

Classification of PsA in the Context of New Criteria for SpA

The seminal work by Moll and Wright in the 1970s in recognizing the common characteristics of a number of hitherto distinct diseases led to the concept of spondyloarthropathies. Exactly how these different disorders relate to each other is still not clear. It is also not obvious whether clinical practice or clinical research would be better served by use of broad criteria that subsumes all these diseases, or by use of criteria for individual diseases. The issue has become more problematic recently because of new criteria that divide patients with SpA somewhat artificially into those with predominantly axial symptoms and those with predominantly peripheral symptoms.

A group of experts in ankylosing spondylitis (ASAS, Assessment of Spondyloarthritis International Society) recently developed new criteria that subsume all forms of SpA into either axial SpA or peripheral SpA, depending mainly on the presence of back symptoms [19, 20]. The original motivation for these new criteria was the problem of studying early ankylosing spondylitis prior to the development of sacroiliitis on plain radiographs, a characteristic necessary for classification as AS by the modified New York (mNY) criteria. Undoubtedly, new criteria were required for this purpose, but in developing new criteria, ASAS also renamed the disease: axial SpA. Notwithstanding the logical contortions required to develop criteria for an as-yet-nonexistent disorder, it is clear that the criteria are not the 'gold-standard' and that expert opinion about which patients have SpA can be in disagreement with the ASAS criteria [21].

The next step was for ASAS to invent another condition: peripheral SpA, for patients with mainly peripheral symptoms to be also classified as SpA [22]. Presumably, this was to allow patients with SpA who did not meet the axial criteria to be also classified as SpA. There is clearly overlap between the conditions, which is even apparent in the way the criteria are constructed: peripheral symptoms can allow a patient with back pain and HLA-B27 to be classified as axSpA; spinal symptoms or imaging evidence of sacroiliitis can allow a patient with peripheral symptoms to be classified as pSpA. It is a little confusing that the same set of characteristics can allow classification as either axSpA or pSpA.

Patients with psoriatic arthritis can be classified as axSpA, pSpA or both depending on whether they also have back pain, HLA-B27, or imaging evidence of sacroiliitis. Interestingly patients with plain radiographic evidence of sacroiliitis without clinical symptoms of back pain would not be classified as axSpA. Non-symptomatic axial disease is not infrequently seen in PsA [23]. It is also clear that the ASAS criteria are less accurate than the CASPAR criteria for the classification of PsA with sensitivity of only 52 % compared with 89 % [24].

The appropriate classification category for patients with PsA with mainly axial symptoms is difficult. Clinical trials of ankylosing spondylitis and axial SpA are designed to include patients who fulfil mNY or ASAS axSpA criteria. Such studies will include a proportion of patients with PsA, or at least people who fulfil CASPAR criteria for PsA. Conversely, all clinical trials of treatment for PsA select on the basis of active peripheral joint disease and hardly ever report spinal outcomes for the subset of patients with concomitant axial disease. It is therefore difficult to know much about treatment response in axial PsA. On the other hand, observational studies have suggested that there are phenotypic differences between AS and axial SpA. This is a problem of classification and more fundamentally, concept of disease – if it thought that PsA patients with axial disease are best considered as a form of axSpA, then it might make more sense that they are included with other axSpA. However, in fact patients with psoriasis or PsA were excluded from the ABILITY-1 trial, which was a study of adalimumab in patients with axial SpA [25]. This might imply that the investigators thought that PsA is not part of axSpA, although a more likely explanation is that adalimumab has already been shown to be effective for PsA and so inclusion of PsA patients might be unethical in a placebo-controlled study. In any case, this study perfectly illustrates that the axSpA criteria are not being used for PsA in exactly the situation for which classification criteria are designed – case-definition for clinical trials.

All in all, is it difficult at this time to recommend the use of ASAS criteria for the classification of PsA [26].

Future Evolution of the CASPAR Criteria

As classification criteria, CASPAR has been very successful and it is doubtful that new criteria for PsA will be markedly more accurate without some novel and profound insights into the fundamental pathophysiology, genetics or aetiology of the disease. Nevertheless, there are three areas of the criteria that might be improved upon: differential weighting of previous vs. current psoriasis, defining psoriasis more carefully and defining inflammatory MSK symptoms more carefully.

The higher weighting for currently apparent psoriasis in CASPAR has been criticized for potentially mis-classifying patients in cross-sectional epidemiological studies, since the skin disease may relapse and remit and not be apparent at all times in many people with disease. In addition, criterion 1(b) gives as much weight to a patient derived history of psoriasis as to a history of physician-diagnosed psoriasis, which may not be appropriate. A suggested modification has been to include a history of physician-diagnosed psoriasis into criterion 1(a) so that currently present or previously documented psoriasis would both attract two points and therefore make it easier for patients whose skin disease was in remission to be classified as having PsA [27]. The authors of this suggestion found that the Moll and Wright criteria were more sensitive than CASPAR, identifying slightly more people with PsA in a Danish twin study (54/34 944 compared to 50/34 944). The modified CASPAR criteria have been directly compared to the original CASPAR criteria in only a single study [28]. In this study of 356 patients with PsA, RA or non-inflammatory musculoskeletal symptoms, the sensitivity of the modified CASPAR criteria was slightly higher (110/120, 92 % versus 114/120, 95 %) and the specificity was almost identical.

As mentioned earlier, psoriasis is usually identified on the basis of physician (usually dermatologist) opinion. For example, in the nine randomized controlled trials of treatment for psoriasis reported in the New England Journal of Medicine over the last 10 years, the case definition for psoriasis in every trial was physician diagnosis for at least 6 months prior to randomization. Thus, there does not appear to be any practical

Table 3.4 Possible features of inflammatory MSK symptoms

Component	Features
Arthritis	Morning stiffness ≥30 min, joint swelling, joint tenderness, pain that improves with activity and worsens with rest, NSAID or steroid responsive, limited joint motion, insidious onset, chronic duration, fatigue, proximal distribution, joint deformity, boggy or spongy joint to palpation, joint erythema or warmth, presence of extra-articular manifestations
Spondylitis	Morning stiffness ≥30 min, chronic back pain >3 months, hip or buttock pain, younger age, pain that improves with activity and worsens with rest, night pain, insidious onset, no prior history of trauma or surgery at site of pain, NSAID responsive, limited spinal motion, sacroiliac joint tenderness
Enthesitis	Pain near the joint, swelling at site of pain, functional limitations, history of plantar fasciitis, younger age, bilateral involvement, tenderness at entheseal insertion sites (Achilles, plantar fascia, quadriceps tendon, patellar ligament, iliac crest)
Dactylitis	Digital swelling, digital warmth, digital erythema, focal or diffuse swelling, tenderness at site of tenderness, decreased mobility of digit, "sausage"-like appearance

Reprinted from Mease et al. [29]. With permission from The Journal of Rheumatology

need for classification criteria for psoriasis since the same information (visual skin examination) is available to every physician and the interpretation of skin examination is likely to be fairly similar across trained dermatologists. It is not clear that this is necessarily the case for rheumatologists who also diagnose psoriasis, sometimes on the basis on fairly minimal disease extent. There has been discussion through GRAPPA, as to whether it would be helpful for non-dermatologists for a standardized approach to identifying psoriasis to be incorporated into the CASPAR criteria, possibly using digital images and textual instructions or guidance. Whether this approach leads to more accurate classification remains to be seen.

Similarly, an initiative through GRAPPA has pursued the idea that more precise definition of the entry criterion (inflammatory MSK disease) would permit classification by non-rheumatologists (for example in primary care, dermatology clinics or even in general population surveys). This is an ambitious task. There are currently no widely accepted standards that define inflammatory arthritis, inflammatory spondylitis or inflammatory enthesitis. Each manifestation is associated with particular definitional issues that are not currently resolved. During the GRAPPA meeting in 2013, a number of clinical features associated with inflammatory MSK symptoms were elicited using a nominal group technique [28] (Table 3.4).

Further work is planned to see which combinations of these features are most discriminatory in patients with inflammatory and non-inflammatory

MSK disorders and to then validate in an external data-set.

There are some conceptual issues with validation of this particular item within the CASPAR criteria. In particular, it is necessary to consider the three-step nature of the validation process. Firstly, there is validation of the new item definition against how the item was previously obtained (that is, rheumatologist evaluation). The new item definition will presumably not perfectly mirror the rheumatologist evaluation, so there will be some misclassification. To determine the effect of that classification error, the overall performance of the modified CASPAR criteria will need to be re-evaluated in a consecutive series of patients with different kinds of inflammatory arthritis. Thirdly, the entry criteria ("stem") will need to be re-defined in order to make clear which population of patients the new criteria should be applied to. At present, the criteria are designed to be applied to people with inflammatory MSK symptoms. However, if this particular criterion becomes a mandatory item rather than an entry stem, then an additional criterion that specifies the target population will be required, such as people with any kind of MSK symptom (joint pain, back pain etc.). The performance of the criteria will then need to be evaluated in that population of interest – people with any kind of MSK symptom (for example, in primary care or dermatology clinic settings). It is not clear that so much work would be justified by the final product. It is also not clear what would be the consequences of discovering worse test characteristics in any new version of the CASPAR criteria. There may be a case for not changing something that works well, even if part of the reason for the accuracy of CASPAR is due to the need for rheumatologists to define inflammatory MSK disease.

References

1. Langley RG, Elewski BE, Lebwohl M, et al. Secukinumab in plaque psoriasis--results of two phase 3 trials. N Engl J Med. 2014;371:326–38.
2. Gladman DD, Shuckett R, Russell ML, Thorne JC, Schachter RK. Psoriatic arthritis (PSA)--an analysis of 220 patients. Q J Med. 1987;62:127–41.
3. Bennett RM. Psoriatic arthritis. In: McCarty DJ, editor. Arthritis and related conditions. 9th ed. Philadelphia: Lea & Febiger; 1979. p. 645.
4. Vasey F, Espinoza LR. Psoriatic arthropathy. In: Calin A, editor. Spondyloarthropathies. Orlando, Florida: Grune & Stratton; 1984. p. 151–85.
5. Dougados M, van der Linden S, Juhlin R, et al. The European Spondyloarthropathy Study Group preliminary criteria for the classification of spondyloarthropathy. Arthritis Rheum. 1991;34:1218–27.
6. McGonagle D, Conaghan PG, Emery P. Psoriatic arthritis: a unified concept twenty years on. Arthritis Rheum. 1999;42:1080–6.
7. Taylor WJ, Marchesoni A, Arreghini M, Sokoll K, Helliwell PS. A comparison of the performance characteristics of classification criteria for the diagnosis of psoriatic arthritis. Semin Arthritis Rheum. 2004;34:575–84.
8. Taylor WJ, Gladman DD, Helliwell PS, Marchesoni A, Mease PJ, Mielants H. Classification criteria for psoriatic arthritis: new criteria from a large international study. Arthritis Rheum. 2006;54:2665–73.
9. Congi L, Roussou E. Clinical application of the CASPAR criteria for psoriatic arthritis compared to other existing criteria. Clin Exp Rheumatol. 2010;28:304–10.
10. Leung YY, Tam LS, Ho KW, et al. Evaluation of the CASPAR criteria for psoriatic arthritis in the Chinese population. Rheumatology (Oxford). 2010;49:112–5.
11. Zlatkovic-Svenda M, Kerimovic-Morina D, Stojanovic RM. Psoriatic arthritis classification criteria: moll and wright, ESSG and CASPAR – a comparative study. Acta Reumatol Port. 2013;38:172–8.
12. Coates LC, Conaghan PG, Emery P, et al. Sensitivity and specificity of the classification of psoriatic arthritis criteria in early psoriatic arthritis. Arthritis Rheum. 2012;64:3150–5.
13. Tillett W, Costa L, Jadon D, et al. The ClASsification for Psoriatic ARthritis (CASPAR) criteria--a retrospective feasibility, sensitivity, and specificity study. J Rheumatol. 2012;39:154–6.
14. D'Angelo S, Mennillo GA, Cutro MS, et al. Sensitivity of the classification of psoriatic arthritis criteria in early psoriatic arthritis. J Rheumatol. 2009;36:368–70.
15. Chandran V, Schentag CT, Gladman DD. Sensitivity and specificity of the CASPAR criteria for psoriatic arthritis in a family medicine clinic setting. J Rheumatol. 2008;35:2069–70; author reply 70.
16. Chandran V, Schentag CT, Gladman DD. Sensitivity of the classification of psoriatic arthritis criteria in early psoriatic arthritis. Arthritis Rheum. 2007;57:1560–3.
17. Hernan MF, Gustavo C, Jose Antonio MC. Prevalence of psoriatic arthritis in psoriasis patients according to newer classification criteria. Clin Rheumatol. 2014;33:243–6.
18. Coates LC, Aslam T, Al Balushi F, et al. Comparison of three screening tools to detect psoriatic arthritis in patients with psoriasis (CONTEST study). Br J Dermatol. 2013;168:802–7.
19. Rudwaleit M, Landewe R, van der Heijde D, et al. The development of Assessment of SpondyloArthritis international Society classification criteria for axial spondyloarthritis (part I): classification of paper patients by expert opinion including uncertainty appraisal. Ann Rheum Dis. 2009;68:770–6.
20. Rudwaleit M, van der Heijde D, Landewe R, et al. The development of Assessment of SpondyloArthritis international Society classification criteria for axial spondyloarthritis (part II): validation and final selection. Ann Rheum Dis. 2009;68:777–83.
21. Braun J, Baraliakos X, Kiltz U, Heldmann F, Sieper J. Classification and diagnosis of axial spondyloarthritis – what is the clinically relevant difference? J Rheumatol. 2014;42(1):31–8.
22. Rudwaleit M, Taylor WJ. Classification criteria for psoriatic arthritis and ankylosing spondylitis/axial spondyloarthritis. Bailliere's Best Pract Res Clin Rheumatol. 2010;24:589–604.
23. Battistone MJ, Manaster BJ, Reda DJ, Clegg DO. Radiographic diagnosis of sacroiliitis – are sacroiliac views really better? J Rheumatol. 1998;25: 2395–401.
24. van den Berg R, van Gaalen F, van der Helm-van Mil A, Huizinga T, van der Heijde D. Performance of classification criteria for peripheral spondyloarthritis and psoriatic arthritis in the Leiden early arthritis cohort. Ann Rheum Dis. 2012;71:1366–9.
25. Sieper J, van der Heijde D, Dougados M, et al. Efficacy and safety of adalimumab in patients with non-radiographic axial spondyloarthritis: results of a randomised placebo-controlled trial (ABILITY-1). Ann Rheum Dis. 2013;72:815–22.
26. Taylor WJ, Robinson PC. Classification criteria: peripheral spondyloarthropathy and psoriatic arthritis. Curr Rheumatol Rep. 2013;15:1–7.
27. Pedersen OB, Junker P. On the applicability of the CASPAR criteria in psoriatic arthritis. Ann Rheum Dis. 2008;67:1495–6.
28. Zlatkovic, Svenda MI, Kerimovic, Morina D, Stojanovic RM. Psoriatic arthritis criteria evaluation: CASPAR and Modified CASPAR. Clin Exp Rheumatol 2011;29:899-900
29. Mease PJ, Garg A, Helliwell PS, Park JJ, Gladman DD. Development of criteria to distinguish inflammatory from noninflammatory arthritis, enthesitis, dactylitis, and spondylitis: a report from the GRAPPA 2013 Annual Meeting. J Rheumatol. 2014;41:1249–52.

Epidemiology of Psoriasis and Psoriatic Arthritis

4

Rodolfo Perez-Alamino, Hisham Sharlala, Ade Adebajo, and Luis R. Espinoza

Abstract

Psoriatic arthritis (PsA) is a unique type of chronic inflammatory arthritis that occurs in association with the skin manifestations of psoriasis, commonly presenting with extra articular manifestations which includes nail involvement, enthesitis and dactilitis. It is also important to note that like rheumatoid arthritis PsA has been shown to have significant cardiovascular comorbidities.

Studying the epidemiology of PsA has been limited by the lack of a universally agreed classification criteria. Since the introduction of the CASPAR classification criteria, we are seeing a promising trend towards the acceptance of this criteria as an internationally agreed method for present and future epidemiological and research work in the field of PsA.

In this chapter we present the available data on the incidence and prevalence of Psoriasis, PsA and the possible associated CVD comorbidities. The data show the extent of variabilities of PsA incidence and prevalance between different ethnic and population groups. The highest reported prevalence of Psoriasis worldwide (11.8 %) came from Kazakhastan, and generally believed to be higher in populations of European ethnicity and lowest in West Africa and East Asia.

The prevalance of PsA in the general population ranged from the highest reported in Italy 0.42 % to the lowest in Japan at 0.001 %. On the other hand the prevalence of PsA in Psoriasis patients increases to the range of 6–40 %. The incidence of reported cases of PsA is gradually increasing due to the improved awareness of the condition amongst primary care physicians.

R. Perez-Alamino, MD (✉)
Department of Rheumatology, Hospital Avellaneda,
2000 Catamarca Street, San Miguel De Tucuman
4000, Argentina
e-mail: ofo_pa@hotmail.com

H. Sharlala, MRCP (Rheumatology)
Department of Rheumatology, Barnsley District
General Hospital, Barnsley, South Yorkshire, UK

A. Adebajo, FRCP, FACP, FAcMed
Faculty of Medicine, Dentistry and Health,
University of Sheffield, Sheffield, UK

L.R. Espinoza, MD
Internal Medicine, Section of Rheumatology,
LSU Health Sciences Center,
New Orleans, LA, USA

© Springer International Publishing Switzerland 2016
A. Adebajo et al. (eds.), *Psoriatic Arthritis and Psoriasis: Pathology and Clinical Aspects*,
DOI 10.1007/978-3-319-19530-8_4

Keywords

Prevalence • Subgroups • Demographics • Psoriasis • Psoriatic arthritis

Introduction

Psoriasis (PsO) and psoriatic arthritis (PsA) are systemic inflammatory disorders with a complex etiopathogenesis that involve the interplay of environmental, genetic, and innate and adaptive immune system factors. Psoriatic arthritis (PsA) is a unique type of inflammatory arthritis that is associated with skin psoriasis. Current evidence on molecular, cellular, and tissue levels suggest that PsA is a distinctive form of inflammatory arthritis compared with rheumatoid arthritis (RA), the most common form of inflammatory arthritis [1]. PsA is a common systemic inflammatory arthropathy, which in addition to skin and nail involvement may be associated with peripheral and axial joint involvement, enthesitis, dactylitis, and important comorbidities – especially cardiovascular morbidity. Early diagnosis and treatment help prevent progressive joint involvement and disabilities [2]. However, PsA is underdiagnosed in PsO patients, which may be due in part to under-recognition of PsA symptoms and a lack of effective screening tools.

Epidemiology is the study of the distribution and the determinants of diseases in human populations. Like the clinical findings and pathology, the epidemiology of a disease is an integral part of its basic description and the most important determinant of the burden of a disease in a population. Decisions in policy and health care use are often influenced by prevalence and incidence of chronic diseases [3]. However, most of these studies are observational and the evidence is generally considered low [4].

A few limitations when determining the epidemiology of a disease should be noted. The frequency of diseases reported in studies depends on which criteria are used for confirmation in the individual patients. In addition, numbers on prevalence and incidence may vary due to different study design and approach to assess the disease criteria. In the last 40 years, major advances have

been made in the recognition and classification of PsA as an entity. In 1973, the first criteria for PsA were proposed by Moll and Wright, which required the presence of inflammatory arthritis, psoriasis and absence of rheumatoid factor (RF) [5]. One major limitation of this criteria is the poor sensitivity for discrimination between RA and psoriasis. In addition, the pattern of disease may change overtime and, therefore, is not useful for classification.

Later, different diagnostic criteria were proposed by Vasey and Espinoza, McGonagle et al., and Gladman, although none of them have been widely adopted [6]. In 2006, the Classification for Psoriatic Arthritis (CASPAR) group, an international group gathered to develop classification criteria for PsA, proposed a new set of criteria, which were found easier to use in epidemiologic studies. The sensitivity and specificity of these criteria are 91.4 % and 98.7 %, respectively [7]. Other studies have simply used the combination of psoriasis and (inflammatory) arthritis as a definition, not distinguishing or excluding other diagnoses, such as RA with coincidental psoriasis.

In this chapter we aim to review the epidemiology of PsO and PsA throughout the world by reviewing the literature on incidence and prevalence of PsO and PsA.

Prevalence of Psoriatic Arthritis in General Population

Psoriatic arthritis can develop at any time, but it appears most often between the ages of 30 and 50. Unlike other types of inflammatory arthritis, which have a large female predominance, PsA seems to affect men at about the same or slightly higher rate compared to women [8, 9]. Male-to-female ratio is from 0.7:1–2.1:1 [10]. There are minor ethnic variabilities in the presentation of PsA. In a study by Roussou et al. [70] on the population of north east London, it was shown that Asian patients developed PsA at a younger age [40.7 years +, −11.7] compared to Caucasian patients [46.7+, −15.8] which was statistically significant, the study also has shown that the Asian females but not males had more aggressive disease and more severe disease course in terms of ESR readings, BASDAI and BASFI scores.

Old studies have shown that there is a significantly increased familial recurrence risk of PsA which is more than what is reported for rheumatoid arthritis or psoriasis alone [66]. Interestingly a study has shown that there is an excessive paternal transmission of PsA, patients who have affected parent are more likely to have affected father than mother [67].

It should be noted that the exact prevalence of PsA in general population is unknown. Estimates from 16 published studies ranged between 0.001 % (from Japan) to 0.42 % (Italian population) (Table 4.1). This variation may be related to the absence of a valid classification criteria for the disease and also the different case definitions used in previous studies. Remarkably, most of the studies come from United States and Europe. Some of them used administrative databases, others population surveys and others used clinical observations within hospital admissions. Cross-sectional population surveys that collect data directly from subjects reported a higher prevalence than retrospective studies, which were based on medical record review [11–27]. Most studies used the coexistence of psoriasis and arthritis, others used the Vasey and Espinoza criteria, and others the European Spondylarthropathy Study Group (ESSG) criteria, which have had lower sensitivity (0.55) than, for example, the Moll and Wright criteria (sensitivity 0.95) in comparative studies [15].

The study from Japan shown the lowest prevalence of PsA in general population: 0.001 %. In this study including patients from 134 medical Japanese institutes, authors defined the presence of PsA by ESSG/Amor criteria (clinical and radiographic features) [16]. On the other hand, De Angelis et al. in a large cohort of Italian patients showed the higher prevalence of PsA reported: 0.42 % [20]. In a North American study

that used the CASPAR criteria (the Rochester Epidemiology Project), Scheeb et al. found a prevalence of 0.16 % [14]. Ogdie et al. [68] conducted an important population based study of The Health Improvement Network (THIN) in the UK which included 4.8 million patients and estimated the prevalence of PsA at 0.19 % (95 % CI 0.19 %, 0.19 %).

Recently, a study from Argentina including patients from a private health system (based on the CASPAR criteria) found a prevalence of 0.07 % [26]. It should be noted that relevant information on PsA epidemiology from Africa, Asia, and South America is still scarce.

Prevalence of Psoriatic Arthritis in Psoriasis Patients (Table 4.2)

Estimates of the prevalence of PsA among patients with PsO ranged between 6 and 40 % [28, 29]. Most studies were also conducted in Europe and United States, although rates were found lower in Asian population (1–9 %) [30]. Divergent distribution of HLA in different ethnic groups and other genetic determinants may account for these differences in prevalence. A Chinese study found a prevalence of 5.8 % of PsA in patients with PsO. It should be recognized that the underdiagnosis of PsA is probably high in this part of the world [31].

Recently, a systematic review of the incidence and prevalence of PsA conducted by Alamanos et al. reported a marked variability on the incidence and prevalence estimates of PsA in the general population among countries and areas of the world. It was noted that several methodological issues, including different definitions for case identification of the disease and geography variability, were important limitations on the interpretation of the epidemiological data [32]. A large cross-sectional observational study was conducted in European dermatology clinics, including a large number of patients (n = 1560) with PsO (psoriasis vulgaris). This study estimated that prevalence of PsA (by CASPAR criteria) increased with time since diagnosis of PsO, reaching 20.5 % after 30 years. In addition, it has

Table 4.1 Summary of studies on prevalence of PsA in general population

Year/author	Country	Sample	Diagnosis method	Criteria	Prevalence (%, 95 % CI)
1994, Boyer et al. [11]	Alaskan Eskimos	Population from Alaska Area Native Health Service	Records review + medical evaluation	ESSG/Amor	<0.1
1994, Alexeeva et al. [12]	Russia	People from two settlements	Questionnaire + medical evaluation	Not defined	0.3
1998, Braun et al. [13]	Germany	Blood donors (HLA-B27 +/−)	Questionnaire + medical evaluation	ESSG	0.29
1999, Shbeeb et al. [14]	USA	All registered patients	Medical records review	Psoriasis + arthritis	0.10 (0.08–0.12)
2001, Hukuda et al. [16]	Japan	Patients from medical institutes	Questionnaire for medical record review	ESSG/Amor	0.001
2005, Saraux et al. [17]	France	Random sample of phone numbers	Screening question + phone rheum interview	Diagnosis by phone or medical examination	0.19 (0.09–0.35)
2005, Trontzas et al. [18]	Greece	Nine regions	Visiting households for interview	ESSG + psoriasis	0.17 (0.10–0.24)
2005, Madland et al. [19]	Norway	All PsA patients seen at rheumatology centers	Patients records, four rheumatology centers	Psoriasis + arthritis	0.2 (1.8–2.1)
2007, De Angelis et al. [20]	Italy	Random sample of patients	Questionnaire + medical evaluation	mNY	0.42 (0.31–0.61)
2007, Love et al. [21]	Iceland	Psoriasis database + hospital records	Interview + medical evaluation	Swe PsA	0.14 (0.11–0.17)
2009, Liao et al. [22]	China	All residents of Dalang Town	Questionnaire + medical evaluation	ESSG	0.02
2009, Wilson et al. [23]	USA	All registered patients	Medical records review	CASPAR	0.16 (0.13–0.19)
2010, Hanova et al. [24]	Czech Republic	All referred patients	Medical evaluation by rheumatologist	Vasey and Espinoza	0.05 (0.04–0.06)
2011, Haglund et al. [25]	Sweden	All registered patients	ICD-10 codes from health care register	ICD-10 code	0.25 (0.24–0.26)
2011, Soriano et al. [26]	Argentina	Patients from a private health system	Medical records review	CASPAR	0.07 (0.06–0.09)
2011, Alverez-Nemegyei [27]	Mexico	Random sample	Screening COPCORD questionnaire + medical evaluation	mNY	0.02

Table 4.2 Summary of studies on prevalence of PsA in patients with psoriasis

Year/author	Country	Sample	Diagnosis method	Criteria	Prevalence (%, 95 % CI)
2005, Gelfand et al. [29]	USA	Random sample (n=27,220)	Screening question+phone rheum interview	Diagnosis by phone	11 (9–14)
2009, Reich et al. [34]	Germany	Consecutive psoriasis patients from 48 community-acad centers (n=1,511)	Screening question+medical evaluation	CASPAR	20.6
2009, Ibrahim et al. [35]	UK	Two UK general practices (n=22,500)	Screening question+medical evaluation	CASPAR	13.8
2010, Christophers [33]	Five European countries	Consecutive psoriasis patients from derm clinics (n=1,560)	Questionnaire+medical evaluation	CASPAR	20.5
2011, Yang et al. [31]	China	Consecutive psoriasis patients from derm clinics (n=1,928)	Questionnaire+medical evaluation	CASPAR	5.8
2013, Haroon et al. [37]	Canada	Consecutive psoriasis patients from derm clinics (n=100)	Screening question+medical evaluation	CASPAR	29
2014, Maldonado-Ficco et al. [38]	Argentina	Consecutive psoriasis patients from derm clinics (n=100)	Screening question+medical evaluation	CASPAR/ASAS peripheral criteria	17

been shown that the risk of developing PsA did not decrease with time [33].

Another large study (n = 1511 patients) with PsO (psoriasis vulgaris) from academic and community dermatology practices in Germany investigated the prevalence and clinical pattern of PsA in a daily practice population of patients with PsO. The study identified 21 % of the patients as having PsA (by Moll and Wright criteria), with a recent diagnosis in 85 % of these patients. In addition, more than 95 % had active arthritis and 53 % of the patients had a polyarticular involvement. The findings of the study were consistent with a high prevalence of undiagnosed cases of active PsA among patients with PsO seen by dermatologists [34]. By using the CASPAR criteria, the estimated prevalence of PsA among patients with PsO from two large United Kingdom general practices, was found to be 13.8 % [35]. Other studies shown that up to 30 % of psoriasis patients had PsA when assessed carefully by rheumatologist, a significant percentage of these patients were not given the diagnosis of PsA prior to these assessments, which points to the need for increasing the awareness about this condition among primary care physicians [69].

A diagnosis of PsA may also occur in patients initially presenting with undifferentiated arthritis. In a large cohort (n = 1018) of British patients with early arthritis, a diagnosis of PsA was made in 13 % of patients, where almost 90 % of the patients had PsO at initial presentation [36].

Two studies investigated the presence of PsA (defined by CASPAR criteria) in a cohort of 100 consecutive PsO patients. In the first study, conducted by Haroon et al., the disease was diagnosed in 29 % [37]. In the second study from Argentina, authors found a prevalence of 17 %. Remarkably, these patients had significantly higher PsO duration and nail involvement as compared with those without arthritis [38]. Well before the introduction of CASPAR classification criteria, Marsal et al. studied the clinical, radiological and HLA association with PsA and concluded that axial PsA with or without peripheral joints involvement, was associated with HLA B27 in 43 % of cases while only 11 % of PsA presenting with peripheral disease had a positive

HLA B27 association [71]. Queiro et al. has shown in his study that males with Spondyloarthropathy were more susceptible to a more severe spinal disease while females are more likely to have peripheral joint disease [72].

Incidence of Psoriatic Arthritis (Table 4.3)

Several studies have investigated the incidence of PsA. Estimates ranged between 0.1/100,000 (Japanese study) to 23/100,000 from a Finnish study. Hukuda et al. reported the lowest incidence of PsA (defined by ESSG criteria), based on a screening questionnaire and medical records review to all medical Japanese institutions seeking patients with SpA [16]. On the other hand, Savolainen et al. found the highest incidence of PsA reported so far. In this report, information about the study was given through a local newspaper in Finland, and classification was based on the presence of psoriasis and arthritis, excluding RF positive polyarthritis or spondylitis with psoriasis [41]. However, contradictory results have been reported in a previous study from the same country. In 1996, Kaipiainen et al. based on insurance claims and hospital records, reported a lower incidence of PsA (6/100,000) between 1990 and 1995, using the same criteria followed by Savoilainen [39].

A prospective study from Toronto including patients with PsO who did not have PsA at baseline found an incidence of newly diagnosed PsA, also based upon the CASPAR criteria, of almost 2 % per year. Clinical variables associated with increased risk of PsA development in this study were the severity of PsO, the presence of scalp and intergluteal lesions, and the presence of nail lesions [43].

The incidence rates reported in several studies from Sweden, Greece, USA, Czech Republic and Argentina were uniform, ranging from 3.0/100,000 to 8/100,000 [23, 40–42]. Using the resources from the population-based Rochester Epidemiology Project to identify all cases of inflammatory arthritis in a period between 1980 and 1990, with a definite diagnosis of psoriasis,

Table 4.3 Summary of studies on incidence of PsA

Year/author	Country	Sample	Diagnosis method	Criteria	Period	Incidence (/100,000)
1996, Kaipiainen et al. [39]	Finland	All patients receiving drug reimbursm	Insurance claims and hospital records	Psoriasis + arthritis	1990	6
1999, Shbeeb et al. [15]	USA	All patients registered	Medical records review	Psoriasis + arthritis	1982–1991	6.6 (5–8.2)
2001, Hukuda et al. [17]	Japan	Patients from medical institutes	Questionnaire for medical records review	ESSG/Amor		0.1
2002, Söderlin et al. [40]	Sweden	All referred patients	Medical evaluation by rheumatologist	Psoriasis + seronegative arthritis	1999–2000	8 (4–15)
2003, Savolainen et al. [41]	Finland	All referred patients	Medical evaluation by rheumatologist	Psoriasis + seronegative arthritis	2000	23.1 (13.2–37.5)
2003, Alamanos et al. [42]	Greece	Hospitals and private practice	Medical records review	ESSG	1982–2001	3.02 (1.55–4.49)
2009, Wilson [23]	USA	All medical records	Medical records review	CASPAR	1970–1999	7.2 (6–8.4)
2010, Hanova et al. [24]	Czech Republic	All referred patients	Medical evaluation by rheumatologist	Vasey and Espinoza	2002–2003	3.6 (1.4–7.6)
2011, Soriano et al. [26]	Argentina	Patients from a private health system	Medical records review	CASPAR	2000–2006	6.3 (4.2–8.3)
2011, Eder et al. [43]	Canada	All psoriasis patients (n=313)	Medical evaluation by rheumatologist	CASPAR	2006–2009	1.87/100 psoriasis patients

Shbeeb et al. reported a PsA incidence rate of 6.6/100,000 [14]. Another study from the same population reported a population-based incidence of PsA (by CASPAR criteria), between 1970 and 1999. In this study, the overall age-adjusted and sex-adjusted incidence of PsA per 100,000 significantly increased from 3.6 between 1970 and 1979 to 9.8 between 1990 and 2000 [23].

Prevalence of Psoriasis

The population prevalence of psoriasis has been reported to range from 0 to 11.8 % [44] although it should be noted that there are no validated classification criteria for psorais. Psoriasis is considered as a prevalent worldwide disease. However, it has been reported some geographic differences, being generally more common in the colder north than in the tropics. The highest prevalence was reported among Northern Europeans, while the lowest prevalence was seen in aboriginal populations of South America [45].

In general, clinic-based prevalence estimates are consistently higher than population-based estimates. In a population-based study including about 10,000 inhabitants from Faroe Islands, Lomholt et al. reported a psoriasis prevalence of 2.8 % [47]. A recent population-based study from Norway reported an overall psoriasis prevalence of 4.8 %, although the diagnosis was patient-reported so the prevalence could be overestimated [48]. The psoriasis prevalence rates reported in different studies including Northern Europeans are fairly uniform: 4.2 % in a population-based health survey from Norway [49]; in Sweden, the population prevalence was estimated to be 1.4 %; in Denmark the prevalence found was 3.2 % for men and 2.5 % for women [46]. The most recent study from West Yorkshire (United Kingdom) reported that 633 people in a combined general practice database of 22,500 had one of the psoriasis diagnostic labels indicated, thus equating to a prevalence of 2.8 % [35]. Two studies from Germany, based on surveys followed by clinical examination found a psoriasis prevalence between 2.5 and 3.5 % [50]. Studies from Western European countries

(Italy, France, Spain) also reported an uniform psoriasis prevalence rates between (2.9 and 5.2 %) [51–54]. Thus, in Europe the prevalence of psoriasis varies anywhere from 0.6 to 6.5 %. It should be noted that the prevalence estimates vary based on the method of assessment, geographic location and ethnicity.

In North America, two population-based surveys based on patient report of physician diagnosis reported a psoriasis prevalence of 2.2 and 2.6 %, respectively [55, 56]. Recently, Kurd et al. using the National Health and Nutrition Examination Survey (NHANES) 2003–2004, reported a higher prevalence of 3.15 % [57].

However, African-Americans population have reported a lower prevalence of psoriasis compared to Caucasian counterparts. Gelfand et al., based on patient report of physician diagnosed psoriasis, showed a prevalence of 1.3 % in African-Americans, significantly lower than in Whites (2.5 %) [58]. Most African-Americans trace their origins from West Africa where the prevalence of psoriasis is lower than elsewhere in Africa. Estimates of psoriasis prevalence in West Africa (Nigeria, Mali, Ghana, Angola) ranged between 0.08 and 0.9 % [59, 60], significantly lower than the prevalance reported from East Africa (Egypt) and South Africa: 3–4 % [61]. Studies from Central America (Nicaragua, Guatemala, Honduras) have found a lower prevalence of psoriasis, ranged between 0.2 and 0.7 % [44]. Prevalence reported from other American countries is higher: Brazil 1.3 %, Jamaica 1.3 %, Venezuela 2 %, Paraguay 4.2 % and Trinidad and Tobago 6 % [44].

The highest prevalence of psoriasis worldwide (11.8 %) was reported by Eckes et al. from Kazakhstan [46]. However, studies from other Asia countries such as Japan, Taiwan, Malaysia, Kuwait, Saudi Arabia and China have reported a lower prevalence, ranged between 0.05 and 5.5 % [62–64]. Remarkably in two studies including indigenous population, no case of psoriasis have been reported. The first was a survey-based study including a large sample (25,000) of natives from the Andean region in South America [45]. Similar data was reported in a study including more than 3000 Australian Aborigens, were no case of psoriasis was found in natives from central, northern, and southern Australia [44]. However, contrary to what has been reported in the literature, Toloza et al. recently reported the presence of both psoriasis and PsA in aboriginal people from the Andean Mountains of Peru. Of the 16 aboriginal patients in this report, five were natives of Quechua ancestry and one was native Aymara [65].

In summary, although psoriasis is prevalent worldwide, is rare in certain indigenous populations. The prevalence is higher in those with European ethnicity, especially northern European. The prevalence is similar in North and East Africa, but lower in West Africa and in East Asia.

The Epidemiology of CVD Comorbidities in Psoriatic Arthritis

Psoriatic disease is a chronic, systemic inflammatory disease that is not confined to the skin and joint manifestations but also has serious comorbid conditions; epidemiological studies have shown a significant association with number of the CVD risk factors.

Smoking is known to increase the risk of ACPA positive rheumatoid arthritis, but until recently it was not known if it has any relationship to PsA. Wenging et al. investigated this in an interesting study of a population of nearly 95,000 females from the Nurses Health Study 2 over a period of 14 years (1991–2005) and found that smokers had a significantly higher risk of developing PsA, the relative risk for past smokers was 1.54 (95 % CI 1.06–2.24) and for current smokers was even higher at 3.13 (95 % CI 2.08–4, 71). There was also a very clear association between the number of years smoked or the number of cigarettes packs consumed over the years with the increasing risk of developing PsA (P value for the trend was <0.0001), the final conclusion was that the risk of PsA among psoriasis patients was monotonically elevated with smoking intensity and duration [73].

There is conflicting evidence regarding the association between diabetes and patients with psoriasis or PsA, but in at least one large population study by Soloman et al., there was an increased risk of diabetes in patients with psoriasis and PsA compared to a non-rheumatic control group. The incidence of DM among patients with PsA was 8, 2 per 1000 persons years and for non-rheumatic control group it was 5.8 per 1000 persons years. The adjusted hazard ratio was 1.4 (95 % CI 1.3–1.5) [74].

It is possible that the apparent association between smoking, DM, obesity and PsA is contributing to the increased risk of CVD in patients with PsA. Miller et al. conducted a meta-analysis of papers on CVD risk in patients with psoriasis and PsA and found that the strongest association was seen in hospital based studies with an odds ratio of 1.8. No significant association with CVD was found in population based studies, and he postulated that the risk of CVD is more in severe PsA but not in the mild skin manifestations [75].

A young man with severe psoriasis or PsA is approximately three times more likely to develop a myocardial infarction when compared to an age and sex matched control, indicating a major link between CVD risk and severity of psoriasis [76].

Framingham risk factor score (FRS) is a widely used measure to identify individuals at high risk of developing CV events within 10 years. The FRS incorporates age, gender, smoking, hypertension, total cholesterol and HDL but it does not take in consideration the potential effect of chronic inflammatory conditions like PsA. Eder et al. has shown in a study of 226 patients with PsA that the FRS underestimates the extent of subclinical atherosclerosis in patients with PsA and recommended the addition of US assessment to improve the risk stratification in these patients [77].

Conclusions

Psoriasis and PsA are chronic systemic diseases that have a major impact on health and quality of life. The prevalence and incidence estimates of these related diseases show ethnic and geographic variations, being generally more common in the colder north than in the tropics. Psoriasis is a worldwide disease, where the highest prevalence was reported among Northern Europeans, while the lowest prevalence was seen in aboriginal populations. The epidemiology of PsA is difficult and has lagged behind the study of other arthropathies, particularly RA and ankylosing spondylitis. Large variations in the population incidence and prevalence rates of PsA were also seen when reviewing the literature, being highest in people of European descent and lowest in the Japanese. Although these variations could in part be attributed to geographic distribution of genetic and environmental factors, different study methodology and case definition may also explain some of the variations. These caveats put important limitations on the interpretation of epidemiological data. In PsA, the introduction of standardized criteria for diagnosis and classification is needed for valid investigation of the disease epidemiology.

References

1. Gladman DD, Antoni C, Mease P, et al. Psoriatic arthritis: epidemiology, clinical features, course, and outcome. Ann Rheum Dis. 2005;64 Suppl 2:ii14–7.
2. Cuchacovich R, Perez-Alamino R, Garcia-Valladares I, et al. Steps in the managament of psoriatic arthritis: a guide for clinicians. Ther Adv Chronic Dis. 2012;3(6):259–69.
3. Fox DM. Evidence of evidence-based health policy: the politics of systematic reviews in coverage decisions. Health Aff. 2005;24(1):114–22.
4. Mallen C, Peat G, Croft P. Quality assessment of observational studies is not common place in systematic reviews. J Clin Epidemiol. 2006;59(8):765–9.
5. Moll JM, Wright V. Psoriatic arthritis. Semin Arthritis Rheum. 1973;3(1):55–78.
6. Helliwell PS, Taylor WJ. Classification and diagnostic criteria for psoriatic arthritis. Ann Rheum Dis. 2005;64(2):ii3–8.
7. Taylor W, Gladman D, Helliwell P, et al. Classification criteria for psoriatic arthritis: development of new criteria from a large international study. Arthritis Rheum. 2006;54(8):2665–73.
8. Gladman D. Epidemiology. Psoriatic arthritis. In: Gordon GB, Ruderman E, editors. Psoriasis and psoriatic arthritis: an integrated approach. Heidelberg: Springer; 2005. p. 57–65.
9. Gladman D, Shuckett R, Russell M, et al. Psoriatic arthritis PsA- an analysis of 220 patients. Q J Med. 1987;62:127.
10. Torre-Alonso JC, Rodriguez-Perez A, Arribas-Castrillo JM, et al. Psoriatic arthritis (PA): a clinical, immunological and radiological study of 180 patients. Br J Rheumatol. 1991;30:245–50.
11. Boyer G, Templin D, Cornoni-Huntley J, et al. Prevalence of spondyloarthropathies in Alaskan Eskimos. J Rheumatol. 1994;21(12):2292–7.
12. Alexeeva L, Krylov M, Vturin V, et al. Prevalence of spondyloarthropathies and HLA-B27 in the native population of Chukotka, Russia. J Rheumatol. 1994;21(12):2298–300.
13. Braun J, Bollow M, Remlinger G, et al. Prevalence of spondylarthropathies in HLAB27 positive and negative blood donors. Arthritis Rheum. 1998;41(1):58–67.
14. Shbeeb M, Uramoto KM, Gibson LE, et al. The epidemiology of psoriatic arthritis in Olmsted County, Minnesota, USA, 1982–1991. J Rheumatol. 2000; 27(5):1247–50.
15. Taylor WJ, Marchesoni A, Arreghini M, et al. A comparison of the performance characteristics of classification criteria for the diagnosis of psoriatic arthritis. Semin Arthritis Rheum. 2004;34:575–84.
16. Hukuda S, Minami M, Saito T, et al. Spondyloarthropathies in Japan: nationwide questionnaire survey performed by the Japan Ankylosing Spondylitis Society. J Rheumatol. 2001;28(3):554–9.
17. Saraux A, Guillemin F, Guggenbuhl P, et al. Prevalence of spondyloarthropathies in France: 2001. Ann Rheum Dis. 2005;64(10):1431–5.
18. Trontzas P, Andrianakos A, Miyakis S, et al. Seronegative spondyloarthropathies in Greece: a population-based study of prevalence, clinical pattern, and management. The ESORDIG study. Clin Rheumatol. 2005;24(6):583–9.
19. Madland TM, Apalset EM, Johannessen AE, et al. Prevalence, disease manifestations, and treatment of psoriatic arthritis in Western Norway. J Rheumatol. 2005;32(10):1918–22.
20. De Angelis R, Salaffi F, Grassi W. Prevalence of spondyloarthropathies in an Italian population sample: a regional community-based study. Scand J Rheumatol. 2007;36(1):14–21.
21. Love TJ, Gudbjornsson B, Gudjonsson JE, et al. Psoriatic arthritis in Reykjavik, Iceland: prevalence, demographics, and disease course. J Rheumatol. 2007;34(10):2082–8.
22. Liao ZT, Pan YF, Huang JL, et al. An epidemiological survey of low back pain and axial spondyloarthritis in a Chinese Han population. Scand J Rheumatol. 2009;38(6):455–9.
23. Wilson FC, Icen M, Crowson CS, et al. Time trends in epidemiology and characteristics of psoriatic arthritis over 3 decades: a population-based study. J Rheumatol. 2009;36(2):361–7.
24. Hanova P, Pavelka K, Holcatova I, et al. Incidence and prevalence of psoriatic arthritis, ankylosing spondylitis, and reactive arthritis in the first descriptive population-based study in the Czech Republic. Scand J Rheumatol. 2010;39(4):310–7.
25. Haglund E, Bremander AB, Petersson IF, et al. Prevalence of spondyloarthritis and its subtypes in southern Sweden. Ann Rheum Dis. 2011;70(6): 943–8.

26. Soriano ER, Rosa J, Velozo E, et al. Incidence and prevalence of psoriatic arthritis in Buenos Aires, Argentina: a 6-year health management organization based study. Rheumatology (Oxford). 2011;50(4): 729–34.

27. Alvarez-Nemegyei J, Pelaez-Ballestas I, Sanin LH, et al. Prevalence of Musculoskeletal pain and rheumatic diseases in the southeastern region of Mexico. A COPCORD-based community survey. J Rheumatol Suppl. 2011;86:21–5.

28. Zacharie H. Prevalence of joint disease in patients with psoriasis: implications for therapy. Am J Clin Dermatol. 2003;4:441.

29. Gelfand JM, Gladman DD, Mease PJ, et al. Epidemiology of psoriatic arthritis in the population of the United States. J Am Acad Dermatol. 2005;53: 573.

30. Tam LS, Leung YY, Li EK. Psoriatic arthritis in Asia. Rheumatology (Oxford). 2009;48(12):1473–7.

31. Yang Q, Qu L, Tian H, et al. Prevalence and characteristics of psoriatic arthritis in Chinese patients with psoriasis. J Eur Acad Dermatol Venereol. 2011;25(12): 1409–14.

32. Alamanos Y, Voulgari PV, Drossos AA. Incidence and prevalence of psoriatic arthritis: a systematic review. J Rheumatol. 2008;35(7):1354–8.

33. Christophers E, Barker JN, Griffiths CE, et al. The risk of psoriatic arthritis remains constant following initial diagnosis of psoriasis among patients seen in European dermatology clinics. J Eur Acad Dermatol Venereol. 2010;24:548.

34. Reich K, Kruger K, Mossner R, et al. Epidemiology and clinical pattern of psoriatic arthritis in Germany: a prospective interdisciplinary epidemiological study of 1511 patients with plaque-type psoriasis. Br J Dermatol. 2009;160:1040.

35. Ibrahim G, Waxman R, Helliwell PS. The prevalence of psoriatic arthritis in people with psoriasis. Arthritis Rheum. 2009;61:1373.

36. Kane D, Stafford L, Bresnihan B, et al. A prospective, clinical and radiological study of early psoriatic arthritis: an early synovitis clinic experience. Rheumatology (Oxford). 2003;42:1460.

37. Haroon M, Kirby B, Fitzgerald O. High prevalence of psoriatic arthritis in patients with severe psoriasis with suboptimal performance of screening questionnaires. Ann Rheum Dis. 2013;72(5):736–40.

38. Maldonado-Ficco H, Citera G, Maldonado-Cocco JA. Prevalence of psoriatic arthritis in psoriasis patients according to newer classification criteria. Clin Rheumatol. 2014;33:1489–93.

39. Kaipiainen-Seppanen O. Incidence of psoriatic arthritis in Finland. Br J Rheumatol. 1996;35(12): 1289–91.

40. Soderlin MK, Borjesson O, Kautiainen H, et al. Annual incidence of inflammatory joint diseases in a population based study in southern Sweden. Ann Rheum Dis. 2002;61(10):911–5.

41. Savolainen E, Kaipiainen-Seppanen O, Kroger L, et al. Total incidence and distribution of inflammatory joint diseases in a defined population: results from the Kuopio 2000 arthritis survey. J Rheumatol. 2003; 30(11):2460–8.

42. Alamanos Y, Papadopoulos NG, Voulgari PV, et al. Epidemiology of psoriatic arthritis in northwest Greece, 1982–2001. J Rheumatol. 2003;30(12):2641–4.

43. Eder L, Chandran V, Shen H, et al. Incidence of arthritis in a prospective cohort of psoriasis patients. Arthritis Care Res (Hoboken). 2011;63:619.

44. Raychaudhuri SP, Farber EM. The prevalence of psoriasis in the world. J Eur Acad Dermatol Venereol. 2001;15:16–7.

45. Gutierrez E, Galarza C, Ramos W, et al. Skin diseases in the Peruvian Amazonia. Int J Dermatol. 2010;49: 794–800.

46. Farber EM, Nall L. Epidemiology: natural history and genetics. In: Roenigk Jr HH, Maibach HI, editors. Psoriasis. New York: Dekker; 1998. p. 107–57.

47. Lomholt G. Psoriasis: prevalence, spontaneous course and genetics: a census study on the prevalence of skin diseases on the Faroe Islands. GEC Gad: Copenhagen; 1963.

48. Gudjonsson JE, Elder JT. Psoriasis: epidemiology. Clin Dermatol. 2007;25:535e46.

49. Olsen AO, Grjibovski A, Magnus P, et al. Psoriasis in Norway as observed in a population-based Norwegian twin panel. Br J Dermatol. 2005;153:346e51.

50. Schäfer T. Epidemiology of psoriasis. Review and the German perspective. Dermatology. 2006;212:327e37.

51. Saraceno R, Mannheimer R, Chimenti S. Regional distribution of psoriasis in Italy. J Eur Acad Dermatol Venereol. 2008;22:324–9.

52. Wolkenstein P, Grob JJ, Bastuji-Garin S, et al. French people and skin diseases: results of a survey using a representative sample. Arch Dermatol. 2003;139: 1614–9.

53. Wolkenstein P, Revuz J, Roujeau JC, et al. Psoriasis in France and associated risk factors: results of a case–control study based on a large community survey. Dermatology. 2009;218:103–9.

54. Ferrándiz C, Bordas X, García-Patos V, et al. Prevalence of psoriasis in Spain (Epiderma Project: phase I). J Eur Acad Dermatol Venereol. 2001;15:20e.

55. Stern RS, Nijsten T, Feldman SR, et al. Psoriasis is common, carries a substantial burden even when not extensive, and is associated with widespread treatment dissatisfaction. J Investig Dermatol Symp Proc. 2004;9:136–9.

56. Koo J. Population-based epidemiologic study of psoriasis with emphasis on quality of life assessment. Dermatol Clin. 1996;14:485–96.

57. Kurd SK, Gelfand JM. The prevalence of previously diagnosed and undiagnosed psoriasis in US adults: results from NHANES 2003–2004. J Am Acad Dermatol. 2009;60:218–24.

58. Gelfand J, Stern R, Nijsten T, et al. The prevalence of psoriasis in African-Americans: results from a population-based study. J Am Acad Dermatol. 2005;52:23–6.

59. Ogunbiyi A, Daramola O, Alese O. Prevalence of skin diseases in Ibadan, Nigeria. Int J Dermatol. 2004;43: 31–6.

60. Doe PT, Asiedu A, Acheampong JW, et al. Skin diseases in Ghana and the UK. Int J Dermatol. 2001;40:323–6.
61. Chandran V, Raychaudhuri S. Geoepidemiology and environmental factors of psoriasis and psoriatic arthritis. J Autoimmun. 2010;34:J314–21.
62. Chang Y, Chen T, Liu P, et al. Epidemiological study of psoriasis in the national health insurance database in Taiwan. Acta Derm Venereol. 2009;89:262–6.
63. Kaur I, Handa S, Kumar B. Natural history of psoriasis: a study from the Indian subcontinent. J Dermatol. 1997;24:230–4.
64. Fatani M, Abdulghani M, Al-Afif K. Psoriasis in the eastern Saudi Arabia. Saudi Med J. 2002;23:213–7.
65. Toloza S, Vega-Hinojosa O, Chandran V, et al. Psoriasis and psoriatic arthritis in peruvian aborigines: a report from the GRAPPA 2011 annual meeting. J Rheumatol. 2012;39:2216–9.
66. Baker H, Golding DN, Thompson M. Psoriasis and arthritis. Ann Intern Med. 1963;58:909–25.
67. Rahman P, Schentag CT, Gladman DD. Excessive paternal transmission in psoriatic arhritis. Arthritis Rheum. 1999;42:1228–31.
68. Ogdie A. Prevalence and treatment patterns of PsA in the UK. Rheumatology. 2013;52(3):568–75.
69. Mease P. Prevalence of rheumatologist diagnosed PsA in patients with psoriasis. J Am Acad Dermatol. 2013;69:729–35.
70. Roussou E, Chopra S, Ngandu DL. Phenotypic and clinical differences between Caucasian and South Asian patients with PsA living in North East London. Clin Rheumatol. 2013;32:591–9.
71. Marsal S, Martinez M, Armadans-Gil L, Gallado D, Ribera A, Lience E. Clinical, radiological and HLA associations as markers for different patterns of PsA. Rheumatology. 1999;38:332–7.
72. Queiro R, Tejon P, Coto P, Alonso S, Alperi M, Sarasqueta C, Gonzalez S, Martinez-Borra J, Lopez-Larrea C, Ballina J. Clinical differences between men and women with PsA. Clin Dev Immunol. 2013;article ID 482691:7.
73. Li W, Han J, Qureshi AA. Smokingand the risk of incident psoriatic arthritis in US women. Ann Rheum Dis. 2012;71:804–8.
74. Soloman DM, Love TJ, Canning C, Scheeweiss S. Risk of diabetes among patients with rheumatoid arthritis, PsA and psoriasis. Ann Rheum Dis. 2010;69: 2114–7.
75. Miller IM, Ellervik C, Yazdanyar S, Gregor B, Jemec E. Meta-analysis of psoriasis, CVD and associated risk factors. J Am Acad Dermatol. 2013;69(6): 1014–24.
76. Gelfand JM, Neimann AL, Shin DB. Risk of myocardial infarction inpatients with psoriasis. JAMA. 2006;296:1735–41.
77. Eder L, Chander V, Gladman DD. The Framingham risk score underestimates the extent of subclinical atherosclerosis in patients with psoriatic disease. Ann Rheum Dis. 2014;73:1990–6.

The Natural History of Psoriatic Arthritis

5

William Tillett and Philip H. Helliwell

Abstract

Psoriatic arthritis is an inflammatory arthritis that usually appears after, or synchronously with, the onset of psoriasis. The disease may manifest in a variety of phenotypes, follows a relapsing and remitting course, with articular damage and functional impairment accumulating over time. Delay to diagnosis results on worse clinical, functional and radiographic outcome. The natural history of disease in the modern era of novel biological treatments and tighter disease control has yet to be determined.

Keywords

Psoriatic arthritis • Phenotype • Outcome • Radiography • Physical Function • Quality of Life • Treatment

In recent years improved classification criteria and the development of large, well classified longitudinal cohort studies have led to a better understanding of the clinical course of psoriatic arthritis. Originally considered a benign form of inflammatory arthritis we now recognise psoriatic arthritis to be more severe, progressive and destructive [1–3], with a significantly negative impact on physical function, quality of life and ability to work [4, 5].

Psoriatic arthritis appears after, or synchronously with, the onset of psoriasis in the majority of patients [1, 6]. In a minority (18 – 13 %) the arthritis precedes the onset of psoriasis [1, 6, 7]. Disease activity of skin psoriasis follows a relapsing and remitting course which is often divergent from joint disease. Early studies of PsA recognised different disease phenotypes; polyarticular (15 %), oligoarticular (70 %), distalinterphalangeal (5 %), spondyloarthritis (5 %) or mutilans pattern (5 %) [8]. Larger cohort studies have confirmed these clinical patterns but it has become apparent that most patients have polyarticular

W. Tillett, MBChB, BSc, PhD, MRCP (✉)
Department of Rheumatology,
Royal National Hospital for Rheumatic Diseases,
Upper Borough Walls, Bath BA11RL, UK
e-mail: w.tillett@nhs.net

P.H. Helliwell, MD, PhD
Leeds Institute of Rheumatic and Musculoskeletal Medicine, University of Leeds, Chapel Allerton Hospital, 2nd Floor, Harehills Lane,
Leeds LS7 4SA, UK
e-mail: p.helliwell@leeds.ac.uk

© Springer International Publishing Switzerland 2016
A. Adebajo et al. (eds.), *Psoriatic Arthritis and Psoriasis: Pathology and Clinical Aspects*,
DOI 10.1007/978-3-319-19530-8_5

(~60 %) disease [9]. The pattern of joint involvement itself may also change during an individual's disease course. In one longitudinal study of 100 patients with mean disease duration of 20 years 64 changed disease phenotype during follow up [6]. Dactylitis (sausage digit) will occur in approximately 50 % of patients with psoriatic arthritis at some point in their disease course [1]. Little is known about the clinical course of psoriatic spondyloarthritis, in part because there is a burden of subclinical disease that is only just being recognised. Current estimates of the prevalence range between 6 and 43 % [9].

Articular damage from active arthritis accumulates over time [9]. Risk factors at diagnosis for progressive disease include high erythrocyte sedimentation rate (ESR) [10] or C reactive protein (CRP) [11], polyarticular disease (≤ four joints) [12], poor functional status (HAQ) and existing radiographic damage (erosions) [10]. It is generally accepted that, with the exception of the psoriatic arthritis mutilans phenotype, radiographic damage is not as severe as seen in RA [13]. However one study identified similar degrees of radiographic destruction similar to RA [14]. Nonetheless there is a large burden of joint destruction in PsA with radiographic damage present in early disease. Recent data from the TICOPA study identified 27 % patients with erosive disease at presentation rising to 31 % at 1 year [15]. Observational cohorts have identified nearly half patients developing radiographic damage in the first 2 years of disease [16] and progressive damage from erosions, joint space narrowing, osteoproliferation and ankylosis continue in established disease [2, 3, 17].

Ultrasound studies of lower limb entheses have demonstrated that enthesitis is more common than is clinically evident and more common in those with psoriasis than in healthy individuals [18, 19]. Nail pitting and onycholysis is indistinguishable from that seen in psoriasis [20]. However nail lesions are more common in patients with PsA than those with psoriasis alone [21] and in those with DIP joint disease [20]. Uveitis is recognised in PsA and is reported in approximately 7 % patients. Two studies of ocular involvement in PsA identified increased uveitis in those positive to HLAB27 and higher rates of insidious onset, bilateral and posterior involvement [22, 23].

Evidence on whether psoriatic arthritis leads to increased risk of death is conflicted. Two studies have not identified an increased risk of death [24, 25]. However in a study from North America of patients followed over 20 years identified higher mortality rates than the general population with an increased risk for death with an SMR of 1.59 (male) 1.65 (female) [26].

Delay to diagnosis is now recognised to adversely affect disease outcome including physical function, articular damage and work disability [27–29]. Impairment in physical function among patients with PsA is considerably worse than the healthy population and at a level comparable with rheumatoid arthritis [30]. Physical function fluctuates with disease activity and in the majority deteriorates with increasing disease duration with a minority (28 %) resistant to long term disability [5]. Work disability in PsA is high with unemployment levels estimated at between 20 and 50 % of unemployment (20–50 %) and work disability (encompassing preesetneeism and productivity loss) at 16–39 %. Work disability is associated with high disease activity and longer disease duration as well as employer and socioeconomic factors [31–33].

It is worthy of note that much of our understanding of the natural history of PsA comes from cohort study data from the 'pre-biologic' era (pre 2001). The impact of biological disease modifying anti rheumatic drugs (bDMARDS) on the natural history of disease has yet to be determined. The last decade has also seen a paradigm shift in treatment strategy from gradual step up drug treatment towards tight control of disease, the concept of minimal disease activity and treatment to target [34]. The clinical course of PsA a modern era of early diagnosis and aggressive treatment with biologic agents will inevitably impact on the clinical course of PsA in years to come.

In summary psoriatic arthritis follows a relapsing and remitting course that is ultimately progressive and destructive in most leading to high levels of physical, functional and work impairment. The natural history of disease in the modern era of novel biological treatments and tighter disease control has yet to be determined.

References

1. Gladman DD, Shuckett R, Russell ML, Thorne JC, Schachter RK. Psoriatic arthritis (PSA) – an analysis of 220 patients. Q J Med. 1987;62:127–41.
2. Ravindran J, Cavill C, Balakrishnan C, Jones SM, Korendowych E, McHugh NJ. A modified Sharp score demonstrates disease progression in established psoriatic arthritis. Arthritis Care Res (Hoboken). 2010;62:86–91.
3. Gladman DD, Stafford-Brady F, Chang CH, Lewandowski K, Russell ML. Longitudinal study of clinical and radiological progression in psoriatic arthritis. J Rheumatol. 1990;17:809–12.
4. Tillett W, de-Vries C, McHugh NJ. Work disability in psoriatic arthritis: a systematic review. Rheumatology. 2012;51:275–83.
5. Husted JA, Tom BD, Farewell VT, Schentag CT, Gladman DD. Description and prediction of physical functional disability in psoriatic arthritis: a longitudinal analysis using a Markov model approach. Arthritis Rheum. 2005;53:404–9.
6. Jones SM, Armas JB, Cohen MG, Lovell CR, Evison G, McHugh NJ. Psoriatic arthritis: outcome of disease subsets and relationship of joint disease to nail and skin disease. Br J Rheumatol. 1994;33:834–9.
7. Yang Q, Qu L, Tian H, Hu Y, Peng J, Yu X, et al. Prevalence and characteristics of psoriatic arthritis in Chinese patients with psoriasis. J Eur Acad Dermatol Venereol. 2011;25:1409–14.
8. Moll JM, Wright V. Psoriatic arthritis. Semin Arthritis Rheum. 1973;3:55–78.
9. Gladman DD, Antoni C, Mease P, Clegg DO, Nash P. Psoriatic arthritis: epidemiology, clinical features, course, and outcome. Ann Rheum Dis. 2005;64 Suppl 2:ii14–7.
10. Bond SJ, Farewell VT, Schentag CT, Gladman DD. Predictors for radiological damage in psoriatic arthritis: results from a single centre. Ann Rheum Dis. 2007;66:370–6.
11. Gladman DD, Mease PJ, Choy EH, Ritchlin CT, Perdok RJ, Sasso EH. Risk factors for radiographic progression in psoriatic arthritis: subanalysis of the randomized controlled trial ADEPT. Arthritis Res Ther. 2010;12:R113.
12. Simon P, Pfoehler C, Bergner R, Schreiber M, Pfreundschuh M, Assmann G. Swollen joint count in psoriatic arthritis is associated with progressive radiological damage in hands and feet. Clin Exp Rheumatol. 2012;30:45–50.
13. Sokoll KB, Helliwell PS. Comparison of disability and quality of life in rheumatoid and psoriatic arthritis. J Rheumatol. 2001;28:1842–6.
14. Rahman P. Comparison of radiological severity in psoriatic arthritis and rheumatoid arthritis. J Rheumatol. 2001;28:1041–4.
15. Coates L, Helliwell P. Low level of erosive change is found in early psoriatic arthritis. EULAR. 2014: SAT0409.
16. Kane D, Stafford L, Bresnihan B, FitzGerald O. A prospective, clinical and radiological study of early psoriatic arthritis: an early synovitis clinic experience. Rheumatology (Oxford). 2003;42:1460–8.
17. Siannis F, Farewell VT, Cook RJ, Schentag CT, Gladman DD. Clinical and radiological damage in psoriatic arthritis. Ann Rheum Dis. 2006;65:478–81.
18. De Simone C, Guerriero C, Giampetruzzi AR, Costantini M, Di Gregorio F, Amerio P. Achilles tendinitis in psoriasis: clinical and sonographic findings. J Am Acad Dermatol. 2003;49:217–22.
19. Gisondi P, Tinazzi I, El-Dalati G, Gallo M, Biasi D, Barbara LM, et al. Lower limb enthesopathy in patients with psoriasis without clinical signs of arthropathy: a hospital-based case-control study. Ann Rheum Dis. 2008;67:26–30.
20. Williamson L, Dalbeth N, Dockerty JL, Gee BC, Weatherall R, Wordsworth BP. Extended report: nail disease in psoriatic arthritis – clinically important, potentially treatable and often overlooked. Rheumatology. 2004;43:790–4.
21. Gladman DD, Anhorn KA, Schachter RK, Mervart H. HLA antigens in psoriatic arthritis. J Rheumatol. 1986;13:586–92.
22. Lambert JR, Wright V. Eye inflammation in psoriatic arthritis. Ann Rheum Dis. 1976;35:354–6.
23. Paiva ES, Macaluso DC, Edwards A, Rosenbaum JT. Characterisation of uveitis in patients with psoriatic arthritis. Ann Rheum Dis. 2000;59:67–70.
24. Shbeeb M, Uramoto KM, Gibson LE, O'Fallon WM, Gabriel SE. The epidemiology of psoriatic arthritis in Olmsted County, Minnesota, USA, 1982–1991. J Rheumatol. 2000;27:1247–50.
25. Buckley C, Cavill C, Taylor G, Kay H, Waldron N, Korendowych E, et al. Mortality in psoriatic arthritis – a single-center study from the UK. J Rheumatol. 2010;37:2141–4.
26. Wong K, Gladman DD, Husted J, Long JA, Farewell VT. Mortality studies in psoriatic arthritis: results from a single outpatient clinic. I. Causes and risk of death. Arthritis Rheum. 1997;40:1868–72.
27. Tillett W, Jadon D, Shaddick G, Cavill C, Korendowych E, de Vries CS, et al. Smoking and delay to diagnosis are associated with poorer functional outcome in psoriatic arthritis. Ann Rheum Dis. 2013;72:1358–61.
28. Gladman DD, Thavaneswaran A, Chandran V, Cook RJ. Do patients with psoriatic arthritis who present early fare better than those presenting later in the disease? Ann Rheum Dis. 2011;70:2152–4.
29. Haroon M, Gallagher P, Fitzgerald O. Diagnostic delay of more than 6 months contributes to poor radiographic and functional outcome in psoriatic arthritis. Ann Rheum Dis. 2015;74(6):1045-50.

30. Husted JA, Gladman DD, Farewell VT, Cook RJ. Health-related quality of life of patients with psoriatic arthritis: a comparison with patients with rheumatoid arthritis. Arthritis Rheum. 2001;45:151–8.

31. Walsh JA, McFadden ML, Morgan MD, Sawitzke AD, Duffin KC, Krueger GG, et al. Work productivity loss and fatigue in psoriatic arthritis. J Rheumatol. 2014;41:1670–4.

32. Tillett W, de-Vries C, McHugh NJ. Work disability in psoriatic arthritis: a systematic review. Rheumatology (Oxford). 2012;51:275–83.

33. Tillett W, Shaddick G, Askari A, Cooper A, Creamer P, Clunie G, et al. Factors influencing work disability in psoriatic arthritis: first results from a large UK multicentre study. Rheumatology (Oxford). 2014;54(1): 157–62.

34. Coates LC, Anna M, McParland L, Brown S, Collier H, Brown SR, Navarro-Coy N, Emery P, Conaghan P, Helliwell P. Effect of tight control of inflammation in early psoriatic arthritis (TICOPA): a multicenre, open-label, randomised controlled trial. Lancet. 2014;383:S36.

Part III

Pathological and Genetic Aspects

Oliver FitzGerald

Immunopathogenesis of Psoriasis Skin and Nail

6

Ami R. Saraiya and Alice B. Gottlieb

Abstract

In this chapter, an overview will be presented of the current understanding of the immunopathogenesis of psoriatic skin disease, nail pathology, and the important clinical and therapeutic implications. Psoriasis is an immune-mediated disorder with varying global prevalence and is associated with environmental triggers, including stress, trauma, medications, and infections.

Plaque psoriasis or psoriasis vulgaris, characterized clinically by erythematous plaques with silvery scale, is the most common type of psoriasis affecting 85–90 % of all patients with the disease.

Keywords

Psoriasis • Immunopathogenesis • Cytokines • Th17 cells • Enthesis • Biologics • Therapeutics

Introduction

In this chapter, an overview will be presented of the current understanding of the immunopathogenesis of psoriatic skin disease, nail pathology, and the important clinical and therapeutic implications. Psoriasis is an immune-mediated disorder with varying global prevalence [1] and is associated with environmental triggers, including stress, trauma, medications, and infections.

Plaque psoriasis or psoriasis vulgaris, characterized clinically by erythematous plaques with silvery scale, is the most common type of psoriasis affecting 85–90 % of all patients with the disease [2].

Immunopathology of the Skin

The maturation cycle from the basal to cornified skin layer in the epidermis is 28 days, but in psoriatic skin cells this process is only 5 days resulting in disrupted terminal differentia-

Alice B. Gottlieb, MD, PhD • A.R. Saraiya, MD (✉)
Department of Dermatology, Tufts Medical Center,
800 Washington Street, Boston, MA, 02111, USA
e-mail: agottlieb@tuftsmedicalcenter.org;
Asaraiya@tuftsmedicalcenter.org

A. Adebajo et al. (eds.), *Psoriatic Arthritis and Psoriasis: Pathology and Clinical Aspects*,
DOI 10.1007/978-3-319-19530-8_6

tion of keratinocytes [3]. Basal keratinocytes produce keratins 5 and 14 and can differentiate to produce keratins 1 and 10, the major keratins of the mature interfollicular epidermis. Keratins 1 and 10 are underexpressed in psoriasis [2]. Keratins 6 and 16, seen in cells with fast turnover, are markers of the active state during inflammation and are increased in lesional and perilesional epidermis of psoriatic plaques [4].

Skin biopsy findings in psoriasis include epidermal acanthosis or thickening, elongated rete ridges, incomplete cornification, parakeratosis or retention of nuclei in the stratum corneum, decreased extracellular lipid resulting in poorly adherent stratum corneum and formation of scales, loss of the granular cell layer, dilation of dermal blood vessels, and cell infiltration by T cells, dendritic cells, neutrophils, and other leukocytes [5]. Munro's microabscesses are neutrophilic granules that infiltrate from the papillary dermis into the stratum corneum [6]. In the stratum spinosum, neutrophils form spongiform pustules of Kogoj [7].

Using scanning laser-Doppler velocimeter, increase in blood flow within plaques is four times that of background blood flow [8]. Local factors responsible for vascular growth are increased at the active edge [9]. Vascular changes are mediated by increased vascular endothelial growth factor (VEGF) expression [10]. Upon cytokine stimulation, adhesion molecules (P and E-selectin, ICAM-1, and VCAM-1) are increased on vascular endothelium to allow leukocyte transmigration into tissues [11]. Transgenic mice that over express VEGF develop skin changes similar to psoriasis [12].

In the late twentieth century, the understanding of the pathogenesis of psoriasis shifted from being primarily keratinocyte mediated to immune mediated. Researchers observed that in vitro T cell clones from psoriasis skin lesions could promote keratinocyte proliferation [13]. Other studies were done with T cell modulating drugs, including anti-CD4 antibodies to treat psoriasis [14, 15], a fusion protein of human interleukin-2 and diphtheria toxin to treat psoriasis [16], and cytotoxic T lymphocyte-associated antigen 4 (CTLA-4)-immunoglobulin [17], suggesting that T helper cells are predominant.

Psoriasis is mediated by both the adaptive and innate immune system. The adaptive immune system is acquired immunity that provides long-term protection through immunologic memory upon re-exposure to an infectious agent. Adaptive immunity players are T and B lymphocytes and antibodies. The innate immune system is the first line of defense against bacterial, fungal and viral infections. Innate immunity players are neutrophils, macrophages, natural killer cells, mast cells, cytokines, antimicrobial peptides, and the complement system. Dendritic cells serve as mediators between the adaptive and innate immune system [10].

Plasmacytoid dendritic cells are increased in psoriatic lesions and produce type 1 interferon after sensing DNA through Toll-like receptors [18]. Interferon alpha treatment has been shown to induce and worsen psoriasis [19]. Toll-like receptors are located on cells such as macrophages and dendritic cells and recognize microbial components [20]. Psoriatic keratinocytes release antimicrobial peptides such as beta-defensins, cathelicidins, and psoriasin (S100A7), which have a chemotactic effect on dendritic cells and T cells [21]. The antimicrobial peptide LL37 binds self-DNA and activates plasmacytoid dendritic cells to produce interferon through toll-like-receptor 9 [20].

TNF alpha, a potent proinflammatory cytokine, is produced by dermal macrophages, dendritic cells, activated keratinocytes, and T-lymphocytes and is implicated in the pathogenesis of psoriasis [22]. TNF alpha is found to be in higher concentration in psoriatic lesions than uninvolved skin [23]. TNF alpha increases production of the pro-inflammatory cytokines IL-1, IL-6, IL-8, the adhesion molecules ICAM-1, P-selectin, and E-selectin thus enabling leukocyte infiltration into the skin, and the transcription factor NFκB, which may inhibit TNF alpha induced apoptosis in psoriatic lesions [24]. Active NFκB/RelA is up regulated in the epidermis of psoriatic plaques and of non-lesional skin from psoriasis patients and is downregulated after treatment with etanercept [25]. In psoriatic lesions, IL-1 increases production of cytokines and expression of cytokeratin 6, IL-6 increases production of acute phase proteins, and IL-8 activates lymphocytes and is a

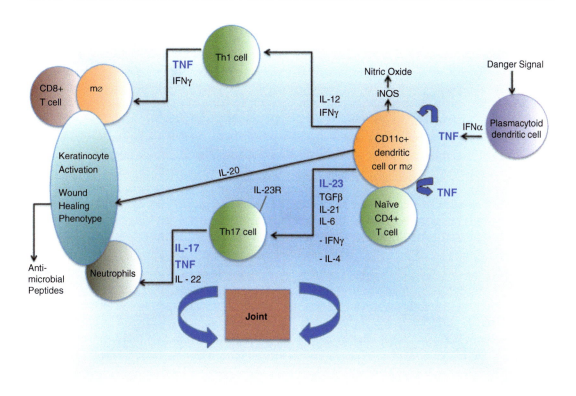

Fig. 6.1 Cytokine signaling in psoriasis and psoriatic arthritis

neutrophil chemoattractant [26]. TNF alpha also induces the skin-specific memory T-cell attractant CCL27 [27].

Mast cells have been associated with psoriatic inflammation and release IFN gamma upon stimulation [28]. Mast cells can also release pro-inflammatory mediators selectively without degranulation [29]. Lin AM, et al. observed IL-17+ mast cells and neutrophils at higher densities in psoriatic lesions than IL-17+ T cells [30]. Furthermore, mast cells form extracellular traps in psoriatic lesions that are associated with IL-17 release, and IL-23 and IL-1β can induce mast cell extracellular trap formation and degranulation [30]. Recently, mast cells have been found to produce IL-33, which has been observed in the epidermis of patients with psoriasis [31].

The release of proinflammatory cytokines by innate immune cells and plasmacytoid dendritic cells stimulates myeloid dendritic cells in the skin. Myeloid dermal dendritic cells are increased in psoriatic lesions and induce autoproliferation of T cells and type 1 helper T cell (Th1) cytokines [32], and more recently type 17 helper T cell (Th17) cells and cytokines have been identified [33].

In the Th1 pathway, antigen-presenting cells (APCs) release IL-12 and IFNg, which promotes differentiation of naïve T cells into Th1 cells via Stat4 signaling and Stat1 signaling, respectively. This induces expression of T-box 21 and secretion of pro-inflammatory cytokines, including IFN-g [34, 35].

In the Th17 pathway (Fig. 6.1), activated dendritic cells present antigen and through cytokines such as IL-23 (a heterodimer of p40 and IL-12 and p19 subunit), TGFß, IL-21, and IL-6, Th17 cells are promoted via Stat3 signaling, inducing expression of transcription factor RORyt and secretion of cytokines including IL-17, IL-21, and IL-22 [36–40].

IL-22, IL-17A, and TNF alpha induce IL-20 production in keratinocytes [41]. IL-17A, IL-17 F and IL-22 in normal human epithelial keratinocytes induced expression of the genes encoding ß-defensin 2, ß-defensin 3, S100A8 and S100A9 [40].

Additionally, a subset of CD4+ effector T cells called Th22 cells produce IL-22, but not IL-17 or IFNg and have low or undetectable expression of Th17 and Th1 transcription factors [42]. IL-22 induces keratinocyte proliferation and epidermal hyperplasia, inhibits keratinocyte terminal differentiation, and promotes antimicrobial protein [43].

Activated dendritic cells, T-helper 1 and T-helper 17 cells produce TNF alpha. Response to psoriasis is observed after treatment with TNF alpha inhibitors such as infliximab [44, 45], adalimumab [46], and etanercept [47]. After treatment with etanercept, psoriatic skin has a decreased Th17 response and reduced epidermal hyperplasia [33]. Psoriatic skin has down regulation of phosphorylated NF-kappaB/RelA after treatment with etanercept [25]. Additionally, treatment with etanercept at 1 month has been observed to selectively induce apoptosis of pathogenic dermal dendritic cells in psoriatic plaques of responding patients [48]. Golimumab and certolizumab are anti-TNF agents, in addition to infliximab, adalimumab, and etanercept, which are approved for treatment of psoriatic arthritis [49].

Due to increased understanding of the immune mediated mechanisms in psoriasis, newer biologic therapy has been developed. IL-23, a key cytokine for Th17 effector cells, and its receptor are increased in tissues of patients with psoriasis, and injection of a monoclonal antibody against IL-23 has shown inhibition of psoriasis in a xenotransplant mouse model [50]. Ustekinumab, a human monoclonal antibody to IL12/23, has shown therapeutic efficacy for the treatment of psoriasis [51–53]. Ustekinumab targets the p40 subunit shared by both IL-12 and IL-23 [51], thus affecting both the Th17 and Th1 responses. Tildrakizumab and guselkumab are IL-23 inhibitors, secukinumab and ixekizumab inhibit IL-17A, and brodalumab is an IL-17-receptor blocker [54].

Therapies that block T cell activation have been studied. Lymphocyte function-associated antigen 3 (LFA-3) on APCs binding with CD2 on the T cell membrane is important for T cell activation [55]. Alefacept, a drug that blocks CD2 from binding with LFA-3, inhibits activation of both CD4 and CD8 cells and was previously studied for psoriasis [56]. T cell activation requires the interaction between the T-cell receptor (TCR) on the surface of T cells and the antigen peptide bound to the major histocompatibility complex (MHC) on the surface of APCs, and the costimulatory signal between the CD28 receptor on T cells and CD80 (B7-1) and CD86 (B7-2) on activated APCs, such as dendritic cells, B cells, and macrophages [57, 58]. When CD28 interacts with B7-1 and B7-2, full T cell activation occurs, including cytokine production, clonal expansion, enhanced T cell survival, and up regulation of CTLA-4, a molecule that is structurally similar to CD28 that binds both B7–1 and B7–2 [59].

Abatacept, a human fusion protein of the extracellular domain of CTLA-4 linked to a modified Fc portion of human IgG1, prevents T cell activation by binding to CD80/CD86 on the surface of APCs [57, 60]. Siplizumab is an anti-CD2 monoclonal antibody that interferes with the costimulatory signal necessary for T cell activation and proliferation [61].

Modern oral anti-psoriatic medications currently under investigation include dimethyl fumarate, apremilast, and janus kinase (JAK) inhibitors [54]. Apremilast, a phosphodiesterase type 4 (PDE4) inhibitor, elevates intracellular camp levels and decreases pro-inflammatory cytokines like IL-23 and TNF alpha, and enhances anti-inflammatory cytokines like IL-10 [62]. Dimethyl fumarate improves multiple sclerosis and psoriasis by interacting with nuclear factor kappa B (NFκB) and interfering with IL-12 and IL-23 expression [54, 63]. The JAK-STAT signaling pathway is fundamental for cytokine receptor signaling [64]. Tofacitinib, a JAK1 and JAK3 inhibitor, and ruxolitinib, a JAK1 and JAK2 have been studied for psoriasis [64, 65].

Immunopathology of the Nails

Psoriatic nail dystrophy has been associated with development of psoriatic arthritis [66]. The prevalence of psoriatic arthritis in the US population

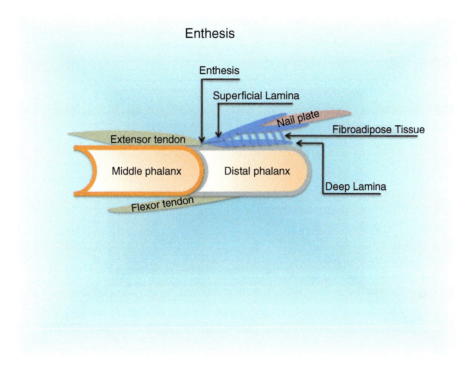

Fig. 6.2 Enthesis anatomy

was reported to be 0.25 %, and the prevalence of psoriatic arthritis among patients with psoriasis in the US population was reported to be 11 % [67].

Normal nail anatomy includes the nail unit, which is composed of the nail plate, and 4 epithelial structures: proximal nail fold, matrix, nail bed, hyponychium [68]. Clinical manifestations of psoriatic nail changes include pitting, discoloration, onycholysis, subungual hyperkeratosis, splinter hemorrhages, and varying other signs based on the extent of psoriasis in the nail matrix [69].

Pitting occurs in the nail plate, which is formed from keratin. Clusters of parakeratotic cells in the stratum corneum in the nail matrix disrupt normal keratinization, and as the nail plate grows outwards there is gradual sloughing of the parakeratotic areas leaving depressions in the nail plate [69]. Discoloration occurs when psoriatic lesions are in the underlying nail bed, onycholysis occurs when the lesions involve the hyponychium, and subungual hyperkeratosis results from the deposition of cells under the nail plate that have not undergone desquamation [69]. Splinter hemorrhages occur in the dermis and pool longitudinally between the epidermal-dermal ridges [70].

The immunopathogenesis of psoriatic nail disease was thought to be similar to psoriatic skin disease. APCs capture antigen, travel to local lymph nodes and activate T cells, and T cells migrate into skin and induce keratinocyte changes through cytokines [69]. In normal skin foreign antigen would be removed, but in psoriatic skin this mechanism continues [71].

However, McGonagle D, et al. describe the origin of pathology to occur at the joint enthesis, or insertion point of ligament and tendon to the bone (Fig. 6.2), an area subject to microdamage and integrated to the nail via the distal phalanx, linking psoriatic skin and joint disease [72]. Histological sections from cadaveric specimens have demonstrated that the distal interphalangeal joint capsule is closely linked with the nail complex, and MRI studies on patients with psoriatic arthritis have shown that the dorsal capsular enthesis is the center of inflammatory reactions and can extend to involve the soft tissues near the nail [73]. A prior study looking at plantar fascia conducted fat suppression MRI tests of the plantar fascia insertion site and adjacent bone, and researchers observed that enthesitis was occasionally associated with osteitis and bone changes [74].

The predominant infiltrating cell at the enthesis fibrocartilage was demonstrated to be the macrophage [75], suggesting the importance of the innate immune system in psoriatic nail disease and psoriatic arthritis [72]. Further studies may elucidate the immunopathogenesis of psoriatic nail disease and psoriatic arthritis.

Conclusion

Psoriasis is a complex skin disorder mediated by immune dysregulation. Through clinical and translational research into the immunopathogenesis of psoriasis, therapeutic options have been developed. As more understanding is gained into the involved cellular signaling and cytokine pathways, new therapeutics may be discovered in the future.

References

1. Parisi R, Symmons DP, Griffiths CE, Ashcroft DM. Identification and Management of Psoriasis and Associated Comorbidity (IMPACT) project team. Global epidemiology of psoriasis: a systematic review of incidence and prevalence. J Invest Dermatol. 2013;133(2):377–85.
2. Griffiths CE, Barker JN. Pathogenesis and clinical features of psoriasis. Lancet. 2007;370(9583):263–71.
3. Sabat R, Sterry W, Philipp S, Wolk K. Three decades of psoriasis research: where has it led us? Clin Dermatol. 2007;25(6):504–9.
4. Komine M, Karakawa M, Takekoshi T, Sakurai N, Minatani Y, Mitsui H, et al. Early inflammatory changes in "perilesional" skin of psoriatic plaques: is there interaction between dendritic cells and keratinocytes? J Invest Dermatol. 2007;127(8):1915–22.
5. Krueger JG, Bowcock A. Psoriasis pathophysiology: current concepts of pathogenesis. Ann Rheum Dis. 2005;64 Suppl 2:ii30–6.
6. Bos JD, Hulsebosch HJ, Krieg SR, Bakker PM, Cormane RH. Immunocompetent cells in psoriasis. In situ immunophenotyping by monoclonal antibodies. Arch Dermatol Res. 1983;275(3):181–9.
7. Chowaniec O, Jablonska S, Beutner EH, Proniewska M, Jarzabek-Chorzelska M, Rzesa G. Earliest clinical and histological changes in psoriasis. Dermatologica. 1981;163(1):42–51.
8. Speight EL, Essex TJ, Farr PM. The study of plaques of psoriasis using a scanning laser-Doppler velocimeter. Br J Dermatol. 1993;128(5):519–24.
9. Goodfield M, Hull SM, Holland D, Roberts G, Wood E, Reid S, et al. Investigations of the 'active' edge of plaque psoriasis: vascular proliferation precedes changes in epidermal keratin. Br J Dermatol. 1994;131(6):808–13.
10. Nestle FO, Kaplan DH, Barker J. Psoriasis. N Engl J Med. 2009;361(5):496–509.
11. Barker JN. Adhesion molecules in cutaneous inflammation. Ciba Found Symp. 1995;189:91–101.
12. Xia YP, Li B, Hylton D, Detmar M, Yancopoulos GD, Rudge JS. Transgenic delivery of VEGF to mouse skin leads to an inflammatory condition resembling human psoriasis. Blood. 2003;102(1):161–8.
13. Prinz JC, Gross B, Vollmer S, Trommler P, Strobel I, Meurer M, et al. T cell clones from psoriasis skin lesions can promote keratinocyte proliferation in vitro via secreted products. Eur J Immunol. 1994;24(3):593–8.
14. Nicolas JF, Chamchick N, Thivolet J, Wijdenes J, Morel P, Revillard JP. CD4 antibody treatment of severe psoriasis. Lancet. 1991;338(8762):321.
15. Prinz J, Braun-Falco O, Meurer M, Daddona P, Reiter C, Rieber P, et al. Chimaeric CD4 monoclonal antibody in treatment of generalised pustular psoriasis. Lancet. 1991;338(8762):320–1.
16. Gottlieb SL, Gilleaudeau P, Johnson R, Estes L, Woodworth TG, Gottlieb AB, et al. Response of psoriasis to a lymphocyte-selective toxin (DAB3891L-2) suggests a primary immune, but not keratinocyte, pathogenic basis. Nat Med. 1995;1(5):442–7.
17. Abrams JR, Kelley SL, Hayes E, Kikuchi T, Brown MJ, Kang S, et al. Blockade of T lymphocyte costimulation with cytotoxic T lymphocyte-associated antigen 4-immunoglobulin (CTLA4Ig) reverses the cellular pathology of psoriatic plaques, including the activation of keratinocytes, dendritic cells, and endothelial cells. J Exp Med. 2000;192(5):681–94.
18. Nestle FO, Conrad C, Tun-Kyi A, Homey B, Gombert M, Boyman O, et al. Plasmacytoid predendritic cells initiate psoriasis through interferon-alpha production. J Exp Med. 2005;202(1):135–43.
19. Funk J, Langeland T, Schrumpf E, Hanssen LE. Psoriasis induced by interferon-alpha. Br J Dermatol. 1991;125(5):463–5.
20. Lande R, Gregorio J, Facchinetti V, Chatterjee B, Wang YH, Homey B, et al. Plasmacytoid dendritic cells sense self-DNA coupled with antimicrobial peptide. Nature. 2007;449(7162):564–9.

21. Buchau AS, Gallo RL. Innate immunity and antimicrobial defense systems in psoriasis. Clin Dermatol. 2007;25(6):616–24.

22. Victor FC, Gottlieb AB, Menter A. Changing paradigms in dermatology: tumor necrosis factor alpha (TNF-alpha) blockade in psoriasis and psoriatic arthritis. Clin Dermatol. 2003;21(5):392–7.

23. Ettehadi P, Greaves MW, Wallach D, Aderka D, Camp RD. Elevated tumour necrosis factor-alpha (TNF-alpha) biological activity in psoriatic skin lesions. Clin Exp Immunol. 1994;96(1):146–51.

24. Victor FC, Gottlieb AB. TNF-alpha and apoptosis: implications for the pathogenesis and treatment of psoriasis. J Drugs Dermatol. 2002;1(3):264–75.

25. Lizzul PF, Aphale A, Malaviya R, Sun Y, Masud S, Dombrovskiy V, et al. Differential expression of phosphorylated NF-kappaB/RelA in normal and psoriatic epidermis and downregulation of NF-kappaB in response to treatment with etanercept. J Invest Dermatol. 2005;124(6):1275–83.

26. Brotas AM, Cunha JM, Lago EH, Machado CC, Carneiro SC. Tumor necrosis factor-alpha and the cytokine network in psoriasis. An Bras Dermatol. 2012;87(5):673–81.

27. Homey B, Alenius H, Müller A, Soto H, Bowman EP, Yuan W, et al. CCL27-CCR10 interactions regulate T cell-mediated skin inflammation. Nat Med. 2002;8(2): 157–65.

28. Ackermann L, Harvima IT, Pelkonen J, Ritamaki-Salo V, Naukkarinen A, Harvima RJ, et al. Mast cells in psoriatic skin are strongly positive for interferon-gamma. Br J Dermatol. 1999;140(4):624–33.

29. Theoharides TC, Alysandratos KD, Angelidou A, Delivanis DA, Sismanopoulos N, Zhang B, et al. Mast cells and inflammation. Biochim Biophys Acta. 2012;1822(1):21–33.

30. Lin AM, Rubin CJ, Khandpur R, Wang JY, Riblett M, Yalavarthi S, et al. Mast cells and neutrophils release IL-17 through extracellular trap formation in psoriasis. J Immunol. 2011;187(1):490–500.

31. Kritas SK, Saggini A, Varvara G, Murmura G, Caraffa A, Antinolfi P, et al. Impact of mast cells on the skin. Int J Immunopathol Pharmacol. 2013;26(4):855–9.

32. Nestle FO, Turka LA, Nickoloff BJ. Characterization of dermal dendritic cells in psoriasis. Autostimulation of T lymphocytes and induction of Th1 type cytokines. J Clin Invest. 1994;94(1):202–9.

33. Zaba LC, Cardinale I, Gilleaudeau P, Sullivan-Whalen M, Suárez-Fariñas M, Fuentes-Duculan J, et al. Amelioration of epidermal hyperplasia by TNF inhibition is associated with reduced Th17 responses. J Exp Med. 2007;204(13):3183–94.

34. Afkarian M, Sedy JR, Yang J, Jacobson NG, Cereb N, Yang SY, et al. T-bet is a STAT1-induced regulator of IL-12R expression in naïve CD4+ T cells. Nat Immunol. 2002;3(6):549–57.

35. Szabo SJ, Kim ST, Costa GL, Zhang X, Fathman CG, Glimcher LH. A novel transcription factor, T-bet, directs Th1 lineage commitment. Cell. 2000;100(6): 655–69.

36. Muranski P, Restifo NP. Essentials of Th17 cell commitment and plasticity. Blood. 2013;121(13): 2402–14.

37. Harrington LE, Hatton RD, Mangan PR, Turner H, Murphy TL, Murphy KM, et al. Interleukin 17-producing CD4+ effector T cells develop via a lineage distinct from the T helper type 1 and 2 lineages. Nat Immunol. 2005;6(11):1123–32.

38. Oppmann B, Lesley R, Blom B, Timans JC, Xu Y, Hunte B, et al. Novel p19 protein engages IL-12p40 to form a cytokine, IL-23, with biological activities similar as well as distinct from IL-12. Immunity. 2000;13(5):715–25.

39. Langrish CL, Chen Y, Blumenschein WM, Mattson J, Basham B, Sedgwick JD, et al. IL-23 drives a pathogenic T cell population that induces autoimmune inflammation. J Exp Med. 2005;201(2):233–40.

40. Wilson NJ, Boniface K, Chan JR, McKenzie BS, Blumenschein WM, Mattson JD, et al. Development, cytokine profile and function of human interleukin 17-producing helper T cells. Nat Immunol. 2007;8(9): 950–7.

41. Wolk K, Witte E, Warszawska K, Schulze-Tanzil G, Witte K, Philipp S, et al. The Th17 cytokine IL-22 induces IL-20 production in keratinocytes: a novel immunological cascade with potential relevance in psoriasis. Eur J Immunol. 2009;39(12):3570–81.

42. Duhen T, Geiger R, Jarrossay D, Lanzavecchia A, Sallusto F. Production of interleukin 22 but not interleukin 17 by a subset of human skin-homing memory T cells. Nat Immunol. 2009;10(8):857–63.

43. Fujita H. The role of IL-22 and Th22 cells in human skin diseases. J Dermatol Sci. 2013;72(1):3–8.

44. Chaudhari U, Romano P, Mulcahy LD, Dooley LT, Baker DG, Gottlieb AB. Efficacy and safety of infliximab monotherapy for plaque-type psoriasis: a randomised trial. Lancet. 2001;357(9271):1842–7.

45. Reich K, Nestle FO, Papp K, Ortonne JP, Evans R, Guzzo C, et al. Infliximab induction and maintenance therapy for moderate-to-severe psoriasis: a phase III, multicentre, double-blind trial. Lancet. 2005; 366(9494):1367–74.

46. Menter A, Tyring SK, Gordon K, Kimball AB, Leonardi CL, Langley RG, et al. Adalimumab therapy for moderate to severe psoriasis: a randomized, controlled phase III trial. J Am Acad Dermatol. 2008;58(1):106–15.

47. Papp KA, Tyring S, Lahfa M, Prinz J, Griffiths CE, Nakanishi AM, et al. A global phase III randomized controlled trial of etanercept in psoriasis: safety, efficacy, and effect of dose reduction. Br J Dermatol. 2005;152(6):1304–12.

48. Malaviya R, Sun Y, Tan JK, Wang A, Magliocco M, Yao M, et al. Etanercept induces apoptosis of dermal dendritic cells in psoriatic plaques of responding patients. J Am Acad Dermatol. 2006;55(4):590–7.

49. Kivelevitch D, Mansouri B, Menter A. Long term efficacy and safety of etanercept in the treatment of psoriasis and psoriatic arthritis. Biologics. 2014;17(8): 169–82.

50. Tonel G, Conrad C, Laggner U, Di Meglio P, Grys K, McClanahan TK, et al. Cutting edge: a critical functional role for IL-23 in Psoriasis. J Immunol. 2010;185(10):5688–91.

51. Krueger GG, Langley R, Leonardi C, Yeilding N, Guzzo C, Wang Y, et al. A human interleukin-12/23 monoclonal antibody for the treatment of psoriasis. N Engl J Med. 2007;356(6):580–92.

52. Leonardi CL, Kimball AB, Papp KA, Yeilding N, Guzzo C, Wang Y, et al. Efficacy and safety of ustekinumab, a human interleukin-12/23 monoclonal antibody, in patients with psoriasis: 76-week results from a randomised, double-blind, placebo-controlled trial (PHOENIX 1). Lancet. 2008;371(9625):1665–74.

53. Papp KA, Langley RG, Lebwohl M, Krueger GG, Szapary P, Yeilding N, et al. Efficacy and safety of ustekinumab, a human interleukin-12/23 monoclonal antibody, in patients with psoriasis: 52-week results from a randomised, double-blind, placebo-controlled trial (PHOENIX 2). Lancet. 2008;371(9625):1675–84.

54. Belge K, Brück J, Ghoreschi K. Advances in treating psoriasis. F1000Prime Rep. 2014;6:4.

55. Miller GT, Hochman PS, Meier W, Tizard R, Bixler SA, Rosa MD, et al. Specific interaction of lymphocyte function-associated antigen 3 with CD2 can inhibit T cell responses. J Exp Med. 1993;178(1):211–22.

56. Krueger GG, Papp KA, Stough DB, Loven KH, Gulliver WP, Ellis CN. A randomized, double-blind, placebo-controlled phase III study evaluating efficacy and tolerability of 2 courses of alefacept in patients with chronic plaque psoriasis. J Am Acad Dermatol. 2002;47(6):821–33.

57. Iannone F, Lapadula G. The inhibitor of costimulation of T cells: abatacept. J Rheumatol Suppl. 2012;89:100–2.

58. Sayegh MH, Turka LA. The role of T-cell costimulatory activation pathways in transplant rejection. N Engl J Med. 1998;338(25):1813–21.

59. Yamada A, Salama AD, Sayegh MH. The role of novel T cell costimulatory pathways in autoimmunity and transplantation. J Am Soc Nephrol. 2002;13(2): 559–75.

60. Moreland L, Bate G, Kirkpatrick P. Abatacept. Nat Rev Drug Discov. 2006;5(3):185–6.

61. Bissonnette R, Langley RG, Papp K, Matheson R, Toth D, Hultquist M, et al. Humanized anti-CD2 monoclonal antibody treatment of plaque psoriasis: efficacy and pharmacodynamic results of two randomized, double-blind, placebo-controlled studies of intravenous and subcutaneous siplizumab. Arch Dermatol Res. 2009;301(6):429–42.

62. Schafer P. Apremilast mechanism of action and application to psoriasis and psoriatic arthritis. Biochem Pharmacol. 2012;83(12):1583–90.

63. Ghoreschi K, Brück J, Kellerer C, Deng C, Peng H, Rothfuss O, et al. Fumarates improve psoriasis and multiple sclerosis by inducing type II dendritic cells. J Exp Med. 2011;208(11):2291–303.

64. Meyer DM, Jesson MI, Li X, Elrick MM, Funckes-Shippy CL, Warner JD, et al. Anti-inflammatory activity and neutrophil reductions mediated by the JAK1/JAK3 inhibitor, CP-690,550, in rat adjuvant-induced arthritis. J Inflamm (Lond). 2010;7:41.

65. Hsu L, Armstrong AW. JAK inhibitors: treatment efficacy and safety profile in patients with psoriasis. J Immunol Res. 2014;2014:283617. Epub 2014 May 5.

66. Wilson FC, Icen M, Crowson CS, McEvoy MT, Gabriel SE, Kremers HM. Incidence and clinical predictors of psoriatic arthritis in patients with psoriasis: a population-based study. Arthritis Rheum. 2009; 61(2):233–9.

67. Gelfand JM, Gladman DD, Mease PJ, Smith N, Margolis DJ, Nijsten T, et al. Epidemiology of psoriatic arthritis in the population of the United States. J Am Acad Dermatol. 2005;53(4):573.

68. Zaias N. Embryology of the human nail. Arch Dermatol. 1963;87:37–53.

69. Jiaravuthisan MM, Sasseville D, Vender RB, Murphy F, Muhn CY. Psoriasis of the nail: anatomy, pathology, clinical presentation, and a review of the literature on therapy. J Am Acad Dermatol. 2007;57(1):1–27.

70. Zaias N. Psoriasis of the nail. A clinical-pathologic study. Arch Dermatol. 1969;99(5):567–79.

71. Krueger JG. The immunologic basis for the treatment of psoriasis with new biologic agents. J Am Acad Dermatol. 2002;46(1):1–23.

72. McGonagle D, Benjamin M, Tan AL. The pathogenesis of psoriatic arthritis and associated nail disease: not autoimmune after all? Curr Opin Rheumatol. 2009;21(4):340–7.

73. Tan AL, Benjamin M, Toumi H, Grainger AJ, Tanner SF, Emery P, et al. The relationship between the extensor tendon enthesis and the nail in distal interphalangeal joint disease in psoriatic arthritis--a high-resolution MRI and histological study. Rheumatology (Oxford). 2007;46(2):253–6.

74. McGonagle D, Marzo-Ortega H, O'Connor P, Gibbon W, Pease C, Reece R, et al. The role of biomechanical factors and HLA-B27 in magnetic resonance imaging-determined bone changes in plantar fascia enthesopathy. Arthritis Rheum. 2002;46(2):489–93.

75. McGonagle D, Marzo-Ortega H, O'Connor P, Gibbon W, Hawkey P, Henshaw K, et al. Histological assessment of the early enthesitis lesion in spondyloarthropathy. Ann Rheum Dis. 2002;61(6):534–7.

Immunopathology of the Psoriatic Arthritis Musculoskeletal Lesions

7

Kurt de Vlam

Abstract

Psoriatic arthritis is a complex inflammatory joint disease associated with psoriasis. The immunopathology of the skin and joint involvement resembles each other in some aspects but not all of them. Joint involvement is characterized by hypervascularity, cellular hypertrophy and inflammatory cellular infiltrate. Lymphocytes and dendritic cells play an important role in the pathogenesis of psoriasis and psoriatic arthritis; Their role in the early and late phase of the disease has still to be elucidated. Among the lymphocytes there is an important role for the Th17 cells linking the innate and adaptive immune systems. Future therapies are focusing on these effector cells and their products. Pre-osteoclasts and mature osteoclasts are other important players in the disease process, especially in psoriatic arthritis.

The immunopathology of psoriatic arthritis is just at the early beginning of unravelling its secrets.

Keywords

Immunopathology • Psoriatic arthritis • Inflammation • Synovitis • Enthesitis • Osteitis • Th17 lymphocytes • Osteoclasts • Dendritic cells

Psoriatic arthritis (PsA) is a chronic inflammatory disease of joints, enthesis and bone in patients with psoriasis (PsO). Locomotor involvement occurs simultaneously or subsequent to the skin manifestations in the majority of the patients. A minority of the patients develops joint involvement before the appearance of psoriasis. This could suggest that the pathological inflammatory processes in the skin may play a role in the development of the joint disease. Besides joint and skin manifestations, numerous patients also have co-morbidities such as cardiovascular disease, metabolic syndrome, diabetes, hyperlipidemia, liver diseases

K. de Vlam, MD, PhD
Department of Rheumatology,
University Hospitals Leuven, Leuven, Belgium
e-mail: Kurt.devlam@uzleuven.be

© Springer International Publishing Switzerland 2016
A. Adebajo et al. (eds.), *Psoriatic Arthritis and Psoriasis: Pathology and Clinical Aspects*,
DOI 10.1007/978-3-319-19530-8_7

and mood disturbances. The association of these different diseases in the same patient led to the development of the concept of "psoriatic disease" [1, 2].

Is Psoriatic Arthritis an Autoimmune Disease or Auto Inflammatory Disease?

PsA has been viewed as an archetypical autoimmune disorder and by extension psoriasis and psoriatic nail disease also. Classical autoimmune diseases are characterised by the presence of autoantibodies, often present in the preclinical phase which suggest the possible development of overt autoimmune disease. Rheumatoid arthritis (RA), primary biliary cirrhosis, Hashimoto's thyroiditis and systemic lupus erythematosus are classic examples. Other characteristics of autoimmune diseases include MHC class II association, tissue related autoantigens and extra-articular involvement. The disease can be induced in animal models by injection of specific autoantigens. The acquired immune system plays an important role in the pathogenesis of autoimmune diseases [3].

In PsA, tissue-specific autoantibodies have not yet been identified. Psoriasis and psoriatic arthritis are associated with MHC Class 1. PsA cannot be induced by injection by autoantigens in animal models but by overexpression or deletion of specific growth factors, cytokines or proteins in specific signaling pathways.

Inflammatory Process in Psoriatic Disease Including Psoriatic Arthritis and Psoriasis

An important distinction must be made in psoriasis and psoriatic arthritis natural history by identifying 2 phases: an initiation phase where inflammation starts and a maintenance phase that perpetuates the inflammatory process. This distinction is actually clearer in psoriasis than in psoriatic arthritis. This conceptual distinction can help to divide cellular and molecular events

that initiate and trigger the disease and events that induce a self-perpetuating inflammatory process.

Psoriatic arthritis is a complex disease resulting from an interplay of environmental factors and genetic susceptibility, mainly in genes related to innate and acquired immunity but also to genes in the different metabolic pathways. Psoriatic arthritis may be initiated by triggering events that are not yet fully understood. In any case, the most important event or biomarker is the presence or history of skin psoriasis itself [4].

The immunopathology in psoriatic arthritis can be studied by analyzing the immunopathologic differences between inflammation in the psoriatic skin and synovitis. Organ specific reactions between skin and synovial tissue can partly explains these differences. An alternative approach compares the key differences between PsA and RA, a different inflammatory arthritis.

The inflammatory process in PsA is not limited to the synovial membrane, as in RA but affects also the enthesis, juxta-articular bone, tendon sheaths and fat pads.

Synovitis

The key features of both psoriasis and psoriatic arthritis are increased vascularity, tissue proliferation and infiltration by inflammatory cells.

Angiogenesis is a prominent early event in psoriasis and psoriatic arthritis. Macroscopically PsA synovitis is characterised by tortuous hypervascularity and the presence of hyperemic villi. To some extent thin fibrinoid deposits are also present. Arthroscopic evaluation in RA shows a more straight vessel pattern. Elongated and tortuous vessel are a specific feature and suggest dysregulated angiogenesis. Factors associated with angiogenesis such as VEGF and TGFbeta are present in the synovial fluid of PsA patients. Angiopoetins are present in both skin and synovial lesions [5, 6]. The degree of vascularity is higher in PsA compared to RA but has similar levels of VEGF in the synovial fluid but less VEGF mRNA and Ang2 mRNa in the perivascular regions [7–9].

Hypertrophy of cellular layers is recognized in both psoriasis and psoriatic arthritis.

Psoriatic skin shows acanthosis (uniform elongation of the rete ridges), parakeratosis and orthokeratosis, loss of the granular cell layer and the formation of spongiform pustules and parakeratotic microabscesses. Mitotic activity, commonly seen only in the basal cells, is typically increased in psoriasis.

In psoriatic arthritis hypertrophy of the synovial layer is omnipresent but to a lesser extent than in rheumatoid arthritis [10].

In psoriatic arthritis there is a marked **infiltration** of mononuclear cells (T and B lymphocytes as well as macrophages and plasmacells) and polymorphonuclear cells. The cellular infiltrate is predominantly in the perivascular regions and may migrate to the lining layers of the joint or epidermis. Follicular aggregates of lymphocytes, both of T cells and B cells, resembling lymphoid follicles are a marked feature of RA but have also been described in PsA. More extensive analysis of synovial tissue in PsA showed frequent ectopic lymphoid neogenesis with typical highly organized structure responding upon effective treatment [11].

Enthesitis

The enthesis or site of ligamentous attachment adjacent to the joint is hardly studied in PsA. The few available materials originate mostly from patients with Spondyloarthropathy, including some specimens from PsA patients.

Enthesitis is an important feature in psoriatic arthritis. Recent studies have suggested that inflammation in psoriatic arthritis (PsA) may arise at the enthesis based on imaging and anatomical data and might be present in the subclinical phase of the disease [12]. In the earliest clinical phase, peri-entheseal edema has been demonstrated on MRI. Inflammation at the enthesis might be accompanied by an exuberant repair response that results in new bone formation or even ankylosis.

Biopsy material from Achilles tendon or anterior cruciate entheses have shown disruption of the normal enthesis architecture within its fibrous part with disorganisation of the normal fibrillar architecture, increased vascularity and cellular infiltration [13].

Histological analysis shows that the enthesis architecture is abnormal in the SpA group, with increased vascularity in the fibrous part of the enthesis and cellular infiltration compared with normal subjects. On immunohistochemical analysis the predominant immune cells at the enthesis were CD68 positive macrophages, mainly found at the sites of increased vascularity and cellularity. Neither the fibrous part of the enthesis nor the fibrocartilaginous parts were infiltrated by lymphocytes (either CD3 or CD8) but T lymphocytes could be detected in the bone marrow near the enthesis (predominantly CD8) [13, 14].

Osteitis and Juxta Articular Bone Involvement

In PsA there are different manifestations of dynamic bone involvement including large eccentric erosions, tuft resorption, periostitis, ankylosis and acro-osteolysis. Two striking features of peripheral involvement in PsA are subchondral perientheseal edema and diffuse bone edema, which are not present in RA [15, 16].

In RA edema is considered to be a pre-erosive lesion. It is not clear if bone edema in PsA reflects the same process or might be related to osteoproliferation also seen in spontaneous arthritis model in caged DBA1 mice. This model shows some striking characteristics of PsA such as ankylosing enthesitis, dactylitis and onychoperiostitis. The morphological changes in this model are BMP-driven [17].

The subchondral bone adjacent to the joint or enthesis is hardly studied in psoriatic arthritis. The few available materials originate mostly from patients with spondyloarthropathy, including some specimens from PsA patients.

The sub-enthesis bone is disorganised with increased vascularity. Hyperosteoclastic erosive lesions are found. The bone marrow shows edema and inflammatory cellular infiltrate including T cells (CD4+ and CD8+) and CD68+ macrophages, proliferating fibroblasts. There is an increased expression of TNFα and transforming growth factor β mRNA. In less destructive areas, cellular hyperplasia and fibrillation of the chondroid matrix occurs in the cartilaginous zone. Fibrous tissue proliferation is observed in some cases [13, 14].

Cellular and Molecular Compartments Involved in Psoriatic Arthritis

lymphocytes

T lymphocytes

The role of T lymphocytes is somewhat controversial. While T lymphocytes are present in the synovial tissue in PsA among other cell types, some groups reported a lower prevalence than compared to rheumatoid arthritis. From clinical trials it is clear that T cell targeted therapies may be beneficial but far less effective than recent cytokine-targeted approaches. This does not mean than T cell may not be important. A specific subset could still promote the inflammatory process and T regulatory cells may play a role in controlling the inflammatory process. In the synovial infiltrate, T cells are present among other cell types, and oligoclonal T-cell expansions have been demonstrated in the synovium, suggesting that an antigen-driven T-cell response could be promoting ongoing inflammation [18, 19]. It remains to be elucidated which antigen may be driving these T cells.

T lymphocytes are the most frequent cellular population in both PsO and PsA.

In both tissues there is a prominent lymphocytic infiltrate, localised to the dermal papillae in skin and to the sub-lining layer stroma in the joint [10].

CD4+ cells are the most frequent population in skin and synovial tissue but in synovial fluid and enthesis the CD8+ population is more predominant. The latter may be the driving force for the arthritis. This is supported by the known association of PsA with MHC class 1 molecules and the increased frequency of PsA in HIV patients upon CD4 depletion.

B lymphocytes

Interestingly the skin of patients with psoriatic arthritis compared to the skin of those with psoriasis alone showed differences in the presence of B-lymphocyte and there were significantly more DR+ cells in the psoriatic arthritis epidermis compared with psoriasis alone [20]. With B cells also abundant in synovial tissue, the exact role of B cells in PsA and PsO remains to be elucidated.

Th17 Lymphocytes

Recent characterisation of a new subset of T cells: Th17, may shed a new light on the role and the importance of T cells in the inflammatory process in PsA. Th17 are a new type of effector T lymphocytes producing IL17, TNF-α, IL-21 and IL-22 upon stimulation with IL-23. The latter is abundantly present in the psoriatic skin lesions. Th17 cells develop from naïve CD4 cells upon stimulation by IL-23 in the presence of IL-6 and TGF-β [21]. Activated Th17 cells migrate to the inflamed tissue. They overexpress CCL2 and its receptor CCR 6. Hereby neutrophils are attracted to the site of inflammation [22]. Increased frequencies of IL-17+ and IL-22+ CD4+ T cells are seen in PB of patients with PsA and Ps. A higher proportion of the CD4+ cells, making IL-17 or IL-22, expressed IL-23R and frequencies of IL-17+, CCR6+ and CCR4+ T cells are elevated in patients with Ps and those with PsA. In patients with PsA, CCR6+ and IL-23R+T cells numbers are elevated in SF compared to PB [23]. In the synovial fluid of PsA patients both the IL-17+CD8+ and IL-17+CD4+ compartments are enriched compared to the peripheral blood whereas in the synovial fluid of RA patients showed only in increase in IL-17+CD4+ T cells compared to the peripheral blood. In PsA these T cell subset also correlated with disease activity and erosion status after 2 years of treatment.

Dendritic Cells

In psoriatic skin the dendritic cell population is overall increased in the epidermis and dermis. Different types of DC are present in the dermis: myloied DC, plasmacytoid DC's and Slan DC(6-sulfo LacNAc dendritic cells, a less common type of DC). But plasmacytoid DCs, microbial infection, autoantigens such as LL37 and mechanical stress are other inducers of DC and innate immune mechanisms. LL37 seems to be the missing link between the innate immune reaction and the adaptive immune reaction in PsO. The aggregation of LL37 with autogenous DNA activates Toll like receptor-9 on plasmacytoid DCs resulting in production of TNF-α, IL23, IL-6 and IFN-γ by myeloid DCs. Together with cytokines produced by macrophages, this promotes Th17 polarisation and naïve CD 4 cells [24].

DCs in synovial tissue in PsA are poorly studied. They are equally present in the synovial fluid of RA and PsA patients but almost absent in the SF of osteoarthritis patients [25]. DCs are more prevalent in the synovial tissue of RA patients than PsA [7]. In PsA mostly plasmacytoid DCs are present but seems to be in an immature state [26]. Stimulation by mycobacterium and TLR 2 ligands results in a disturbed immune response towards some mycobacteria and in turn impaired clearance of these bacteria, setting the stage for the chronic inflammation of joints, entheses, skin, and the gut [27].

Macrophages

There is some controversy about the role and presence of macrophages. Initially immunohistological analysis showed fewer macrophages invading the stroma and migrating to the lining layer in PsA SM than in RA SM [10]. More recent analysis showed that macrophages are abundantly present in the synovial tissue in PsA compared to RA. Both CD68+ and CD163+ macrophages are present. But recent data shows no difference for CD68+ macrophages but a clear increase in the CD163+ subset in PsA compared to RA [7, 10]. Macrophages are the source of pro-inflammatory cytokines such as TNF-α and synergizes the effect of myeloid DCs promoting the polarization of TH17 cells.

Patients with PsA have increased levels of S100A8/A9 possibly because of the activated monocyte/macrophage system, thereby reflecting disease activity [28].

Macrophage derived chemokine (MDC) is present in the synovial fluid and tissue in PsA. It binds to CCR4 which is expressed by memory T cells in the skin of Ps patients. This may suggest that MDC plays an important role in attracting these memory cells into the joints.

Osteoclasts/Pre-osteoclasts

Altered bone remodeling is a key feature of psoriatic arthritis but can present with varying degrees in the individual patient. The altered bone remodeling is a combination of bone formation and bone resorption, represented by the presence of bone erosions. Those erosions result from bone resorption by osteoclasts [29].

Blood samples from PsA patients, particularly those with bone erosions visible on plain radiographs, exhibit a marked increase in osteoclast precursors (OCPs) compared with those from healthy controls. Moreover, PsA PBMCs readily formed osteoclasts in vitro without exogenous receptor activator of NF-kappaB ligand (RANKL) or MCSF. Blocking osteoprotegerin (OPG) and TNF-α with their specific antibodies inhibits osteoclast formation. The osteoclast (OC) formation in PsA patients is supported by data showing the production of osteoclastogenic cytokines, such as RANKL, TNF-α and IL -7 by lymphocytes and fibroblasts [30].

Immunohistochemical analysis of subchondral bone and synovium revealed RANK-positive perivascular mononuclear cells and osteoclasts in PsA specimens. RANKL expression was dramatically up-regulated in the synovial lining layer, while OPG immunostaining was restricted to the endothelium. These results suggest a model for understanding the pathogenesis of aggressive bone erosions in PsA.

OCP's arise from CD14 + mononuclear cell lineage upon stimulation with RANK and, MCSF and express CD16+ marker. The expression of CD16+ is associated with a higher bone erosion score [31].

Monocytes need to express DC-stamp in order to differentiate into OCPs. The bone marrow (BM) of patients with PsA harbors a subset of DC-STAMP+CD45intermediate monocytes

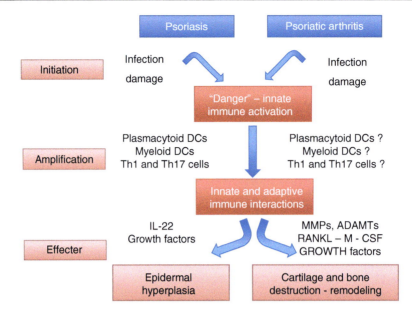

Fig. 7.1 Parallels between psoriasis and psoriatic arthritis. In both diseases, initiation, amplification, and effecter phases can be distinguished. Innate immune mechanisms appear essential in the initiation of the cascades, but in the further development of the chronic inflammatory reaction, adaptive immune mechanisms also contribute. In the effecter phase, tissue specificity of the reaction may be a critical factor in determining the outcome of the disease.

ADAMTS a disintegrin and metalloproteinase with thrombospondin motifs. *DC* dendritic cell, *IL* interleukin, *M-CSF* monocyte colony-stimulating factor, *MMP* matrix metalloproteinase, *RANKL* receptor activator of nuclear factor-kB ligand, *Th* T-helper cell (Reprinted from Lories and de Vlam [34]. With permission from Springer Science)

which was absent in the blood. In general, more OCPs are found in the BM than in the peripheral blood supporting the BM as the major source of circulating OCP's [32].

In vivo, OCP frequency, correlates with joint scores and disability scores and declined substantially in PsA patients following treatment with anti-TNF agents [33].

Summary

Immunopathological studies show that psoriatic arthritis is immunological disease with different cells contributing to the immunopathogenesis. Formerly considered as a pure autoimmune disease recent immunopathological findings are shifting insights towards a disease with autoimmune and autoinfammatory characteristics. In this concept some aspects of the disease are addressed by innate immune mechanisms and others by acquired immune reactions with their respective cell populations (Fig. 7.1).

References

1. Scarpa R, Ayala F, Caporaso N, Olivieri I. Psoriasis, psoriatic arthritis, or psoriatic disease? J Rheumatol. 2006;33(2):210–2.
2. Ritchlin C. Psoriatic disease--from skin to bone. Nat Clin Pract Rheumatol. 2007;3(12):698–706. Review.
3. McGonagle D, McDermott MF. A proposed classification of the immunological diseases. PLoS Med. 2006;3(8):e297.
4. McGonagle D, Ash Z, Dickie L, McDermott M, Aydin SZ. The early phase of psoriatic arthritis. Ann Rheum Dis. 2011;70 Suppl 1:i71.
5. Fearon U, Reece R, Smith J, Emery P, Veale DJ. Synovial cytokine and growth factor regulation of MMPs/TIMPs: implications for erosions and angiogenesis in early rheumatoid and psoriatic arthritis patients. Ann N Y Acad Sci. 1999;878:619–21.

6. Kuroda K, Sapadin A, Shoji T, Fleischmajer R, Lebwohl M. Altered expression of angiopoietins and Tie2 endothelium receptor in psoriasis. J Invest Dermatol. 2001;116(5):713–20.

7. Kruithof E, Baeten D, De Rycke L, Vandooren B, Foell D, Roth J, Cañete JD, Boots AM, Veys EM, De Keyser F. Synovial histopathology of psoriatic arthritis, both oligo- and polyarticular, resembles spondyloarthropathy more than it does rheumatoid arthritis. Arthritis Res Ther. 2005;7(3):R569–80.

8. Gudbjörnsson B, Christofferson R, Larsson A. Synovial concentrations of the angiogenic peptides bFGF and VEGF do not discriminate rheumatoid arthritis from other forms of inflammatory arthritis. Scand J Clin Lab Invest. 2004;64(1):9–15.

9. Fearon U, Griosios K, Fraser A, Reece R, Emery P, Jones PF, Veale DJ. Angiopoietins, growth factors, and vascular morphology in early arthritis. J Rheumatol. 2003;30(2):260–8.

10. Veale D, Yanni G, Rogers S, Barnes L, Bresnihan B, Fitzgerald O. Reduced synovial membrane ELAM-1 expression, macrophage numbers and lining layer hyperplasia in psoriatic arthritis as compared with rheumatoid arthritis. Arthritis Rheum. 1993;36: 893–900. 2.

11. Cañete JD, Santiago B, Cantaert T, Sanmartí R, Palacin A, Celis R, Graell E, Gil-Torregrosa B, Baeten D, Pablos JL. Ectopic lymphoid neogenesis in psoriatic arthritis. Ann Rheum Dis. 2007;66(6):720–6.

12. Emad Y, Ragab Y, Gheita T, Anbar A, Kamal H, Saad A, Darweesh H, El-Shaarawy N, Azab A, Ismail A, Rasker JJ, Knee Enthesitis Working Group. Knee enthesitis and synovitis on magnetic resonance imaging in patients with psoriasis without arthritic symptoms. J Rheumatol. 2012;39(10):1979–86.

13. Laloux L, Voisin MC, Allain J, Martin N, Kerboull L, Chevalier X, Claudepierre P. Immunohistological study of entheses in spondyloarthropathies: comparison in rheumatoid arthritis and osteoarthritis. Ann Rheum Dis. 2001;60(4):316–21.

14. McGonagle D, Marzo-Ortega H, O'Connor P, Gibbon W, Hawkey P, Henshaw K, Emery P. Histological assessment of the early enthesitis lesion in spondyloarthropathy. Ann Rheum Dis. 2002;61:534–7.

15. McGonagle D, Gibbon W, O'Connor P, Green M, Pease C, Emery P. Characteristic magnetic resonance imaging entheseal changes of knee synovitis in spondylarthropathy. Arthritis Rheum. 1998;41(4): 694–700.

16. Jevtic V, Watt I, Rozman B, Kos-Golja M, Demsar F, Jarh O. Distinctive radiological features of small hand joints in rheumatoid arthritis and seronegative spondyloarthritis demonstrated by contrast-enhanced (Gd-DTPA) magnetic resonance imaging. Skeletal Radiol. 1995;24(5):351–5.

17. Lories RJ, Matthys P, de Vlam K, Derese I, Luyten FP. Ankylosing enthesitis, dactylitis, and onychoperiostitis in male DBA/1 mice: a model of psoriatic arthritis. Ann Rheum Dis. 2004;63(5):595–8.

18. Tassiulas I, Duncan SR, Centola M, Theofilopoulos AN, Boumpas DT. Clonal characteristics of T cell infiltrates in skin and synovium of patients with psoriaticarthritis. Hum Immunol. 1999;60(6): 479–91. 28.

19. Chang JC, Smith LR, Froning KJ, Schwabe BJ, Laxer JA, Caralli LL, Kurkland HH, Karasek MA, Wilkinson DI, Carlo DJ. CD8+ T-cells in psoriatic lesions preferentially use T-cell receptors V beta 3 and/or V beta 13.1 genes. Ann N Y Acad Sci. 1995;756:370–81.

20. Veale DJ, Barnes L, Rogers S, FitzGerald O. Immunohistochemical markers for arthritis in psoriasis. Ann Rheum Dis. 1994;53:450–4.

21. Lee E, Trepicchio WL, Oestreicher JL, Pittman D, Wang F, Chamian F, Dhodapkar M, Krueger JG. Increased expression of interleukin 23 p19 and p40 in lesional skin of patients with psoriasis vulgaris. J Exp Med. 2004;199(1):125–30.

22. Menon B, Gullick NJ, Walter GJ, Rajasekhar M, Garrood T, Evans HG, Taams LS, Kirkham BW. Interleukin-17+CD8+ T cells are enriched in the joints of patients with psoriatic arthritis and correlate with disease activity and joint damage progression. Arthritis Rheumatol. 2014;66(5):1272–81.

23. Benham H, Norris P, Goodall J, Wechalekar MD, FitzGerald O, Szentpetery A, Smith M, Thomas R, Gaston H. Th17 and Th22 cells in psoriatic arthritis and psoriasis. Arthritis Res Ther. 2013;15(5):R136.

24. Diani M, Altomare G, Reali E. T cell responses in psoriasis and psoriatic arthritis. Autoimmun Rev. 2015;14(4):286–92.

25. Jongbloed SL, Lebre MC, Fraser AR, Gracie JA, Sturrock RD, Tak PP, McInnes IB. Enumeration and phenotypical analysis of distinct dendritic cell subsets in psoriatic arthritis and rheumatoid arthritis. Arthritis Res Ther. 2006;8(1):R15.

26. Lande R, Giacomini E, Serafini B, Rosicarelli B, Sebastiani GD, Minisola G, Tarantino U, Riccieri V, Valesini G, Coccia EM. Characterization and recruitment of plasmacytoid dendritic cells in synovial fluid and tissue of patients with chronic inflammatory arthritis. J Immunol. 2004;173(4):2815–24.

27. Wenink MH, Santegoets KC, Butcher J, van Bon L, Lamers-Karnebeek FG, van den Berg WB, van Riel PL, McInnes IB, Radstake TR. Impaired dendritic cell proinflammatory cytokine production in psoriatic arthritis. Arthritis Rheum. 2011;63(11):3313–22.

28. Aochi S, Tsuji K, Sakaguchi M, Huh N, Tsuda T, Yamanishi K, Komine M, Iwatsuki K. Markedly elevated serum levels of calcium-binding S100A8/A9 proteins in psoriatic arthritis are due to activated monocytes/macrophages. J Am Acad Dermatol. 2011;64(5):879–87.

29. Ritchlin CT, Haas-Smith SA, Li P, Hicks DG, Schwarz EM. Mechanisms of TNF-alpha- and RANKL-

mediated osteoclastogenesis and bone resorption in psoriatic arthritis. J Clin Invest. 2003;111(6):821–31.

30. Colucci S, Brunetti G, Cantatore FP, Oranger A, Mori G, Quarta L, Cirulli N, Mancini L, Corrado A, Grassi FR, Grano M. Lymphocytes and synovial fluid fibroblasts support osteoclastogenesis through RANKL, TNFalpha, and IL-7 in an in vitro model derived from human psoriatic arthritis. J Pathol. 2007;212(1): 47–55.

31. Chiu YG, Shao T, Feng C, Mensah KA, Thullen M, Schwarz EM. Ritchlin CT.CD16 (FcRgammaIII) as a potential marker of osteoclast precursors in psoriatic arthritis. Arthritis Res Ther. 2010;12(1):R14.

32. Chiu YG, Ritchlin CT. Characterization of DC-STAMP+ Cells in Human Bone Marrow. J Bone Marrow Res. 2013;1:1–14

33. Anandarajah AP, Schwarz EM, Totterman S, Monu J, Feng CY, Shao T, Haas-Smith SA, Ritchlin CT. The effect of etanercept on osteoclast precursor frequency and enhancing bone marrow oedema in patients with psoriatic arthritis. Ann Rheum Dis. 2008;67(3): 296–301.

34. Lories RJ, de Vlam K. Is psoriatic arthritis a result of abnormalities in acquired or innate immunity? Curr Rheumatol Rep. 2012;14(4):375–82.

Innate and Acquired Cellular Immune Responses in Psoriasis and Psoriatic Arthritis

8

Bruce Kirkham

Abstract

Concepts of psoriasis and psoriatic arthritis pathogenesis are changing due to new knowledge of their immunopathology. Originally considered a disease of abnormal keratinocyte function, psoriasis was then considered an autoimmune Th1 T cell mediated condition due to the large number of interferon-γ secreting T cells in the skin. Recent findings showing a key role for cytokines such as interleukin 17 (IL-17) and IL-23, produced by a variety of resident skin cells, has led to the current concept that psoriasis is due to dysregulated immune function. Findings in psoriatic arthritis have generated similar changes in thought. A key factor in this change was the increased number of cell types capable of producing IL-17 and IL-23. IL-17 was originally described as a CD4 T cell product, then found to define the Th17 specific CD4 lineage. Interleukin 23, an antigen presenting cell product, plays a central role in the differentiation and stabilisation of Th17 cells. Subsequently, IL-17 was found to be produced by many immune cells of both the adaptive and the innate immune systems, including CD8 T cells, NK and innate lymphoid cells, gamma-delta T cells and neutrophils. Innate immune cells respond to pathogen or cell damage signals, with immediate cytokine responses providing early defence. Innate cell interaction with the acquired or adaptive immune system links the responses. The skin as the primary interface with the external environment, provides the first line of host defence against injury and infection, and is rich in cells of both the innate and adaptive immune system. This chapter will review the current evidence of innate and adaptive immune function in psoriasis and psoriatic arthritis, with an emphasis on recent reports.

B. Kirkham, BA, MD, FRACP, FRCP
Department of Rheumatology, Guy's & St Thomas'
NHS Foundation Trust, Guy's Hospital,
Great Maze Pond, London SE1 9RT, UK
e-mail: bruce.kirkham@gstt.nhs.uk

© Springer International Publishing Switzerland 2016
A. Adebajo et al. (eds.), *Psoriatic Arthritis and Psoriasis: Pathology and Clinical Aspects*,
DOI 10.1007/978-3-319-19530-8_8

Keywords

Innate immunity • Adaptive immunity • Acquired immunity • Cytokines •
Interleukin 17 • IL-17 • IL-23 • CD8 cells • NK cells • Innate lymphoid
cells • Gamma delta cells • Neutrophils • Mast cells • Dendritic cells

Introduction

This chapter will review cellular immunity of
the adaptive and innate immune systems,
emphasising the new knowledge that interaction
of these systems could play a central role in the
pathogenesis of psoriasis (PsO) and psoriatic
arthritis (PsA). It will review how current theories of disease pathogenesis have been influenced by increasing knowledge, in particular,
the rapid accumulation of knowledge of IL-17
biology.

Cellular Composition of PsO and PsA

As has been well described in earlier chapters,
healthy skin is an immune-competent tissue, consisting of three major compartments, with a dedicated T cell population. The superficial epidermis
mainly made of keratinocytes, also has a resident
population of dendritic antigen-presenting cells
called Langerhans cells. The next layer, the dermis, is a collagenous connective tissue with
blood vessels, containing many immune cells
and structures including hair follicles, sweat and
sebaceous glands, above the third adipose layer
called the subcutis [1]. Psoriasis is a complex
condition resulting from a combination of genetic
predisposition and environmental triggers. The
three main histological features of psoriasis are
epidermal hyperplasia, dilatation and proliferation of dermal blood vessels and accumulation of
inflammatory cells, particularly neutrophils and
T lymphocytes in the dermis [2]. Keratinocytes,
key skin cells mediating many of the functional
properties of skin, can also respond to pro-
inflammatory cytokines and generate pro-inflammatory activation loops. Tissue resident dendritic
and Langerhans cells, produce pro-inflammatory

cytokines such as interleukin (IL) -12 and 23,
which mediate immune cell activation [3].

Synovial tissue in normal joints has few resident immune cells. It consists of an intimal lining
layer made up of fibroblast-like synoviocytes and
intimal lining layer macrophages, resting on a
subsynovial layer of loose connective tissue,
which contains blood vessels, nerve endings,
fibroblasts, adipocytes, and a small number of
immune cells including mast cells and macrophages [4]. Inflamed joints are characterised by
increased synovial lining cell numbers, increased
sublining vascularity, with large numbers of cells
within this sub-synovial layer, including T and B
lymphocytes, macrophages, dendritic cells, fibroblasts, neutrophils and mast cells [5]. The difference in cellularity was quantified by counting
leucocytes obtained from digesting arthroscopic
synovial biopsies of inflammatory arthritis joints
compared to non-inflamed joints. The median
cell yield was 2286 cells/mg tissue in the non-
inflamed group vs. 20,222 cells/mg in the arthritis group [6].

Several studies have compared the synovial
cell types in PsA with the most common inflammatory arthritis, rheumatoid arthritis (RA) [7–
10]. Although these studies all reported
differences between PsA and RA, many patient
groups were not matched for disease duration
and therapy, key factors which might influence
cellular composition. To address this deficit, van
Kuijk and colleagues investigated synovial
pathology in patients with RA and PsA, matched
for disease duration and therapy [11]. The numbers of fibroblast-like synoviocytes and macrophages was similar, but synovial T cell numbers
were considerably lower in PsA, and plasma
cell numbers trended lower in patients with
PsA. The expression of TNF-α, IL-1β, IL-6 and
IL-18 was similar in PsA and RA, as was
the expression of matrix metalloproteinases,

adhesion molecules and vascular markers. Many differences were numerically but not statistically different, which could relate to the small number of subjects studied, 19 patients with PsA (eight oligoarthritis,11 polyarthritis) and 24 patients with RA. This study has set a standard for comparative studies which require similar clinical factors to enable valid comparisons of immunopathology.

PsA is one of a group of arthritides called the spondyloarthropathies (SpA), which also includes ankylosing spondylitis (AS), reactive arthritis, inflammatory bowel disease (Crohn's Disease and Ulcerative Colitis) related arthritis and a less well defined group called undifferentiated SpA (uSpA). Although smaller studies suggested that synovial membrane immunopathology of the different component sub-types are very similar, Baeten and colleagues reported one of the largest studies to date [12]. They analyzed if synovial histopathological features reflect specific phenotypes compared to RA, and also if they could predict global disease activity in SpA. Synovial biopsies obtained from 99 SpA and 86 RA patients with active knee synovitis were analyzed for 15 histological and immuno-histochemical markers. The first group of 82 SpA patients was made up of 19 AS, 33 PsA, 24 undifferentiated SpA (USpA), 4 SpA associated with inflammatory bowel disease, and 2 reactive arthritis, with a validation group of 4 patients with AS, 5 with PsA and 8 with USpA. They report no differences between the SpA subgroups using the study parameters, so considered the SpA group as a single entity. SpA synovitis was characterized by higher vascularity and CD163+ macrophages and polymorphonuclear leukocytes (PMNs) and lower values for lining-layer hyperplasia, lymphoid aggregates, CD1a + cells, intracellular citrullinated proteins, and MHC–HC gp39 complexes compared to RA synovitis. Global disease activity correlated significantly with lining-layer hyperplasia, synovial infiltrate of macrophages, especially the CD163+ subset, and PMNs. However, multiparameter models based on synovial histopathology were relatively poor predictors of disease activity in individual patients.

More recently, Yeremenko and colleagues used synovial gene expression analysis, to compare synovial molecular and cellular processes in SpA compared to RA [13]. They identified differentially expressed genes by pan-genomic microarray and confirmed these findings by quantitative polymerase chain reaction and immunohistochemical analyses of synovial tissue biopsy samples from patients with SpA (n = 63), RA (n =28), and gout (n =9). Microarray analysis identified 64 up-regulated transcripts in SpA synovitis compared to RA. Pathway analysis revealed a myogene signature specific for SpA, which was independent of disease duration, treatment, and SpA subtype (non-psoriatic versus psoriatic). Synovial tissue staining identified the myogene expressing cells as vimentin-positive, prolyl4-hydroxylase–positive, CD90+, CD146+ mesenchymal cells that were significantly over-represented in the intimal lining layer and sublining areas. Samples from a small number of patients before and after tumor necrosis factor inhibitor therapy showed no change in this SpA specific myogene signature.

These studies confirm and extend earlier studies showing significant differences in the cellular composition of synovitis in SpA and RA. They suggest less B cell activity and more non adaptive cellular immune and mesenchymal pathway dependent immune activation in PsA.

New Concepts of Pathogenesis

As many cells infiltrating psoriatic skin are related to the acquired or adaptive immune system, psoriasis had been considered an 'auto-immune' condition. However the epidemiology and more recently the genetic basis of psoriasis has led to changes in this view [1, 2]. The acute forms of psoriasis, guttate and generalised pustular psoriasis, are associated with infections, such as streptococcal or viral infections. Other environmental factors which can cause psoriasis include trauma (the well known but poorly understood Koebner phenomenon), HIV infection, hypocalcaemia in generalized pustular psoriasis, psychogenic stress and drugs (lithium, beta-blockers, anti-malarials, interferon, NSAIDs, rapid reduction of glucocorticosteroids). This epidemiology, with genetic relationships relating to many non-immune pathways, has produced the current view that psoriasis could be a dysregulated inflammatory response to multiple environmental stimuli [1, 14]. Similarly concepts of the pathogenesis of PsA, previously considered a T cell driven autoimmune condition are also under discussion [15, 16]. The potential mechanisms are similar to those above, with additional recent genome-wide association studies in PsA identifying variants of the *TRAF3IP2* gene, encoding Act-1 (NF-κB activator 1), a key mediator of IL-17 signalling [17], and the *RUNX3* gene [18], a transcription factor that promotes CD8+ T cell development in the thymus, as risk factors for disease development. In addition there has been renewed interest in the role of inflammation at the enthesis, the site where tendons, ligaments and joint capsule structures integrate into bone [19, 20]. In both PsO and PsA, many of these new concepts have been generated by new information relating to the role and type of cells producing interleukin-17 (IL-17) and the related IL-23 pathway [21].

IL-17 Producing Cells

Initially, discovered in CD4+T cells, the Th17 effector cell has dominated research agendas, and a Th1 or Th17 acquired/adoptive immune response was considered the most likely driver of PsO. More recent information that IL-17 is produced by many other cells including CD8+T cells and innate immune system cells, including γδ T cells, natural killer (NK) cells, NKT cells, and several populations of innate lymphoid cells (ILCs), all belonging to a family of IL-17-secreting lymphocytes, as well as neutrophils, has changed this view. It is possible that initial environmental stimulation of innate immune responses could interact with adaptive responses leading to the chronic condition [14].

Immunohistochemical studies of IL-17 expression in psoriasis skin show neutrophils and mast cells are the most frequently stained

cells [22]. Neutrophils had originally been shown to produce IL-17 mRNA in studies of lung pathology [23]. More recently in an animal model of acute ischemia-induced renal reperfusion injury, neutrophil derived IL-17, was shown to play a central early role in the disease process, as well as influencing later natural killer T cell interferon gamma (IFNγ) dependent processes [24]. In a study of immunohistochemical skin changes from patients with PsO treated with an anti-IL-17A monoclonal antibody, secukinumab, neutrophil staining for IL-17A was almost completely lost within 2 weeks, when skin changes were noted, whereas mononuclear cells including lymphocytes and mast cells remained positive up to 12 weeks after therapy started [25]. These findings in skin are replicated to some extent in studies of synovial membrane, where mast cells are the most numerous cells staining for IL-17A in both PsA and RA [26, 27]. A recent study of spinal facet joints from patients with AS compared to osteoarthritis (OA), demonstrated significant bone marrow immune cell infiltrates, with IL-17-secreting cells detected at a higher frequency in AS than OA [28]. Immunofluorescence microscopy revealed the majority of IL-17+ cells were myeloperoxidase-positive (35.84 ± 13.06/high-power field (HPF) and CD15+ (24.25 ± 10.36/HPF) indicative of neutrophils, while CD3+ T cells (0.51 ± 0.49/ HPF) and AA-1+ mast cells (2.28 ± 1.96/HPF) were less often IL-17-positive. The issue of whether mast cells produce IL-17, ie contain detectable IL-17mRNA for Il-17, or absorb Il-17 via IL-17 receptors is as yet unclear. A recent report suggests skin mast cells are positive for IL-17A mRNA, but that most IL-17A is produced by skin CD8+ lymphocytes, with mast cells producing more IL-22 [29].

These immunohistochemical findings led some observers to hypothesise that IL-17+ T lymphocytes may not play a role in PsA or PsO. However, when skin cells from patients with PsO, were investigated by the technique of tissue digestion and preparation of mononuclear cell preparations, followed by short *in vitro* stimulation and flow cytometry, it was clear that IL-17+ T lymphocytes were present [30, 31]. Res and colleagues, noted that in psoriatic plaques, both CD4+IL-17+ and CD8+IL-17+ lymphocytes were detected [32], with the frequency of CD8+IL-17+ cells related to the psoriasis severity. This discrepancy in detection of IL-17+ cells, may relate to the fact that T cells rapidly release cytokines, in contrast to the other cell types which store secretory products for coordinated mediator release in response to a relevant stimulus. CD8+ IL-17+ cells, previously detected in response to bacterial infections had been termed 'Tc17' cells to differentiate them from the well known Th17 cells [33]. They have less cytotoxic capacity compared to the usual CD8+ IFNγ+cytotoxic T cell, and probably have an immune activating role [33]. Preliminary studies of naive CD8 T cells show they follow a similar differentiation pathway to Th17 cells, utilising IL-1β, IL-6 and TGF-β, with a secondary critical role for IL-23 in stabilising the cell type and triggering Il-17 production [34].

Our group recently reported for the first time, that the PsA joint, but not the RA joint, is enriched for IL-17+CD8+ T cells [35]. Mononuclear cells from paired samples of synovial fluid (SF) and peripheral blood (PB) from patients with PsA or RA were stimulated *ex vivo*, and T cells examined by flow cytometry. Within the CD3+T cell compartment, both IL-17+CD4- (predominantly CD8+) and IL-17+CD4+T cells were significantly enhanced in the SF compared to the PB of patients with PsA (n=21), whereas in patients with RA, only IL-17+CD4+T cells were increased in the SF compared to the PB (n =14). The frequency of IL-17+CD4-T cells in PsA SF positively correlated with multiple disease activity measures, including the CRP level, ESR, DAS28 and power Doppler ultrasound score, and was increased in patients with erosive disease compared with non-erosive disease. We also confirmed that levels of CD107a, perforin, and granzyme B were attenuated in IL-17+CD8+ T cells compared to IFNγ+CD8+T cells, indicating these IL-17+CD8+ T cells do not have prototypical cytotoxic function. These findings suggest a similarity in immunopathologic characteristics of PsA and PsO, with a potential pathogenic role for the CD8+ T cells, which has been long suggested particularly in PsA [10], and emphasise the difference to RA.

We also did not detect any differences in the frequencies of PB IL-17+ T cells from patients with PsA, RA or age matched healthy controls. Although several groups have reported this, the recent report from Appell and colleagues cited above [28], using a different *in vitro* stimulatory technique of Staphylococcus aureus Enterotoxin B and phorbol 12-myristate 13-acetate/ionomycin was similar to our findings. They showed the frequency of IL-17+CD4+ T cells in SF was elevated compared to PB in AS and RA, but PB levels were not different in patients with SpA, RA, OA and healthy controls.

The Innate Immune System

Innate immunity plays a key role in the early response to pathological insults especially infections [36]. Cells of the innate immune system are responsive to signals of pathogens or cellular damage, and generate immediate cytokine and cell-to-cell responses. These responses provide early defence and also interact with the acquired immune system to stimulate and direct this system's initial response, connecting and relating the adaptive response to the original stimulus [37]. Mucosal or epidermal surfaces are in direct contact with the external environment, and not surprisingly, are rich in cells of the innate immune system. The skin is the primary interface with the external environment and provides the first line of host defence against injury and infection [38]. Similar to the lung and gut mucosal barrier, the skin is equipped with a diverse set of immune cells which can react to different insults, but which also have the potential to cause abnormal responses and disease. These factors had suggested a potentially important role for the innate immune system in the immunopathology of PsO and perhaps PsA. This interest became increasingly important when these cells were identified as major producers of IL-17.

Many cell types make up the innate immune system, including several lymphoid cell subsets, polymorphonuclear neutrophils, dendritic cells and tissue Langerhans cells [39, 40]. Natural killer (NK) cells, gamma delta (γδ) T-cells and innate lymphoid cells (ILC) are important lymphocyte subsets able both to produce cytokines including IL-17 and to kill cellular targets [41]. NK cells are large granular lymphocytes, defined by their expression of CD56 and the lack of a T-cell receptor (TCR)–CD3 complex, whose functions include killing cells expressing stress-induced molecules. NK cells are part of a group of cells called innate lymphoid cells which do not have rearranged TCR. Instead of relying on the T-cell receptor to mediate effector functions, they react to cytokines and cellular ligands, produced in tissues after infection or injury, as well as to pathogen-associated molecular patterns [42]. NK cells have receptors that recognize and respond to human leucocyte antigen (HLA), including the killer immunoglobulinlike receptors (KIRs). Some KIRs can recognize different forms of HLA-B27 and this pathway has been implicated in spondyloarthritis pathogenesis [43]. HLA-B27 genotype is highly expressed in the PsA subset presenting with axial (spinal) components of the disease, so similar pathogenesis may be involved in this group [44].

Innate lymphoid cells (ILC) are lymphoid cells that do not express the usual markers of the major adaptive cell populations such as T and B cells [45]. Three groups are described in humans, relating to their dependence on the transcriptional repressor Inhibitor of DNA binding 2 (Id2) and on the IL-2Rγ chain. The ILC3 subset, which also includes lymphoid tissue inducer cells (LTi), is dependent on the transcription factor RORγT, as well as expression of the IL-7Rα chain, and can produce IL-17A and/or IL-22 upon stimulation [46]. In humans ILC3 can be subdivided on the basis of the expression of the natural cytotoxicity receptors (NCRs) NKp44, NKp46 and NKp30, which identifies those cells that can produce IL-22 and /or IL-17A.

Gamma delta (γδ) cells are a population of CD3 T-cells that express a TCR comprising γ and δ chains, related but distinct from the usual T cell αβTCR [33, 41]. γδ T-cells are enriched in epithelial and mucosal tissues [47]. Similar to NK cells, γδ T cells are involved in non-MHC-restricted cytotoxicity in cell-mediated immune responses. The γδ TCR does not engage MHC-antigen complexes like αβ T cells but acts more like a pattern recognition receptor, recognizing factors produced by bacterial metabolic pathways, cell damage and inflammatory cytokines produced by macrophages or dendritic cells responding to infectious signals [41]. Most human γδ T cells are either the Vδ1+ (peripheral blood) or Vδ2+ subclasses (epithelial sites).

An interesting insight into integrative functions of immune system has been gained by the increased awareness that cytokine patterns generating functional phenotypes initially seen in adaptive immune lymphocytes, such as Th1 and Th2 subsets, are replicated in innate lymphocytes. These data have been summarised in a recent review suggesting that both innate and adaptive immune responses, can be grouped into three groups, Type 1 (IFNγ dependent), Type 2 (IL-4 etc) and Type 3 (IL-17 pathway) [48].

Innate Immune Cells in Psoriasis and Psoriatic Arthritis

γδ T Cells

γδ T cells mediate rapid tissue responses in murine skin and participate in cutaneous immune regulation including protection against cancer [49]. The role of human γδ cells in cutaneous homeostasis and pathology is poorly characterized. Laggner and colleagues studied γδ T cells in psoriasis skin pathology [50]. They showed that human blood contains a distinct subset of pro-inflammatory cutaneous lymphocyte antigen (CLA) and C-C chemokine receptor (CCR) 6 positive Vγ9Vδ2 T cells, which is rapidly recruited into perturbed human skin. These cells produced pro-inflammatory mediators including IL-17A and activated keratinocytes in a TNF-α and IFN-γ dependent process. Patients with psoriasis had increased Vγ9Vδ2 T cells in psoriatic skin. Peripheral blood levels were lower than healthy controls and patients with atopic dermatitis, but normalized after successful treatment of psoriasis.

In one of the few studies in PsA, Spadero and colleagues investigated γδ TCR antigen and NK surface marker positive cells by flow cytometry in PB and SF (PsA n = 17, RA n =16) lymphocytes in PsA and RA patients, compared to healthy controls [51]. Both PsA and RA patients had lower levels of peripheral blood γδ T cells compared to healthy controls (percentages and absolute numbers), with similar levels in SF and PB. In contrast PB levels of NK and NK-T lymphocytes were similar in all groups, with synovial fluid levels were lower than PB in PsA and RA. There were no significant correlations of the different SF or PB lymphocyte subsets with clinical or serological measures. Our small study of SF IL-17+CD3+ cells in PsA, we found no increase in γδ T cells in SF compared to PB [35].

In a recent study of PB IL-23R+T cells in SpA, Kenna et al studied 17 patients with active AS, 8 PsA, 9 RA and 20 healthy subjects [52]. They reported the proportion of PB IL-23R+T cells was 2-fold higher in AS patients than healthy controls, due to a 3-fold increase in IL-23R+ γδ T cells in AS patients. Similar to studies above, the proportions of IL-17+ CD4+ and CD8+ cells were not significantly different. IL- 23R+γδ T cells had enhanced IL-17 secretion, with no IL-17 production from IL-23R– γδ T cells in AS patients in response to stimulation with IL-23 and/or anti-CD3/CD28. Since IL-23 is a maturation and growth factor for IL-17–producing cells, increased IL-23R expression may regulate the function of this putative pathogenic γδ T cell population.

NK Cells

Natural killer cells are rare in healthy skin. Studies in patients with psoriasis have shown that the frequency of cells expressing NK receptors, such as CD56, is significantly increased in lesional skin, with decreased levels in peripheral blood compared to healthy controls [53, 54]. The functional relevance of these cells is unclear, although injection of peripheral blood NK cells from subjects with psoriasis into human skin grafts in mice can form psoriaform–like changes [55].

Dalbeth and Callan reported on NK cell frequency in paired samples of peripheral blood and synovial fluid from 22 patients with inflammatory arthritis, 5 of whom had SpA (3 PsA, 2 AS) [56]. The overall percentage was similar in PB and SF,, but SF cells showed an entirely different distribution of NK cell phenotypes, with the majority of NK cells expressing high levels of CD56. Most SF NK cells did not express CD16 or KIR/KAR, but expressed high levels of CD94 and NKG2A. The synovial NK cells responded to a combination of IL-12 and IL-15, by rapidly secreting INFγ. They suggested this subset may be preferentially recruited from the periphery and further activated by cytokines in the joint.

A more recent report by Tang et al, studied NK cell function leading on from previous work in which they showed IL-15 is capable of arming CD8 effector T cells to kill independently of their TCR via an NK receptor called natural killer group 2 member D (NKG2D) in a cytosolic phospholipase A2 (cPLA2)-dependent process [57]. As NK cells also express NKG2D, this group investigated if resting NK cells could be primed to the effector phase by IL-15, and studied a possible role for this pathway in the pathogenesis of psoriatic arthritis. They reported that PsA patients had upregulated IL-15 and major histocompatibility complex class I chain-related A (MICA) in synovial tissues, and that this environment enabled NK cell activation and killing via NKG2D and cPLA2. They were able to reproduce the phenotype of joint NK cells from blood NK cells by incubating them with IL-15. These findings, similar to the earlier finding of Dalbeth and Callan above, suggest a pathogenic role for NK cells when activated by environmental stress signals and demonstrate that IL-15 is capable of priming resting NK cells in tissues to the effector phase.

Innate Lymphoid Cells

Recently Villanova and colleagues showed that a substantial proportion of IL-17A and IL-22 producing cells in skin and blood of normal individuals and psoriasis patients are CD3 negative innate lymphocytes [58]. Immunophenotyping of human ILC subsets showed an increased frequency of circulating NKp44+ ILC3 in blood of psoriasis patients compared to healthy individuals or atopic dermatitis patients. More than 50% of circulating NKp44+ ILC3 expressed cutaneous lymphocyte-associated antigen indicating their potential for skin homing. Psoriasis skin had an increased frequency of total ILC compared to blood, and NKp44+ ILC3 were also increased in non-lesional psoriatic skin compared to normal skin.

These results were extended by Teunissen and colleagues [59], who found that healthy peripheral blood CD117$^+$ ILC3, NKp44 negative (NCR$^-$ ILC3), CD117$^-$NCR$^-$CRTH2$^-$CD161$^+$ ILC1, and CRTH2$^+$ ILC2, express the skin-homing receptor cutaneous lymphocyte antigen (CLA). NCR$^+$ ILC3 were scarce in peripheral blood. In normal skin, they detected ILC2 and NCR$^-$ ILC3, a small proportion of CD161$^+$ILC1, but few NCR$^+$ ILC3. Skin ILC2 and NCR$^+$ ILC3 (present in cultured dermal explants) subsets produced IL-13 and IL-22, respectively, after cytokine stimulation. Dermal NCR$^-$ ILC3 converted to NCR$^+$ILC3 when cultured with IL-1β and IL-23. They found increased proportions of NCR$^+$ ILC3 in psoriasis skin and peripheral blood of psoriasis patients compared to skin and blood of healthy individuals. The proportions of ILC2 and CD161$^+$ ILC1 were similar. NCR$^+$ ILC3 from skin and blood of psoriasis patients produced IL-22, suggesting that NCR$^+$ ILC3 may participate in psoriasis pathology.

MAIT Cells

Mucosa-associated invariant T (MAIT) cells are innate T cells that are abundant in humans, which possess an evolutionarily conserved invariant T cell receptor α chain restricted by the nonpolymorphic class Ib major histocompatibility (MHC) molecule, MHC class I-related protein (MR1). MAIT cells are activated by a MR1-bound riboflavin (vitamin B$_2$) metabolite. Mammals lack the capacity to synthesize ribofla-

vin, therefore riboflavin derivatives can act as microbial signals for the immune system to a broad range of pathogens. MAIT cells produce cytokines such as IFN-γ, TNF, and IL-17A [60, 61]. Recent reports have suggested that the majority of IL-17A+ CD8+ T cells in the blood are MAIT cells. MAIT cells are found in psoriatic skin, however they are not increased in abundance. The majority of IL-17A + CD8+ T cells in psoriasis skin plaques are devoid of MAIT cell characteristics [62]. In our study, SF IL-17+ cells from PsA SF showed no increase in MAIT cells in SF compared to PB [35].

Dendritic Cells

Studies in mice have demonstrated that dendritic cells (DCs) play a critical role in the regulation of skin immunity and tissue homeostasis [63]. In human skin, studies have focused on immunostimulatory DCs and their role during skin inflammation [64]. In human skin, myeloid DCs that reside in the dermis represent a major subset of dermal DCs (DDCs) during tissue homeostasis. Subpopulations of DDCs have been described under both normal and pathological conditions. Classically, DDCs are CD1c + with a CD1a + and CD14+ subpopulation [65]. The functional roles of DDC subsets are incompletely understood, particularly if tissue-resident DCs can also have regulatory properties. Zaba et al. [66] showed that CD1a + DDCs were potent inducers of allogeneic CD4+ and CD8 + T cell proliferation, whereas CD14+ DDCs were less immunogenic and might differentiate into Langerhans cells in response to TGF-β [67]. Recently, Chu and colleagues, showed that CD141+ DDCs are a major IL-10–producing skin-resident DC subset [68]. These cells induced T cell hyporesponsiveness and CD25hi regulatory T cells that suppress skin inflammation. Vitamin D3 (VitD3)–induced CD141+ cells generated from blood DCs were also shown to share phenotypic and functional features of skin-resident CD141+ DDCs. They regulate alloimmunity functions, and the authors speculate may have similar role *in vivo*.

Jongbloed and colleagues characterised the immunophenotype and functional characteristics of myeloid DCs (mDCs) and plasmacytoid DCs (pDCs) in patients with PsA and RA [69]. Circulating peripheral blood pDC numbers were significantly reduced in both PsA and RA. The phenotype of peripheral blood DC subsets in PsA and RA was immature compared to healthy controls, with decreased CD62L expression on both subsets. mDCs and pDCs were present in PsA and RA synovial fluid with the mDC:pDC ratio significantly exceeding that in PB. RA and PsA synovial fluid pDCs displayed an immature phenotype comparable with PB pDCs. In contrast, RA and PsA synovial fluid mDCs displayed a more mature phenotype (increased CD80, CD83 and CD86 expression) compared to PB mDCs. Both SF DC subsets matured following toll-like receptor stimulation. pDCs from PB and SF produced INF-γ and TNFα on TLR9 stimulation, but of interest, with the findings above from skin DC, only SF pDCs produced IL-10. Similarly, mDCs from PB and SF produced similar TNFα levels in response to TLR2, but SF mDCs produced more IL-10 than PB controls. These data show the potential for these cells to play a role both in a pro and anti-inflammatory role in skin and joints [70].

Enthesitis in Spondyloarthropathies

The spondyloarthropathies are characterised clinically by inflammation of the enthesis. Increased awareness of sub-clinical and intra-articular enthesitis detected by MRI, prompted McConagle and colleagues to suggest this might be a site of the early inflammation in PsA [71]. With his colleague Benjamin, they coined the term "synovio-entheseal complex", to emphasise the organised anatomy of these structures, with close proximity to synovial tissue at many sites [72]. This theory was given a major stimulus by an animal model of continuous high level IL-23 delivered by minicircle DNA in the context of collagen-induced arthritis, usually a model related to rheumatoid arthritis, where enthesitis was an early lesion [21]. The entheseal cells that responded to IL-23, were CD3+CD4−CD8−IL-23R+ROR-γt+T lymphoid cells, which produced IL-17 and 22, again suggesting a role of innate immune cells in the early activity of PsA [73]. This hypothesis is the subject of a lively debate [44], but does emphasise the role of IL-23 in stimulating SpA-type clinical syndromes. In normal human entheseal tissue, cardaveric studies (mean age 84 years [range 49–101]), showed degenerative changes and infiltrates of small numbers of inflammatory cells, mainly lymphoid cells (typically 10), with venous dilatation in 73% of sites [74]. Macrophage-like cells were sometimes seen, and neutrophils were scarce. Large collections of inflammatory cells were rare and associated with necrosis. Associated synovial tissue, present at many sites, also contained inflammatory infiltrates. Laloux and colleagues compared entheseal cellular immunopathology in pre-specified sites from surgical samples in 8 subjects with AS, compared to 4 with RA, most of whom were taking glucocorticoids, and 3 with OA [75]. Cellular infiltrates were most commonly seen at bone marrow site of the enthesitis, with significantly higher CD3, CD4 and particularly CD8 cells in the patients with AS, compared to RA and OA. Access to human entheseal tissue in early arthritis is difficult. In a study of five subjects with early enthesitis, confirmed by magnetic resonance imaging and ultrasonography, ultrasound guided needle biopsy was carried out [76]. Control tissue was obtained from two subjects undergoing spinal surgery. The enthesis architecture was abnormal in the SpA group, with increased vascularity and cellular infiltration compared with normal subjects. In contrast, to the aging enthesis, the most common infiltrating cells were CD68 positive macrophages, with a few lymphocytes. These early results will be expanded as this topic is now the focus of widespread interest.

Conclusion

The increased knowledge of innate immunity and the important role of IL-17/23 biology in both psoriasis and psoriatic arthritis, have led to substantial changes in theories of immunopathogenesis on both conditions. Many innate immune system cells reside in skin, and these data show several potential pathways that could translate environmental signals into a chronic adaptive immune response mediated by innate immune cells. The joint is less well researched but the new information summarised here will provide important hypotheses for investigation of pathogenic pathways.

Acknowledgements Many thanks to my colleague Professor Leonie Taams, CMCBI, Kings College London, for critical review of this work.

References

1. Lowes MA, Suárez-Fariñas M, Krueger JG. Immunology of psoriasis. Annu Rev Immunol. 2014;32:227–55.
2. Boehncke WH, Schön MP. Psoriasis. Lancet. S0140-6736(14)61909-7. 2015;386:983–94.
3. Lowes MA, Russell CB, Martin DA, et al. The IL-23/T17 pathogenic axis in psoriasis is amplified by keratinocyte responses. Trends Immunol. 2013;34:174–81.
4. Smith MD, Barg E, Weedon H, Papengelis V, Smeets T, Tak PP, Kraan M, Coleman M, Ahern MJ. Microarchitecture and protective mechanisms in synovial tissue from clinically and arthroscopically normal knee joints. Ann Rheum Dis. 2003;62:303–7.
5. Celis R, Planell N, Fernandez-Sueiro JL, Sanmarti R, Ramirez J, Gonzalez-Alvaro I, et al. Synovial cytokine expression in psoriatic arthritis and associations with lymphoid neogenesis and clinical features. Arthritis Res Ther. 2012;14:R93.
6. Van Landuyt KB, JonesE A, McGonagle D, Luyten FP, Lories RJ. Flow cytometric characterization of freshly isolated and culture expanded human synovial cell populations in patients with chronic arthritis. Arthritis Res Ther. 2010;12:R15.
7. Veale D, Yanni G, Rogers S, Barnes L, Bresnihan B, Fitzgerald O. Reduced synovial membrane macrophage numbers, ELAM-1 expression, and lining layer hyperplasia in psoriatic arthritis as compared with rheumatoid arthritis. Arthritis Rheum. 1993;36:893–900.
8. Danning CL, Illei GG, Hitchon C, Greer MR, Boumpas DT, McInnes IB. Macrophage-derived cytokine and nuclear factor kappaB p65 expression in synovial membrane and skin of patients with psoriatic arthritis. Arthritis Rheum. 2000;43(6):1244–56.
9. Kruithof E, Baeten D, De RL, Vandooren B, Foell D, Roth J, et al. Synovial histopathology of psoriatic arthritis, both oligo- and polyarticular, resembles spondyloarthropathy more than it does rheumatoid arthritis. Arthritis Res Ther. 2005;7(3):R569–80.
10. Costello P, Bresnihan B, O'Farrelly C, FitzGerald O. Predominance of CD8+ T lymphocytes in psoriatic arthritis. J Rheumatol. 1999;26:1117–24.
11. van Kuijk AWR, Reinders-Blankert P, Smeets TJM, Dijkmans BAC, Tak PP. Detailed analysis of the cell infiltrate and the expression of mediators of synovial inflammation and joint destruction in the synovium of patients with psoriatic arthritis: implications for treatment. Ann Rheum Dis. 2006;65:1551–7.
12. Baeten D, Kruithof E, De Rycke L, Boots AM, Mielants H, Veys EM, De Keyser F. Infiltration of the synovial membrane with macrophage subsets and polymorphonuclear cells reflects global disease activity in spondyloarthropathy. Arthritis Res Ther. 2005;7:R359–69.
13. Yeremenko N, Noordenbos T, Cantaert T, van Tok M, van de Sande M, Cañete JD, Tak PP, Baeten D. Disease-specific and inflammation-independent stromal alterations in spondylarthritis synovitis. Arthritis Rheum. 2013;65:174–85.
14. Mak RKH, Hundhausen C, Nestle FO. Progress in understanding the immunopathogenesis of psoriasis. Clinical subtypes, histological features and associated comorbidities. Actas Dermosifiliogr. 2009;100 Suppl 2:2–13.
15. Baeten D, Van Damme N, Van den Bosch F, Kruithof E, De Vos M, Mielants H, Veys EM, De Keyser F. Impaired Th1 cytokine production in spondyloarthropathy is restored by anti-TNFalpha. Ann Rheum Dis. 2001;60:750–5.
16. Ambarus C, Yeremenko N, Tak PP, Baeten D. Pathogenesis of spondyloarthritis: autoimmune or autoinflammatory? Curr Opin Rheumatol. 2012;24:351–8.
17. Huffmeier U, Uebe S, Ekici AB, Bowes J, Giardina E, Korendowych E, et al. Common variants at TRAF3IP2 are associated with susceptibility to psoriatic arthritis and psoriasis. Nat Genet. 2010;42:996–9.
18. Apel M, Uebe S, Bowes J, Giardina E, Korendowych E, Juneblad K, et al. Variants in RUNX3 contribute to susceptibility to psoriatic arthritis, exhibiting further common ground with ankylosing spondylitis. Arthritis Rheum. 2013;65:1224–31.
19. McGonagle D, Lories RJ, Tan AL, Benjamin M. The concept of a "synovio-entheseal complex" and its implications for understanding joint inflammation and damage in psoriatic arthritis and beyond. Arthritis Rheum. 2007;56(8):2482–91.
20. McGonagle D, Benjamin M, Tan AL. The pathogenesis of psoriatic arthritis and associated nail disease: not autoimmune after all? Curr Opin Rheumatol. 2009;21(4):340–7.
21. Sherlock JP, Joyce-Shaikh B, Turner SP, et al. IL-23 induces spondyloarthropathy by acting on ROR-γt+CD3+ CD4–CD8– entheseal resident T cells. Nat Med. 2012;18:1069–76.
22. Kirkham BW, Kavanaugh A, Reich K. Interleukin-17A: a unique pathway in immune mediated diseases: psoriasis, psoriatic arthritis, and rheumatoid arthritis. Immunology. 2014;141:133–42.
23. Ferretti S, Bonneau O, Dubois GR, Jones CE, Trifilieff A. IL-17, produced by lymphocytes and neutrophils, is necessary for lipopolysaccharide induced airway neutrophilia: IL-15 as a possible trigger. J Immunol. 2003;170(4):2106–12.
24. Li L, Huang L, Vergis AL, Ye H, Bajwa A, Narayan V, Strieter RM, Rosin DL, Okusa MD. IL-17 produced

by neutrophils regulates IFN-γ–mediated neutrophil migration in mouse kidney ischemia-reperfusion injury. J Clin Invest. 2010;120:331–42.

25. Reich K, Papp KA, Matheson RT, Tu JH, Bissonnette R, Bourcier M, Gratton D, Kunynetz RA, Poulin Y, Rosoph LA, Stingl G, Bauer WM, Salter JM, Falk TM, Blödorn-Schlicht NA, Hueber W, Sommer U, Schumacher MM, Peters T, Kriehuber E, Lee DM, Wieczorek GA, Kolbinger F, Bleul CC. Evidence that a neutrophil-keratinocyte crosstalk is an early target of IL-17A inhibition in psoriasis. Exp Dermatol. 2015;24(7):529–35. doi:10.1111/ exd.12710.

26. Hueber AJ, Asquith DL, Miller AM, Reilly J, Kerr S, Leipe J, et al. Mast cells express IL-17A in rheumatoid arthritis synovium. J Immunol. 2010;184: 3336–40.

27. Noordenbos T, Yeremenko N, Gofita I, van de Sande M, Tak PP, Canete JD, et al. Interleukin-17–positive mast cells contribute to synovial inflammation in spondylarthritis. Arthritis Rheum. 2012;64:99–109.

28. Appel H, Maier R, Wu P, Scheer R, Hempfing A, Kayser R, Thiel A, Radbruch A, Loddenkemper C, Sieper J. Analysis of IL-17+ cells in facet joints of patients with spondyloarthritis suggests that the innate immune pathway might be of greater relevance than the Th17-mediated adaptive immune response. Arthritis Res Ther. 2011;13:R95.

29. Mashiko S, Bouguermouh S, Rubio M, Baba N, Bissonnette R, Sarfati M. Human mast cells are major IL-22 producers in patients with psoriasis and atopic dermatitis. J Allergy Clin Immunol. pii: S0091-6749(15)00175-X. 2015;136:351–9.

30. Kryczek I, Bruce AT, Gudjonsson JE, Johnston A, Aphale A, Vatan L, et al. Induction of IL-17 + T cell trafficking and development by IFN-γ: mechanism and pathological relevance in psoriasis. J Immunol. 2008;181:4733–41.

31. Ortega C, Fernandez AS, Carrillo JM, Romero P, Molina IJ, Moreno JC, et al. IL-17-producing CD8 T lymphocytes from psoriasis skin plaques are cytotoxic effector cells that secrete Th17-related cytokines. J Leukoc Biol. 2009;86:435–43.

32. Res PC, Piskin G, de Boer OJ, van der Loos CM, Teeling P, Bos JD, et al. Overrepresentation of IL-17A and IL-22 producing CD8 T cells in lesional skin suggests their involvement in the pathogenesis of psoriasis. PLoS One. 2010;5:e14108.

33. Andersson J, Samarina A, Fink J, Rahman S, Grundstrom S. Impaired expression of perforin and granulysin in CD8 + T cells at the site of infection in human chronic pulmonary tuberculosis. Infect Immun. 2007;75:5210–22.

34. Huber M, Heink S, Grothe H, Guralnik A, Reinhard K, Elflein K, Hünig T, Mittrücker HW, Brüstle A, Kamradt T, Lohoff M. A Th17-like developmental process leads to CD8(+) Tc17 cells with reduced cytotoxic activity. Eur J Immunol. 2009;39:1716–25.

35. Menon B, Gullick NJ, Walter GJ, Rajasekhar M, Garrood T, Evans HG, Taams LS, Kirkham BW. Interleukin-17 + CD8 + T cells are enriched in the joints of patients with psoriatic arthritis and correlate

with disease activity and joint damage progression. Arthritis Rheum. 2014;66:1272–81.

36. Medzhitov R, Janeway Jr C. Innate immunity. N Engl J Med. 2000;343:338–44.

37. Isailovic N, Daigo K, Mantovani A, Selmi C. Interleukin-17 and innate immunity in infections and chronic inflammation. J Autoimmun. 2015;60:1–11.

38. Diani M, Altomare G, Reali E. T cell responses in psoriasis and psoriatic arthritis. Autoimmun Rev. 2015;14:286–92.

39. Al-Mossawi MH, Ridley A, Kiedel S, Bowness P. The role of natural killer cells, gamma delta T-cells and other innate immune cells in spondyloarthritis. Curr Opin Rheumatol. 2013;25:434–9.

40. Koyasu S, Moro K. Role of innate lymphocytes in infection and inflammation. Front Immunol. 2012; 3:101.

41. Sutton CE, Mielke LA, Mills KHG. IL-17-producing γδ T cells and innate lymphoid cells. Eur J Immunol. 2012;42:2221–31.

42. Spits H, Cupedo T. Innate lymphoid cells: emerging insights in development, lineage relationships, and function. Annu Rev Immunol. 2012;30:647–75.

43. Bowness P, Ridley A, Shaw J, et al. Th17 cells expressing KIR3DL2þ and responsive to HLA-B27 homodimers are increased in ankylosing spondilitis. J Immunol. 2011;186:2672–80.

44. FitzGerald O, Haroon M, Giles JT, Winchester R. Concepts of pathogenesis in psoriatic arthritis: genotype determines clinical phenotype. Arthritis Res Ther. 2015;17(1):115.

45. McKenzie AN, Spits H, Eberl G. Innate lymphoid cells in inflammation and immunity. Immunity. 2014; 41:366–74.

46. Montaldo E, Juelke K, Romagnani C. Group 3 innate lymphoid cells (ILC3s): origin, differentiation and plasticity in humans and mice. Eur J Immunol. 2015;45(8):2171–82. doi:10.1002/eji.201545598.

47. Gray EE, Suzuki K, Cyster JG. Cutting edge: identification of a motile IL-17-producing gammadelta T cell population in the dermis. J Immunol. 2011;186: 6091–5.

48. Annunziato F, Romagnani C, Romagnani S. The 3 major types of innate and adaptive cell-mediated effector immunity. J Allergy Clin Immunol. 2015; 135:626–35.

49. Sumaria N, Roediger B, Ng LG, Qin J, Pinto R, Cavanagh LL, et al. Cutaneous immunosurveillance by self-renewing dermal gammadelta T cells. J Exp Med. 2011;208:505–18.

50. Laggner U, Di Meglio P, Perera GK, Hundhausen C, Ke L, Niwa Ali N, Smith CH, Hayday AC, Nickoloff BJ, Nestle FO. Identification of a novel pro-inflammatory human skin-homing Vγ9Vδ2 T cell subset with a potential role in psoriasis. J Immunol. 2011;187:2783–93.

51. Spadaro A, Scrivo R, Moretti T, Bernardini G, Riccieri V, Taccari E, Strom R, Valesini G. Natural killer cells and gamma/delta T cells in synovial fluid and in peripheral blood of patients with psoriatic arthritis. Clin Exp Rheumatol. 2004;22:389–94.

52. Kenna TJ, Davidson SI, Duan R, Bradbury LA, McFarlane J, Smith M, Weedon H, Street S, Thomas R, Thomas GP, Brown MA. Enrichment of circulating interleukin-17–secreting interleukin-23 receptor–positive γδT cells in patients with active ankylosing spondylitis. Arthritis Rheum. 2012;64:1420–9.

53. Ottaviani C, Nasorri F, Bedini C, et al. CD56 (bright) CD16(-) NK cells accumulate in psoriatic skin in response to CXCL10 and CCL5 and exacerbate skin inflammation. Eur J Immunol. 2006;36:118–28.

54. Luci C, Gaudy-Marqueste C, Rouzaire P, Audonnet S, Cognet C, Hennino A, Nicolas JF, Grob JJ, Tomasello E. Peripheral natural killer cells exhibit qualitative and quantitative changes in patients with psoriasis and atopic dermatitis. Br J Dermatol. 2012;166:789–96.

55. Gilhar A, Ullmann Y, Kerner H, et al. Psoriasis is mediated by a cutaneous defect triggered by activated immunocytes: induction of psoriasis by cells with natural killer receptors. J Invest Dermatol. 2002;119:384–91.

56. Dalbeth N, Callan MFC. A subset of natural killer cells is greatly expanded within inflamed joints. Arthritis Rheum. 2002;46:1763–72.

57. Tang F, Sally B, Ciszewski C, Abadie V, Curran SA, Groh V, FitzGerald O, Winchester RJ, Jabri B. Interleukin 15 primes natural killer cells to kill via NKG2D and cPLA2 and this pathway is active in psoriatic arthritis. PLoS One. 2013;8(9):e76292.

58. Villanova F, Flutter B, Tosi I, Grys K, Sreeneebus H, Perera GK, Chapman A, Smith CH, Di Meglio P, Nestle FO. Characterization of innate lymphoid cells (ILC) in human skin and blood demonstrates increase of NKp44+ ILC3 in psoriasis. J Invest Dermatol. 2014;134:984–91.

59. Teunissen MBM, Munneke JM, Bernink JH, Spuls PI, Res PCM, te Velde A, Cheuk S, Brouwer MWD, Menting SP, Eidsmo L, Spits H, Hazenberg MD, Mjösberg J. Composition of innate lymphoid cell subsets in the human skin: enrichment of NCR⁺ ILC3 in lesional skin and blood of psoriasis patients. J Invest Dermatol. 2014. doi:10.1038/jid.2014.146.

60. Cowley SC. MAIT cells and pathogen defence. Cell Mol Life Sci. 2014;71:4831–40.

61. Dusseaux M, Martin E, Serriari N, Peguillet I, Premel V, Louis D, et al. Human MAIT cells are xenobiotic-resistant, tissue-targeted, CD161hi IL-17-secreting T cells. Blood. 2011;117:1250–9.

62. Johnston A, Gudjonsson JE. Psoriasis and the MAITing game: a role for IL-17A+ invariant TCR CD8+ T cells in psoriasis? J Invest Dermatol. 2014;134:2864–6.

63. Merad M, Manz MG. Dendritic cell homeostasis. Blood. 2009;113:3418–27.

64. Nestle FO, Di Meglio P, Qin J-Z, Nickoloff BJ. Skin immune sentinels in health and disease. Nat Rev Immunol. 2009;9:679–91.

65. Nestle FO, Zheng XG, Thompson CB, Turka LA, Nickoloff BJ. Characterization of dermal dendritic cells obtained from normal human skin reveals phenotypic and functionally distinctive subsets. J Immunol. 1993;151:6535–45.

66. Zaba LC, Fuentes-Duculan J, Eungdamrong NJ, Abello MV, Novitskaya I, Pierson KC, et al. Psoriasis is characterized by accumulation of immunostimulatory and Th1/Th17 cell-polarizing myeloid dendritic cells. J Invest Dermatol. 2009;129:79–88.

67. Klechevsky E, Morita R, Liu M, Cao Y, Coquery S, Thompson-Snipes L, Briere F, Chaussabel D, Zurawski G, Palucka AK, et al. Functional specializations of human epidermal Langerhans cells and CD14+ dermal dendritic cells. Immunity. 2008;29:497–510.

68. Chu C-C, Ali N, Karagiannis P, Di Meglio P, Skowera A, Napolitano L, Barinaga G, Grys K, Sharif-Paghaleh E, Karagiannis SN, Peakman M, Lombardi G, Nestle FO. Resident CD141 (BDCA3)+ dendritic cells in human skin produce IL-10 and induce regulatory T cells that suppress skin inflammation. J Exp Med. 2012;209:935–94.

69. Jongbloed SL, Lebre MC, Fraser AR, Gracie JA, Sturrock RD, Tak PP, McInnes IB. Enumeration and phenotypical analysis of distinct dendritic cell subsets in psoriatic arthritis and rheumatoid arthritis. Arthritis Res Ther. 2006;8:R15.

70. Gaston JS, Jarvis LB, Zhang L, Goodall JC. Dendritic cell: T-cell interactions in spondyloarthritis. Adv Exp Med Biol. 2009;649:263–76.

71. McGonagle D, Gibbon W, O'Connor P, et al. Characteristic magnetic resonance imaging entheseal changes in knee synovitis in spondylarthropathy. Arthritis Rheum. 1998;41:694–700.

72. Benjamin M, Mcgonagle D. Histopathologic changes at "synovio–entheseal complexes" suggesting a novel mechanism for synovitis in osteoarthritis and spondylarthritis. Arthritis Rheum. 2007;56:3601–9.

73. Cua DJ, Tato CM. Innate IL-17-producing cells: the sentinels of the immune system. Nat Rev Immunol. 2010;10:479–89.

74. Benjamin M, Mcgonagle D. The anatomical basis for disease localisation in seronegative spondyloarthropathy at entheses and related sites. J Anat. 2001;199:503–26.

75. Laloux L, Voisin MC, Allain J, Martin N, Kerboull L, Chevalier X, Claudepierre P. Immunohistological study of entheses in spondyloarthropathies: comparison in rheumatoid arthritis and osteoarthritis. Ann Rheum Dis. 2001;60:316–21.

76. McGonagle D, Marzo-Ortega H, O'Connor P, Gibbon W, Hawkey P, Henshaw K, Emery P. Histological assessment of the early enthesitis lesion in spondyloarthropathy. Ann Rheum Dis. 2002;61:534–7.

Cytokine Pathways in Psoriasis and Psoriatic Arthritis

9

Ankit Saxena, Smriti K. Raychaudhuri, and Siba P. Raychaudhuri

Abstract

Psoriatic disease is a systemic autoimmune disease mostly associated with skin and joint involvement (psoriatic arthritis). Strong evidences from clinical studies and experimental models suggest that both innate and adaptive immune responses are involved in its pathogenesis. Psoriatic disease used to be regarded as a Th1-driven disease, now there are substantial evidences to suggest regulatory role of Th17 cells as well in the pathogenesis of psoriasis and psoriatic arthritis. Cytokines play a critical role; besides IFN-γ and TNFα, IL-23/Th17 pathway plays a dominant role in the inflammatory and proliferative cascades of both the skin and joint tissues. Recently in a series of elegant experiments using mouse models and human tissues it has been demonstrated that IL-23 induced Th17 cytokines (IL-17 and IL-22) can contribute to all four pathologic events in a psoriatic disease: development of psoriatic plaque, pannus formation in the joint, joint erosion and new bone formation.

Keywords

Psoriasis • Psoriatic Arthritis • Cytokines • IL-17 • IL-23 • TNFα • Keratinocytes • Osteoclast • Osteoblast

A. Saxena, PhD
Division of Immunology,
Department of Pathology, Johns Hopkins University School of Medicine,
Baltimore, MD, USA
e-mail: asaxena4@jhmi.edu

S.K. Raychaudhuri, MD
Psoriasis Clinic and Division of Rheumatology,
VA Medical Center Sacramento,
Sacramento, CA, USA

S.P. Raychaudhuri, MD (✉)
Psoriasis Clinic and Division of Rheumatology,
VA Medical Center Sacramento,
Sacramento, CA, USA

Division of Rheumatology, Allergy & Clinical immunology, School of Medicine,
University of California Davis, 10535 Hospital Way Mather, Davis, CA, 95655, USA
e-mail: sraychaudhuri@ucdavis.edura,
ysiba@hotmail.com

© Springer International Publishing Switzerland 2016
A. Adebajo et al. (eds.), *Psoriatic Arthritis and Psoriasis: Pathology and Clinical Aspects*,
DOI 10.1007/978-3-319-19530-8_9

Introduction

Psoriasis and psoriatic arthritis (PsA), often termed as 'psoriatic disease' are autoimmune diseases which share certain similar pathological events and clinical features [1, 2]. PsA is a seronegative autoimmune inflammatory joint disease that develops in approximately 25 % of the psoriasis patients usually within 10 years of start of skin manifestations.

Although considerable progress has been made in deciphering the pathogenesis of psoriatic disease, the exact cause still remains a mystery. Psoriatic disease is a multifactorial disease involving a complex interaction of genetic, immunologic and environmental factors that modify the function of lymphocytes, neutrophils epidermal keratinocytes, synovial cells (FLS) and osteoclasts through important cytokines/chemokines and growth factors [2–5].

The inflammation associated with psoriatic disease is a sequel of multiple pathological events. The disease is primarily characterized by hyperplasia of epidermal keratinocytes, angiogenesis and infiltration of immune cells in the affected skin; where as in the joints the primary outcomes are pannus formation, erosion of bone and new bone formation. The immunopathogenesis of psoriatic disease is complex and still evolving. The role of innate and adaptive immune responses is now well established in its pathogenesis. Cytokines are the primary product of immune activation. Various cytokines play a detrimental role in the psoriasis pathogenesis; however, understanding of their role in the disease is still evolving. In this complex milieu, pathogenic T cell subpopulations (Th1, Th17, Th22) and their signature cytokines (IFN-γ, TNF-α, IL-17, IL-22), chemokines, adhesion molecules, growth factors like nerve growth factor (NGF) and neuropeptides act in an integrated way through their corresponding receptors to evolve pathognomonic features of psoriasis and psoriatic arthritis [3, 5–10].

Immunopathogenesis of Psoriatic Disease and the Cytokine Network

Interactions of the Dermal Dendritic Cells (DCs) and T Cells

A current dominant model for the pathogenesis of psoriasis and PsA is that underlying genetic and environmental factors (both exogenous and endogenous) induce dendritic cells (DCs) to release IL-23 and IL-12 and that activate discrete T cell subpopulations such as Th1, Th9, Th17 and Th22 cells [10–12] Raychaudhuri et al. 2014). DCs isolated from psoriasis lesions have been reported to induce the production of IFN-γ and IL-17 by Th1 and Th17 cells, respectively [13, 14]. It has been demonstrated that CD11c + myeloid DCs (BDCA-1+ and BDCA-1−) can stimulate T cells robustly in an allogeneic mixed lymphocyte reaction and similarly induce allogeneic T cells to produce IFN-γ and IL-17. Where as plasmacytoid DCs (pDCs) might play a role in a developing psoriatic lesion. Injury to the skin causes cell death and the production of the antimicrobial peptide LL-37 (cathelicidin or AMP LL37) by keratinocytes. LL-37 forms complexes with self-DNA (released from dying cells). DNA/LL37 complexes bind to TLR9 in pDCs, which leads to production of IFN-α [15]. LL37/RNA complexes can activate plasmacytoid DCs through TLR7, and myeloid DCs can be activated by this complex through TLR8 [15–17]. In PsA also both mDCs and pDCs are present in SF and have been found to be functionally active [18].

Regulatory Role of the T Cells in Psoriatic Disease

Inflammatory infiltrates in the skin and joints have been studied extensively. In both tissues there are prominent lymphocytic infiltrates localized to the dermal papillae in the skin and the sublining layer stroma in the joint. T cells, with a predominance of CD4+ lymphocytes, are the most significant

Fig. 9.1 Immune cell and cytokines in psoriatic keratinocyte inflammation. Myeloid DCs and macrophages produce cytokines that induce IFNγ production by Th1 cells and IL-17 production by Th17 cells. IL-23 also induces production of IL-22 by Th17 and possibly Th22 cells. Cytokines IFNγ, IL-17 and TNFα cooperate to induce the production of anti-microbial peptides (*AMPs*) and chemokines by keratinocytes, thereby enhancing immune-cell recruitment and inflammation in lesions. IL-22 is also involved in promoting epidermal hyperplasia. The IL-20 subfamily cytokines (*IL-19*, *IL-20* and *IL-24*), which are mainly produced by monocytes, also contribute to epidermal hyperplasia

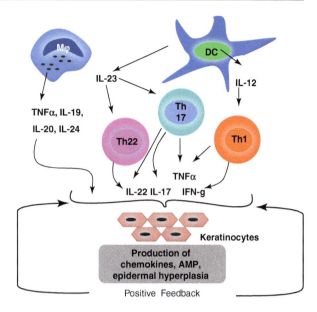

lymphocytes in the tissues; in contrast, this ratio is reversed in the epidermis, SF compartment, and at the enthesis, where CD8+ T cells are more common [19–21]. This differential tropism of CD8+ T cell suggests that CD8+ T cells may be driving the immune response in the joint and skin. This is supported by an association with human leucocyte antigen (HLA) class [22, 23].

The hypothetical Antigen in psoriasis and PsA to which the effector memory T cells are responding remains unknown. However it has been reported that in the peripheral blood T cells reactive to both streptococcal M protein and keratin can be found in psoriasis patients [24–27]. Thus a possible mechanism for autoimmune response in psoriasis could be that streptococcus-specific T cells are cross-reacting with the epidermal keratins (molecular mimicry) [27]. Further an analysis of T cell receptor beta chain variable (TCRβV) gene repertoires revealed common expansions in both skin and synovial inflammatory sites, suggesting an important role for cognate T cell responses in the pathogenesis of psoriatic and that the inciting antigen may be identical or homologous between afflicted skin and synovium [28].

However more direct evidence for psoriatic disease as a T cell mediated autoimmune disease of the skin and joints based comes from series of pre-clinical and clinical studies: (i) CD4+ T cells targeted immunotherapy clears active plaques of psoriasis [6]; (ii) transplanted nonlesional psoriatic skin converts to a psoriatic plaque subsequent to intradermal administration of T cells activated with an antigen cocktail in SCID mice [7, 8]; (iii) blocking of the T cell co-stimulatory molecule improves psoriasis in the SCID mouse-psoriasis xenograft model [8]; (iv) Th17 cell driven cytokines contributes to the pannus formation, osteoclast activation and new bone formation in PsA [6–9].

The cytokine network in the psoriatic skin and synovium is dominated by DCs, monocyte and T-cell derived cytokines: IL-1β, IL-2, IL-10, IFN-γ, TNF-α, Il-17 and IL-22 (Figs. 9.1 and 9.2) [9, 11]. In PsA synovium, higher level of IFN-γ, IL-2, and IL-10 have been detected than in psoriatic skin [29]. Collectively, the cytokines IL-17, IFN-γ, IL-22, and TNF can cause keratinocyte proliferation (Fig. 9.1) as well contributes to the pannus formation in joints (Fig. 9.2). In the next sections we will explain in details about the cytokine net

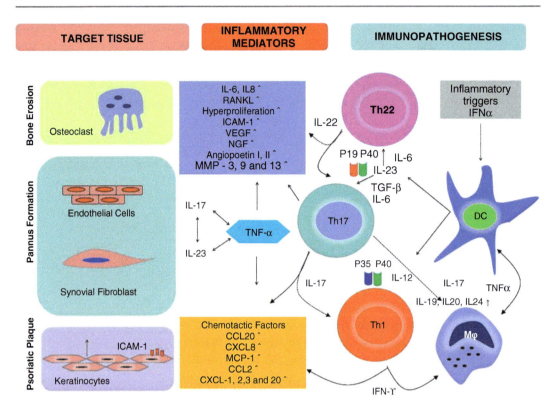

Fig. 9.2 IL-17/IL-23 axis in skin and joint tissues of psoriasis and psoriatic arthritis. The interleukin (IL)-23–IL-17 axis is critical in the regulation of cytokine network and inflammatory mediators contributing in the pathogenesis of psoriasis. Myeloid dendritic cells (DCs) become activated in the presence of inflammatory mediators to produce IL-23 which in turn drives the production of IL-17 and IL-22 by subsets of CD4+ (Th22) and CD8+ (Tc22) cells, whereas IL-12 drives production of interferon (IFN-ϒ). The IL-23 and IL12 are hetrodimer cytokines with commonly shared P40 subunit and unique P19 (IL-23) and P35 (IL-12) subunits. IL-23 and IL-12 are responsible for the differentiation and development of Th1 and Th17 cell subsets. These subunits have emerged as an important drug targets in the treatment of psoriasis. T cell derived cytokines can then activate the target tissues to produce further inflammatory chemokines and cytokines. Some will recruit cells into the skin: IL-8, chemokine CXC ligand (CXCL)1, 2 and 3 are all neutrophil chemotaxins; chemokine CC ligand (CCL)20 attracts chemokine CC receptor (CCR)6+ DCs and T17 cells; and vascular endothelial growth factor (VEGF) is important in inducing the vascular hyperplasia seen in psoriasis. IL-17 and tumor necrosis factor (TNF), as well as IL-17 and IL-22 synergise to orchestrate the damage of joint tissue also. These activated Th-17 cells in the enthesis and in the synovial tissue can promote local inflammation and bone remodeling through a variety of effector mediators such as IL-17 and IL-22; which contribute to inflammation, bone erosion and bone fusion. Abbreviations: *VEGF* vascular endothelial growth factor, *MMP* matrix metalloproteases, *AMP* adenosine monophosphate, *DC* dendritic cell, *Mφ* macrophage, *NGF* nerve growth factor, *GM-CSF* granulocyte macrophage colony stimulating factor, *RANKL* receptor activator of nuclear factor kappa-B ligand, *ICAM-1* intercellular adhesion molecule 1. *Solid lines* show direct effect on the target cell or tissue, *dashed lines* show indirect effect

work in psoriatic disease with a focus on TNF-α and the cytokines of the IL-17/IL-23 axis.

Role of TNF in Psoriasis and Psoriatic Arthritis

TNF-α has been widely studied in psoriasis [30, 31]. TNF-α production is significantly elevated in the lesional skin as compared to nonlesional and healthy skin [32, 33]. Besides keratinocytes, other cell types, such as macrophages, mast cells, and activated T lymphocytes, produce TNF-α in the stimulated skin [34, 35]. The activation of inflammatory mechanisms leads to the production of TNFα which is often facilitated by intervention of other cytokines, such as IL-1, IL-2, GM-CSF, IL-17 and IFN-γ [36, 37].

Overexpressed TNF is localised in the epidermis and around blood vessels in the upper dermis; its sources are KCs, epidermal LCs, dermal dendrocytes (DCs) and macrophages/monocytes [38]. Increased plasma TNF levels are observed in psoriatic patients [32, 39, 40]. However, this cytokine is produced locally as the levels are significantly higher in the blister fluids in comparison to the plasma [41].

Biologically active form of TNFα is a homotrimer consisting of three identical protein chains. TNF exerts its functions by binding to two different receptors: TNFR1/p55 and TNFR2/p75. The latter is expressed solely on immune, endothelial and neuronal cells and is inducible, whereas TNFR1 is expressed ubiquitously and constitutively. Increased levels of TNF are found at the sites of inflammation in several autoimmune diseases and upon neutralization, inflammatory symptoms are generally reduced. This led to the rationale of blocking TNF in patients suffering from autoimmune diseases that are associated with excessive amounts of TNF. Higher levels of TNF, TNFR1 and TNFR2 are observed in psoriatic lesions [33, 41]. Keratinocytes express TNFR1 and are thus responsive to TNF. Stimulation with TNF induces not only immune and inflammatory responses orchestrated by keratinocytes but also tissue remodeling, cell motility, cell cycling, and apoptosis [42]. TNF is produced by a variety of cells involved in the pathophysiology of psoriasis, such as keratinocytes, dendritic cells (DCs), and NKT, Th1, Th17 and Th22 cells. This implies that TNF might be involved in both the initial phase and the chronic phase of psoriasis. Therefore, neutralization of TNF can affect several stages of the disease by interfering with the activation of different cell subtypes. Although TNF-antagonists are extensively prescribed to patients, the exact mechanism underlying psoriasis is not completely understood and the precise role of TNF is yet to be elucidated.

One plausible mechanism is exaggerated TNF signaling, possibly due to genetic polymorphism in predisposed individuals. A recent meta-analysis by Zhuang et al. revealed a significantly decreased risk of psoriasis for the TNF 308G/A polymorphism and an increased risk for TNF 238G/A [43]. In the past years, new sets of cytokines have been added to the pathophysiology of psoriasis. New players such as IL-19, IL-20, IL-22 and IL-24 have also been implicated in psoriasis and psoriatic arthritis [44]. It has also been postulated that TNF might be involved in the induction of these cytokines. For example, the group of Haase used a murine spontaneous psoriasis model to unravel the role of TNF in the induction of IL-24 and suggested that IL-24 is required for the initiation phase of psoriasis and that this early event depends on TNF/TNFR1 signaling [45]. Transgenic expression of this cytokine was sufficient to induce skin inflammation, and up-regulated levels of IL-24 were found in psoriatic epidermis [45].

Synovial tissue in PsA is also characterized by marked expression of TNFα. Several studies have shown that elevated levels of TNFα are found in the synovial fluid and synovium of patients who have PsA. In addition, TNF receptors are elevated in synovial fluid and their level of expression correlates with clinical disease severity [46].

TNFα contributes to several pathologic events in PsA- (a) Angiogenesis and cell trafficking (b) proliferation of FLS, release cytokines (IL-6, IL-8) and MMPs from FLS (c) activation of osteoclasts [47–49]. In transgenic TNF mice over-expression of TNFα induced erosive polyarthritis and hyperplastic synovial pannus; these observations further substantiates the critical role of TNFα in the pathogenesis of PsA [50]. Perhaps the most convincing evidence for an important role for TNFα in psoriatic disease comes from studies demonstrating that TNFα inhibitors are highly therapeutically effective in psoriasis and PsA. It is obvious that anti-TNF agents will antagonize TNFα directly and will inhibit its effect on adhesions molecules, downregulate specific inflammatory cytokines and MMPs and thus will have a marked inhibitory effect on the inflammatory-proliferative cascades of psoriatic disease. In addition an important observation is made that in psoriasis patients treated with etanercept lesional DCs had lower levels of co-stimulatory molecules [51]. Further, etanercept inhibits expression of co-stimulatory molecules (CD86, HLA-DR, CD11c) in DCs. This suggests that clinical benefit seen with TNFα blockade may be linked to inhibition of T cell immune response and suppression of the effector IL-23/IL-17 cytokine pathway [52].

Role of the IL-12/IL-23/IL-17 Cytokine Pathway in Psoriasis and Psoriatic Arthritis

IL-12, IL-23 and IL-17 have emerged as major players in autoimmune diseases and inflammatory disorder. Psoriasis used to be regarded as Th1-driven disease, now there are substantial evidences to suggest regulatory role of Th17 cell as well in the pathogenesis of psoriatic disease [45, 53]. IL-23 was previously assumed to be essential for differentiation of TH17 cells, but is now known to stimulate survival and expansion of Th17 cells [54]. Similarly, IL-12 is produced by dendritic cells and macrophages and is known to play a role in the differentiation of CD4 naive T cells to T-helper 1 (Th1) cell [55]. In psoriasis patients, the IL-23 pathway is activated and characterized by high level production of IL-23 by DCs and keratinocytes and increased numbers of Th17 cells [56, 57]. Wohn and colleagues showed that the IL-23 produced by Langerin-negative conventional DCs is important for the development of psoriatic lesions in mice [58]. Murine models have helped to elucidate the role of IL-12 and IL-23 in psoriasis. Transfer of IL-12 induced pathogenic T cells in SCID mice resulted in psoriasis lesions which was reversible on administration of anti-IL-12 p40 antibody [59]. IL-12p40 is a shared subunit of IL-12 and IL-23, either or both cytokines could potentially be involved in the disease process. However, p40 transgenic mice constitutively produce IL-23, but not IL-12 in basal keratinocytes; further, injections of recombinant IL-23 in nontransgenic littermates resulted in an inflammatory skin disease similar to that of p40 transgenic mice [60]. Collectively, these studies on transgenic p40 mice indicate that IL-23 may be particularly important for the involvement of keratinocytes in inflammation, and led to the suggestion that IL-23 may be an important target in psoriasis.

Studies of human psoriatic lesions also support a role for IL-12 and IL-23 in psoriasis.

Several human studies have demonstrated increased levels of IL12p40 messenger RNA (mRNA) in psoriatic lesions [61]. Similarly, a study of 18 individuals revealed IL-12p40 mRNA expression in psoriatic lesions but not in normal-appearing skin, whereas IL-12 p35 mRNA was expressed similarly in both psoriatic lesions and normal-appearing skin [62]. Lack of increase in IL-12p35 mRNA (the subunit distinctive of IL-12) suggested a role for IL-23 in the pathogenesis of psoriasis.

Compared to healthy controls, psoriasis patients have higher levels of IL-17 in lesional skin and in peripheral circulation. The levels of IL-17 also correlate with disease severity. Several cell types other than Th17 cells can produce IL-17, including neutrophils, mast cells, macrophages, natural killer cells, dendritic cells and Tc17 cells (CD8[+]). Another type of cells, $\gamma\delta$ T cells, produces more IL-17 than Th17 cells. IL-17 producing $\gamma\delta$ T cells and RORγt[+] innate lymphoid cells are necessary and sufficient to induce psoriatic plaques [63, 64].

Th17 cytokines, in particular interleukin IL-17A, have been shown to be critical for sustaining inflammation in psoriatic plaques. IL-17A stimulates the production of antimicrobial peptides by keratinocytes, which in turn promote recruitment of inflammatory cells. As a consequence of the emerging importance of IL-17A in psoriasis pathogenesis, the relevance of IFNγ is now less clear. Analysis of the cutaneous transcriptome in psoriatic skin lesions has indicated an increased expression of IFNγ-regulated genes and the down-regulation of IFNγ gene is consistently observed with response to patient treatment with etanercept [65]. Kryczek et al. have suggested that one of the main effects of IFNγ is activating antigen-presenting cells early in the psoriatic cascade [66]. In particular IFNγ produced by Th1 and other cells would program myeloid dendritic cell to produce CCL20 ligand of CCR6 and secrete IL-23 thus favouring IL-17 producing cell recruitment and activation. In turn IFNγ would synergize with IL-17-producing cells in inducing human β-defensins production [67]. It is however possible to speculate that IL-17A and IFNγ producing cells may play different roles in the different phases of the pathogenesis with IL-17A playing the most relevant role as the amplifying effector arm that causes clinical manifestation of skin inflammation and IFNγ taking part in the generation of T cell-dendritic cell aggregate that initiates the self-perpetuating cycle.

The major pathological roles of IL-17 in psoriasis are: recruiting neutrophils to the epidermis of psoriatic lesion by increasing neutrophil specific chemokines [68, 69]; employing additional pathogenic Th17 cells by regulating CCL20 release from keratinocytes [69, 70]; stimulating expression of significant antimicrobial peptides of psoriasis like β-defensin, S100A7, S100A8, S100A9, which consecutively act as pro-inflammatory stimulus [67, 69]; it also disrupts the skin barrier by downregulating expression of filaggrin and adhesion molecules in keratinocytes [71] and induces TNF-α release from dendritic cells and macrophages [69].

The synovium of psoriatic arthritis is enriched with IL-17 producing CD4+ effector memory T cells and functionally active IL-17RA, the most well recognized receptor for IL-17 [48]. Several reports suggest that IL-17 can influence bone and cartilage destruction in inflammatory arthritis [72, 73]. In animal arthritis model disease severity is less in IL-17-deficient mice [74]. IL-17 receptor deficiency results in impaired synovial expression of IL-1 and MMP-3, MMP-9, and MMP-13 and prevents cartilage destruction during chronic reactivated streptococcal cell wall-induced arthritis [75]. To understand the role of IL-17 in the joint pathology of PsA, we examined the ability of IL-17 to induce MMP3 and cytokines by FLS obtained from PsA synovium and have observed that FLS in PsA are tuned to a robust response with IL-17. There was a marked upregulation of IL-6, IL-8, and MMP-3 upon exposure to IL-17 in cultured FLS from PsA patients [48].

Simultaneous Erosion and New Bone Formation the Pathognomic Joint Manifestations of Psoriatic Arthritis

In addition to synovial inflammation it is essential to understand the pathogenesis of excess bone resorption and new bone formation the hall mark features of bone changes in PsA. Bone resorption mediated by osteoclasts and new bone formation by osteoblasts is an integrated process in healthy bones. An elevated RANKL/osteoprotegerin ratio favors the differentiation of osteoclasts from monocytes and tips the balance towards bone resorption. Joint and bone tissues obtained from surgical samples of PsA joints have demonstrated abundant osteoclasts at the pannus and bone junction. Also marked expression of RANKL and relatively faint staining of osteoprotegerin have been observed in the inflamed PsA synovium [76]. IL-17 also promotes bone erosion through the up-regulation of RANKL [77, 78] a key regulator of osteoclastneogenesis. Thus, the downstream effects of IL-17 are likely to influence both joint inflammation and joint erosion.

In a passive transfer model of collagen-induced arthritis it has been observed that the development of pronounced axial and peripheral inflammation at the site of tendon and ligament attachment to bone could be ameliorated with IL-23 antibody treatment [79]. Further this group observed that injection of IL-23 minicircle in the B10.RIII mice could induce inflammation at regions adjacent to enthesis, and also induced erosive arthritis along with new bone formation. They identified a unique population of CD3+, IL-23R+, CD4−, CD8− and RORγ T cells in the enthesis. Most importantly, this T cell phenotype did not arise in mice treated with an antibody to IL-23 [79]. The researchers have also substantiated that IL-23 secreted by this unique CD3+, CD4− and CD8− T cell subset was associated with pannus formation and joint erosion, presumably via up-regulation of TNF and IL-17; and that IL-22, presumably also induced by IL-23, was associated with new bone formation [80].

Relevance of the unique CD3+, CD4− and CD8− resident T cell as described above in human joints remains unknown. However our research group reported that activated synovial T cells of PsA patients produces significantly more IL-22 than those of OA patients and PsA patients have higher concentration of IL-22 in their synovial fluid compared to OA patients [9]. Further in this study we have observed that IL-22 is functionally active in PsA joints. Putting together our observations [9, 48] along with the report of Sherlock et al. [79] it appears that in human IL-23 induced IL-17 and IL-22 together can contribute to all three components of joint pathology in PsA that is synovial inflammation, joint erosion and new bone formation.

References

1. Raychaudhuri SP. A cutting edge overview: psoriatic disease. Clin Rev Allergy Immunol. 2013;44(2):109–13.
2. Lowes MA, Bowcock AM, Krueger JG. Pathogenesis and therapy of psoriasis. Nature. 2007;445(7130):866–73.
3. Raychaudhuri SP, Farber EM. The prevalence of psoriasis in the world. J Eur Acad Dermatol Venereol. 2001;15(1):16–7.
4. Griffiths CE, Barker JN. Pathogenesis and clinical features of psoriasis. Lancet. 2007;370(9583):263–71.
5. Liu Y, Krueger JG, Bowcock AM. Psoriasis: genetic associations and immune system changes. Genes Immun. 2007;8(1):1–12.
6. Gottlieb AB, Lebwohl M, Shirin S, Sherr A, Gilleaudeau P, Singer G, et al. Anti-CD4 monoclonal antibody treatment of moderate to severe psoriasis vulgaris: results of a pilot, multicenter, multiple-dose, placebo-controlled study. J Am Acad Dermatol. 2000;43(4):595–604.
7. Wrone-Smith T, Nickoloff BJ. Dermal injection of immunocytes induces psoriasis. J Clin Invest. 1996;98(8):1878–87.
8. Raychaudhuri SP, Kundu-Raychaudhuri S, Tamura K, Masunaga T, Kubo K, Hanaoka K, et al. FR255734, a humanized, Fc-Silent, Anti-CD28 antibody, improves psoriasis in the SCID mouse-psoriasis xenograft model. J Invest Dermatol. 2008;128(8):1969–76.
9. Mitra A, Raychaudhuri SK, Raychaudhuri SP. Functional role of IL-22 in psoriatic arthritis. Arthritis Res Ther. 2012;14(2):R65.
10. Lowes MA, Russell CB, Martin DA, Towne JE, Krueger JG. The IL-23/T17 pathogenic axis in psoriasis is amplified by keratinocyte responses. Trends Immunol. 2013;34(4):174–81.
11. Johnson-Huang LM, Lowes MA, Krueger JG. Putting together the psoriasis puzzle: an update on developing targeted therapies. Dis Model Mech. 2012;5(4):423–33.
12. Raychaudhuri SP, Mitra A, Datta Mitra A, Abria C, Raychaudhuri SK. Th9 Cells in Inflammatory Cascades of Autoimmune Arthritis. Arthritis Rheum. 2014; 66 (11-Suppl):S708 (Abstract 1602).
13. Zaba LC, Fuentes-Duculan J, Eungdamrong NJ, Abello MV, Novitskaya I, Pierson KC, et al. Psoriasis is characterized by accumulation of immunostimulatory and Th1/Th17 cell-polarizing myeloid dendritic cells. J Invest Dermatol. 2009;129(1):79–88.
14. Zaba LC, Fuentes-Duculan J, Eungdamrong NJ, Johnson-Huang LM, Nograles KE, White TR, et al.
15. Lande R, Gregorio J, Facchinetti V, Chatterjee B, Wang YH, Homey B, et al. Plasmacytoid dendritic cells sense self-DNA coupled with antimicrobial peptide. Nature. 2007;449(7162):564–9.
16. Gilliet M, Lande R. Antimicrobial peptides and self-DNA in autoimmune skin inflammation. Curr Opin Immunol. 2008;20(4):401–7.
17. Ganguly D, Chamilos G, Lande R, Gregorio J, Meller S, Facchinetti V, et al. Self-RNA-antimicrobial peptide complexes activate human dendritic cells through TLR7 and TLR8. J Exp Med. 2009;206(9):1983–94.
18. Jongbloed SL, Lebre MC, Fraser AR, Gracie JA, Sturrock RD, Tak PP, et al. Enumeration and phenotypical analysis of distinct dendritic cell subsets in psoriatic arthritis and rheumatoid arthritis. Arthritis Res Ther. 2006;8(1):R15.
19. Austin LM, Coven TR, Bhardwaj N, Steinman R, Krueger JG. Intraepidermal lymphocytes in psoriatic lesions are activated GMP-17(TIA-1)+CD8+CD3+ CTLs as determined by phenotypic analysis. J Cutan Pathol. 1998;25(2):79–88.
20. Costello P, Bresnihan B, O'Farrelly C, FitzGerald O. Predominance of CD8+ T lymphocytes in psoriatic arthritis. J Rheumatol. 1999;26(5):1117–24.
21. Laloux L, Voisin MC, Allain J, Martin N, Kerboull L, Chevalier X, et al. Immunohistological study of entheses in spondyloarthropathies: comparison in rheumatoid arthritis and osteoarthritis. Ann Rheum Dis. 2001;60(4):316–21.
22. Gladman DD, Anhorn KA, Schachter RK, Mervart H. HLA antigens in psoriatic arthritis. J Rheumatol. 1986;13(3):586–92.
23. Sakkas LI, Loqueman N, Bird H, Vaughan RW, Welsh KI, Panayi GS. HLA class II and T cell receptor gene polymorphisms in psoriatic arthritis and psoriasis. J Rheumatol. 1990;17(11):1487–90.
24. Prinz JC, Gross B, Vollmer S, Trommler P, Strobel I, Meurer M, et al. T cell clones from psoriasis skin lesions can promote keratinocyte proliferation in vitro via secreted products. Eur J Immunol. 1994;24(3):593–8.
25. Kim SM, Bhonsle L, Besgen P, Nickel J, Backes A, Held K, et al. Analysis of the paired TCR alpha- and beta-chains of single human T cells. PLoS One. 2012;7(5):e37338.
26. Diluvio L, Vollmer S, Besgen P, Ellwart JW, Chimenti S, Prinz JC. Identical TCR beta-chain rearrangements in streptococcal angina and skin lesions of patients with psoriasis vulgaris. J Immunol. 2006;176(11):7104–11.
27. Valdimarsson H, Thorleifsdottir RH, Sigurdardottir SL, Gudjonsson JE, Johnston A. Psoriasis–as an autoimmune disease caused by molecular mimicry. Trends Immunol. 2009;30(10):494–501.
28. Tassiulas I, Duncan SR, Centola M, Theofilopoulos AN, Boumpas DT. Clonal characteristics of T cell

infiltrates in skin and synovium of patients with psoriatic arthritis. Hum Immunol. 1999;60(6):479–91.

29. Ritchlin C, Haas-Smith SA, Hicks D, Cappuccio J, Osterland CK, Looney RJ. Patterns of cytokine production in psoriatic synovium. J Rheumatol. 1998;25(8):1544–52.

30. Olivieri I, D'Angelo S, Palazzi C, Padula A. Advances in the management of psoriatic arthritis. Nat Rev Rheumatol. 2014;10(9):531–42.

31. Schottelius AJ, Moldawer LL, Dinarello CA, Asadullah K, Sterry W, Edwards 3rd CK. Biology of tumor necrosis factor-alpha- implications for psoriasis. Exp Dermatol. 2004;13(4):193–222.

32. Bonifati C, Carducci M, Cordiali Fei P, Trento E, Sacerdoti G, Fazio M, et al. Correlated increases of tumour necrosis factor-alpha, interleukin-6 and granulocyte monocyte-colony stimulating factor levels in suction blister fluids and sera of psoriatic patients–relationships with disease severity. Clin Exp Dermatol. 1994;19(5):383–7.

33. Ettehadi P, Greaves MW, Wallach D, Aderka D, Camp RD. Elevated tumour necrosis factor-alpha (TNF-alpha) biological activity in psoriatic skin lesions. Clin Exp Immunol. 1994;96(1):146–51.

34. Wakefield PE, James WD, Samlaska CP, Meltzer MS. Tumor necrosis factor. J Am Acad Dermatol. 1991;24(5 Pt 1):675–85.

35. Rajzer L, Wojas-Pelc A. The role of cytokines released by keratinocytes in psoriasis pathogenesis. Przegl Lek. 2009;66(3):150–4.

36. Victor FC, Gottlieb AB, Menter A. Changing paradigms in dermatology: tumor necrosis factor alpha (TNF-alpha) blockade in psoriasis and psoriatic arthritis. Clin Dermatol. 2003;21(5):392–7.

37. Arican O, Aral M, Sasmaz S, Ciragil P. Serum levels of TNF-alpha, IFN-gamma, IL-6, IL-8, IL-12, IL-17, and IL-18 in patients with active psoriasis and correlation with disease severity. Mediators Inflamm. 2005;2005(5):273–9.

38. Kristensen M, Chu CQ, Eedy DJ, Feldmann M, Brennan FM, Breathnach SM. Localization of tumour necrosis factor-alpha (TNF-alpha) and its receptors in normal and psoriatic skin: epidermal cells express the 55-kD but not the 75-kD TNF receptor. Clin Exp Immunol. 1993;94(2):354–62.

39. Chodorowska G. Plasma concentrations of IFN-gamma and TNF-alpha in psoriatic patients before and after local treatment with dithranol ointment. J Eur Acad Dermatol Venereol. 1998;10(2):147–51.

40. Mussi A, Bonifati C, Carducci M, D'Agosto G, Pimpinelli F, D'Urso D, et al. Serum TNF-alpha levels correlate with disease severity and are reduced by effective therapy in plaque-type psoriasis. J Biol Regul Homeost Agents. 1997;11(3):115–8.

41. Pietrzak AT, Zalewska A, Chodorowska G, Krasowska D, Michalak-Stoma A, Nockowski P, et al. Cytokines and anticytokines in psoriasis. Clin Chim Acta. 2008;394(1–2):7–21.

42. Banno T, Gazel A, Blumenberg M. Effects of tumor necrosis factor-alpha (TNF alpha) in epidermal keratinocytes revealed using global transcriptional profiling. J Biol Chem. 2004;279(31):32633–42.

43. Zhuang L, Ma W, Cai D, Zhong H, Sun Q. Associations between tumor necrosis factor-alpha polymorphisms and risk of psoriasis: a meta-analysis. PLoS One. 2013;8(12):e68827.

44. Tohyama M, Hanakawa Y, Shirakata Y, Dai X, Yang L, Hirakawa S, et al. IL-17 and IL-22 mediate IL-20 subfamily cytokine production in cultured keratinocytes via increased IL-22 receptor expression. Eur J Immunol. 2009;39(10):2779–88.

45. Grine L, Dejager L, Libert C, Vandenbroucke RE. An inflammatory triangle in psoriasis: TNF, type I IFNs and IL-17. Cytokine Growth Factor Rev. 2014;26(1): 25–33.

46. Partsch G, Wagner E, Leeb BF, Dunky A, Steiner G, Smolen JS. Upregulation of cytokine receptors sTNF-R55, sTNF-R75, and sIL-2R in psoriatic arthritis synovial fluid. J Rheumatol. 1998;25(1):105–10.

47. Fitzgerald O, Winchester R. Psoriatic arthritis: from pathogenesis to therapy. Arthritis Res Ther. 2009;11(1):214.

48. Raychaudhuri SP, Raychaudhuri SK, Genovese MC. IL-17 receptor and its functional significance in psoriatic arthritis. Mol Cell Biochem. 2012;359(1–2): 419–29.

49. Weitz JE, Ritchlin CT. Mechanistic insights from animal models of psoriasis and psoriatic arthritis. Curr Rheumatol Rep. 2013;15(11):377.

50. Keffer J, Probert L, Cazlaris H, Georgopoulos S, Kaslaris E, Kioussis D, et al. Transgenic mice expressing human tumour necrosis factor: a predictive genetic model of arthritis. EMBO J. 1991;10(13):4025–31.

51. Zaba LC, Cardinale I, Gilleaudeau P, Sullivan-Whalen M, Suarez-Farinas M, Fuentes-Duculan J, et al. Amelioration of epidermal hyperplasia by TNF inhibition is associated with reduced Th17 responses. J Exp Med. 2007;204(13):3183–94.

52. Summers deLuca L, Gommerman JL. Fine-tuning of dendritic cell biology by the TNF superfamily. Nat Rev Immunol. 2012;12(5):339–51.

53. Lowes MA, Suarez-Farinas M, Krueger JG. Immunology of psoriasis. Annu Rev Immunol. 2014;32:227–55.

54. Qu N, Xu M, Mizoguchi I, Furusawa J, Kaneko K, Watanabe K, et al. Pivotal roles of T-helper 17-related cytokines, IL-17, IL-22, and IL-23, in inflammatory diseases. Clin Dev Immunol. 2013;2013:968549.

55. O'Garra A. Cytokines induce the development of functionally heterogeneous T helper cell subsets. Immunity. 1998;8(3):275–83.

56. Lee E, Trepicchio WL, Oestreicher JL, Pittman D, Wang F, Chamian F, et al. Increased expression of interleukin 23 p19 and p40 in lesional skin of patients with psoriasis vulgaris. J Exp Med. 2004;199(1): 125–30.

57. Yao Z, Painter SL, Fanslow WC, Ulrich D, Macduff BM, Spriggs MK, et al. Human IL-17: a novel cytokine derived from T cells. J Immunol. 1995;155(12): 5483–6.

58. Wohn C, Ober-Blobaum JL, Haak S, Pantelyushin S, Cheong C, Zahner SP, et al. Langerin(neg) conventional dendritic cells produce IL-23 to drive psoriatic plaque formation in mice. Proc Natl Acad Sci U S A. 2013;110(26):10723–8.

59. Ma HL, Liang S, Li J, Napierata L, Brown T, Benoit S, et al. IL-22 is required for Th17 cell-mediated pathology in a mouse model of psoriasis-like skin inflammation. J Clin Invest. 2008;118(2):597–607.

60. Kopp T, Kieffer JD, Rot A, Strommer S, Stingl G, Kupper TS. Inflammatory skin disease in K14/p40 transgenic mice: evidence for interleukin-12-like activities of p40. J Invest Dermatol. 2001;117(3):618–26.

61. Yawalkar N, Karlen S, Hunger R, Brand CU, Braathen LR. Expression of interleukin-12 is increased in psoriatic skin. J Invest Dermatol. 1998;111(6):1053–7.

62. Cheng J, Tu Y, Li J, Huang C, Liu Z, Liu D. A study on the expression of interleukin (IL)-10 and IL-12 P35, P40 mRNA in the psoriatic lesions. J Tongji Med Univ. 2001;21(1):86–8.

63. Pantelyushin S, Haak S, Ingold B, Kulig P, Heppner FL, Navarini AA, et al. Rorgammat + innate lymphocytes and gammadelta T cells initiate psoriasiform plaque formation in mice. J Clin Invest. 2012;122(6): 2252–6.

64. Cai Y, Shen X, Ding C, Qi C, Li K, Li X, et al. Pivotal role of dermal IL-17-producing gammadelta T cells in skin inflammation. Immunity. 2011;35(4):596–610.

65. Swindell WR, Xing X, Stuart PE, Chen CS, Aphale A, Nair RP, et al. Heterogeneity of inflammatory and cytokine networks in chronic plaque psoriasis. PLoS One. 2012;7(3):e34594.

66. Kryczek I, Bruce AT, Gudjonsson JE, Johnston A, Aphale A, Vatan L, et al. Induction of IL-17+ T cell trafficking and development by IFN-gamma: mechanism and pathological relevance in psoriasis. J Immunol. 2008;181(7):4733–41.

67. Liang SC, Tan XY, Luxenberg DP, Karim R, Dunussi-Joannopoulos K, Collins M, et al. Interleukin (IL)-22 and IL-17 are coexpressed by Th17 cells and cooperatively enhance expression of antimicrobial peptides. J Exp Med. 2006;203(10):2271–9.

68. Nograles KE, Zaba LC, Guttman-Yassky E, Fuentes-Duculan J, Suarez-Farinas M, Cardinale I, et al. Th17 cytokines interleukin (IL)-17 and IL-22 modulate distinct inflammatory and keratinocyte-response pathways. Br J Dermatol. 2008;159(5):1092–102.

69. Girolomoni G, Mrowietz U, Paul C. Psoriasis: rationale for targeting interleukin-17. Br J Dermatol. 2012;167(4):717–24.

70. Homey B, Dieu-Nosjean MC, Wiesenborn A, Massacrier C, Pin JJ, Oldham E, et al. Up-regulation of macrophage inflammatory protein-3 alpha/CCL20 and CC chemokine receptor 6 in psoriasis. J Immunol. 2000;164(12):6621–32.

71. Gutowska-Owsiak D, Schaupp AL, Salimi M, Selvakumar TA, McPherson T, Taylor S, et al. IL-17 downregulates filaggrin and affects keratinocyte expression of genes associated with cellular adhesion. Exp Dermatol. 2012;21(2):104–10.

72. Chabaud M, Lubberts E, Joosten L, van Den Berg W, Miossec P. IL-17 derived from juxta-articular bone and synovium contributes to joint degradation in rheumatoid arthritis. Arthritis Res. 2001;3(3):168–77.

73. Koshy PJ, Henderson N, Logan C, Life PF, Cawston TE, Rowan AD. Interleukin 17 induces cartilage collagen breakdown: novel synergistic effects in combination with proinflammatory cytokines. Ann Rheum Dis. 2002;61(8):704–13.

74. Nakae S, Nambu A, Sudo K, Iwakura Y. Suppression of immune induction of collagen-induced arthritis in IL-17-deficient mice. J Immunol. 2003;171(11): 6173–7.

75. Koenders MI, Kolls JK, Oppers-Walgreen B, van den Bersselaar L, Joosten LA, Schurr JR, et al. Interleukin-17 receptor deficiency results in impaired synovial expression of interleukin-1 and matrix metalloproteinases 3, 9, and 13 and prevents cartilage destruction during chronic reactivated streptococcal cell wall-induced arthritis. Arthritis Rheum. 2005;52(10):3239–47.

76. Ritchlin CT, Haas-Smith SA, Li P, Hicks DG, Schwarz EM. Mechanisms of TNF-alpha- and RANKL-mediated osteoclastogenesis and bone resorption in psoriatic arthritis. J Clin Invest. 2003;111(6): 821–31.

77. Koenders MI, Lubberts E, Oppers-Walgreen B, van den Bersselaar L, Helsen MM, Di Padova FE, et al. Blocking of interleukin-17 during reactivation of experimental arthritis prevents joint inflammation and bone erosion by decreasing RANKL and interleukin-1. Am J Pathol. 2005;167(1):141–9.

78. Kotake S, Udagawa N, Takahashi N, Matsuzaki K, Itoh K, Ishiyama S, et al. IL-17 in synovial fluids from patients with rheumatoid arthritis is a potent stimulator of osteoclastogenesis. J Clin Invest. 1999;103(9): 1345–52.

79. Sherlock JP, Joyce-Shaikh B, Turner SP, Chao CC, Sathe M, Grein J, et al. IL-23 induces spondyloarthropathy by acting on ROR-gammat + CD3 + CD4-CD8- entheseal resident T cells. Nat Med. 2012;18(7):1069–76.

80. Lories RJ, McInnes IB. Primed for inflammation: enthesis-resident T cells. Nat Med. 2012;18(7): 1018–9.

Genetics of Psoriasis

10

Jason E. Hawkes, Bing-Jian Feng,
and Kristina Callis Duffin

Abstract

Psoriasis has long been considered a genetic disorder. The first observation that psoriasis is an inherited, familial skin disorder was made in 1957. Extensive epidemiologic evidence and monozygotic twin concordance studies confirmed familial clustering of this chronic inflammatory disease and drove scientific investigation into the genetic basis of psoriasis. Since 1957, the list of psoriasis-associated genetic polymorphisms, including some rare causal mutations, has grown tremendously due to advanced high-throughput genotyping platforms and statistical methods. Nevertheless, the majority of psoriasis patients lack known psoriasis-associated susceptibility loci and the exact molecular mechanisms by which polymorphisms contribute to psoriasis remains poorly understood. Recent work points to a complex interplay between genetics, epigenetics, and the inflammatory signaling networks of skin and immune cell mediators. In contrast, other mutations appear to be causative, such as the recently identified mutations in *IL36RN* and *CARD14*, and shed light on new immunologic pathways driving pustular psoriasis. Evidence is also rapidly accumulating for the role of epigenetic changes in psoriasis heritability. The decreasing cost and rapid advancements in genetic technologies in combination with the formation of multi-institutional patient registries will likely result in a better understanding of the "missing heritability" in psoriasis and other complex, multigenic diseases.

Keywords

Psoriasis • Genetics • Psoriasis genetics • Susceptibility loci • Genome-wide association studies (GWAS) • Human leukocyte antigen (HLA) • Major histocompatibility complex (MHC)

J.E. Hawkes, MD • B.-J. Feng, PhD
K.C. Duffin, MD (✉)
Department of Dermatology, University of Utah,
30 N. 1900 E. 4A330 SOM, Salt Lake City,
UT 84132, USA
e-mail: Kristina.callis@hsc.utah.edu

© Springer International Publishing Switzerland 2016
A. Adebajo et al. (eds.), *Psoriatic Arthritis and Psoriasis: Pathology and Clinical Aspects*,
DOI 10.1007/978-3-319-19530-8_10

Genetic Epidemiology of Psoriasis

Psoriasis has long been considered a complex genetic disorder based on early observations of familial clustering and supporting evidence from extensive epidemiologic twin studies. Monozygotic twin concordance has regularly been reported to be approximately three times higher than what is observed in dizygotic twins [1]. Monozygotic twin concordance in psoriasis has been reported to be as high as 90 %, in a study where monozygotic and dizygotic twin pairs were examined [2]. Concordant monozygotic twin pairs also tend to have a more similar age of onset, distribution pattern, severity, and course compared to dizygotic twins [2, 3].

A recent survey study of 10,725 twin pairs aged 20–71 years in the Danish Twin Registry suggest showed a monozygotic to dizygotic ratio of 33 % vs. 17 %, respectively [4]. Genetic factors explained 54 % (30–73 %) of the variation in the susceptibility to psoriasis, whereas 12 % (0–29 %) was attributable to shared environmental factors versus 34 % (27–43 %) to non-shared environmental factors [4]. The heritability was estimated to be 68 %, which is comparable with the 66 % found by Grjibovski et al. [5]. Overall, these observations indicate that a monozygotic twin has an approximately eightfold increased risk of psoriasis relative to the general population if the co-twin is affected, whereas a dizygotic twin has an approximately fourfold increased risk. However, with the exception of a few specific cases, the inheritance pattern of disease remains unclear in the majority of families with a strong predilection for psoriasis. This observation has driven epidemiological and immunogenetic studies designed to better understand the genetic basis of psoriasis.

HLA-Cw6 and PSORS1

Genetic associations with several immune-mediated cutaneous and rheumatologic conditions in the human leukocyte antigen (HLA) region of the Major Histocompatibility Complex I (MHC I) were first reported in the 1970s. Psoriasis was originally associated with *HLA-B13* [6]. However, a report in the Finnish population demonstrated that the association of psoriasis with *HLA-B* was attributed to its close linkage with *HLA-C*, specifically the HLA-Cw6 region [7]. The *HLA-C* locus was then identified by linkage analysis in 1997 and replicated in numerous populations.

The major genetic determinant of psoriasis, *HLA-Cw0602* (*HLA-Cw6*), resides in the MHC I region on chromosome 6p21.3 (*PSORS1*) and is believed to confer most of the susceptibility to psoriasis. Although several genes, including *CCHCR1*, *CDSN,* and *PSORS1C3*, were interesting candidates owing to their expression in skin and proximity to *HLA-C*, extensive fine mapping studies of this segment led by Elder and colleagues concluded that *HLA-Cw6* is the *PSORS1* risk variant that confers susceptibility to psoriasis. The Genetic Association Information Network (GAIN) study, a multicenter collaborative genome-wide association study (GWAS) of psoriasis, revealed that the most highly associated single nucleotide polymorphism was *rs12191877* (p-value of 3×10^{-53}) is in high linkage disequilibrium with *HLA-Cw6* [8]. Further refinement of the *PSORS1* locus by examining patterns of linkage disequilibrium has narrowed the susceptibility interval now to a 179 kb region, excluding all other protein coding genes [9].

An additional aspect of the HLA-C region and its relationship to psoriasis is its interaction with killer immunoglobulin-like receptors (KIRs). *HLA-C* is a primary ligand for killer immunoglobulin-like receptors, which are expressed on natural killer (NK)-like cells. KIRs are classified as either inhibitory or activating, and during embryonic implantation in pregnancy the interaction between inhibitory KIRs and HLA-C ligands promotes immune self-tolerance [10]. It is also believed that the balance of inhibitory and activating KIRs is important to psoriasis and psoriatic arthritis susceptibility. In general, any single individual is believed to inherit between 7 and 12 of the 16 known *KIR* and *pseudoKIR* genes, located on chromosome 19p13.4 [11, 12]. In psoriasis, the presence of activating

KIRs, particularly *KIR2DS1* and *KIR2DS2*, are associated with development of the disease [13]. The lack of inhibitory *KIR*s or their corresponding HLA-C ligand is associated with the development of psoriatic arthritis [14, 15].

Genotype-Phenotype Association with *HLA-Cw6*

HLA-Cw6 is associated with several phenotypic features of psoriasis, including early age of onset, presence of streptococcal pharyngitis, guttate psoriasis, and possibly improvement during pregnancy. In an Icelandic population, homozygosity for *HLA-Cw6* is associated with a threefold increase risk of psoriasis, a younger age of onset (15 vs. 17.8 years), and higher likelihood of a positive family history (98 % vs. 86 %) [16]. Despite the additive impact, this study reported that homozygosity is not believed to influence the phenotype or the severity (e.g., body surface area) of the disease. However, a 2014 review of 109 Swedish children ages 0–15 revealed a high prevalence of *HLA-Cw6* positivity (65 %), but a stronger association in pubertal children who also had a higher rate of facial lesions and guttate phenotype [17].

The high prevalence of *HLA-Cw6* in patients with guttate psoriasis and streptococcal infection is perhaps one of the most compelling arguments for the gene-environment trigger of this disease. In one series of 134 British patients with guttate psoriasis, 83 % carried at least one *HLA-Cw6* allele, compared to 15 % of controls [18]. Another series of 29 patients with guttate psoriasis, history of sore throat and/or elevated antistreptolysis O (ASO) titer revealed 100 % carried the *HLA-Cw6* allele [19]. Furthermore, even when both guttate and chronic plaque phenotypes are considered, Mallbris et al. showed that the prevalence of positive streptococcal throat swabs in *HLA-Cw*0602* positive patients was twice the prevalence among *HLA-Cw*0602* negative patients [20]. However, carriers of the *HLA-Cw6* allele and/or presence of streptococcal infection are not necessarily a pre-requisite for guttate psoriasis. A study of 105 Irish patients revealed that 11 % of patients with guttate psoriasis had neither risk factor [21].

There are psoriatic phenotypes that are not associated with *HLA-Cw6*. In contrast to early age of onset, later age of onset is not associated with *HLA-Cw6*. The same group who investigated guttate psoriasis also showed that only 20 % of British patients with palmoplantar psoriasis were carriers of *HLA-Cw6* [18]. Additionally, *HLA-Cw1* and *HLA-B* alleles, rather than *HLA-Cw6*, were associated with generalized pustular psoriasis (GPP) in a Japanese cohort [22].

Other Susceptibility Loci within the MHC

The MHC region has a high density of genes that have a role in immunity and inflammation. Thus, it is hypothesized that there are multiple susceptibility genes for psoriasis within this region. Candidate gene association studies have found that the *octamer transcription factor-3* (*OTF3*, also named *POU5F1*) B allele was more prevalent in patients than in controls, even within the *HLA-Cw6*-negative subset of samples [23]. Moreover, less than 25 kb from this gene, two single nucleotide polymorphisms (SNPs) in the *SEEK1* (*PSORS1C1*) gene retained association with psoriasis upon stratification for *HLA-Cw6* positive/negative status [24]. However, the MHC region is characterized by an extended linkage disequilibrium pattern, thus candidate genes studies are very uninformative with regard to pinpointing the location of a causal gene. Later, the development of SNP genotyping arrays made it possible to fine map a susceptibility locus by covering the whole MHC region with a high density of polymorphisms. By stepwise regression, re-analyses of GWAS data identified several additional association signals that were independent of *HLA-Cw6* [25, 26]. However, the SNP added to the model in each step was only a proxy of the causal gene. To further elucidate the underlying causal allele, a recent large-scale stepwise analysis found that the *HLA-Cw6*-independent risk variants include *HLA-C*1203*,

HLA-B amino acid positions 67 and 9, *HLA-A* amino acid position 95, and *HLA-DQA1* amino acid position 53 [27].

PSORS2-9

Although the association with *HLA-Cw6* is strong, only 50–60 % of patients with psoriasis carry the *HLA-Cw6* allele. This compelled researchers to look outside of the MHC region. Early linkage studies using microsatellite markers identified *PSORS2*, which mapped to distal end of chromosome 17q [28, 29], and were confirmed by Nair et al. in 1997 [30]. Using linkage analysis, eight other non-MHC loci (*PSORS2-9*) were initially identified. Yet, despite a joint effort of International Psoriasis Genetics Consortium, no strong gene candidates were identified until GWAS and whole genome/exome sequencing were employed [31].

Subsequent GWAS have been conducted with increasingly large sample sizes, resulting in the identification of 35 susceptibility loci outside the MHC [8, 32, 33]. Besides confirming or finding new loci related to the TNF, IL-23, and IL-17 signaling pathways (*IL12B, STAT2/IL23A, IL23R, TRAF3IP2, IRF4, RUNX3, TNFRSF9, ETS1, SOCS1, STAT3/STAT5A/STAT5B*), a large proportion of newly discovered loci are involved in the innate immune response (*DDX58, KLF4, ZC3H12C, CARD14, CARM1, IL28RA, LCE3D, NOS2, FBXL19, NFKBIA, RNF114, REL, IFIH1, TNIP1, TNFAIP3, IRF4,* and *ELMO1*). Other loci include *ERAP1, PTTG1, IL13, CSMD1, GJB2, SERPINB8, ZNF816A, B3GNT2, TAGAP, ZMIZ1, RPS6KA4/PRDX5, UBE2L3/YDJC,* and *MBD2/POL1/STARD6*. Notably, some of these loci overlap with previous linkage signals, which include *CARD14* (*PSORS2*) and *LCE3D* (*PSORS4*). Moreover, the associated SNP at the *LCE3D* locus is in linkage disequilibrium with a copy number variation (CNV) found to be associated with psoriasis in a previous candidate gene study [34]. Significant gene-gene interactions were also found between the associated loci, including *HLA-C* with *ERAP1* and *HLA-C* with *LCE3D* [33].

IL12B/IL23R/IL23A

With the availability of the HapMap and high-throughput genotyping, identification of numerous novel genetic variants was made possible with GWAS. The first GWAS studies in large cohorts of psoriasis patients of Northern European decent identified novel variants at *IL12B, IL23R,* and *IL23A* [8, 32, 35]. At the time of this discovery, IL-23 had been identified as a key cytokine in the psoriasis pathogenesis, as it promotes the differentiation and expansion of Th17 cells. Three variants have been identified near the following genes, which encode subunits of the IL-23 ligand-receptor complex: *IL12B* (p40 subunit of IL-12 and IL-23), *IL23A* (p19 subunit of IL-23), and *IL23R* (IL23 specific subunit of the IL-23 receptor). This led to speculation that there may be a genetic basis to aberrant IL-23 signaling, lending susceptibility to an inappropriate immune response. Interestingly, the *IL23R* variant that increases psoriasis risk is also associated with Crohn's disease, and neutralization of IL-23 via ustekinumab has clinical efficacy in both diseases.

IL4, IL5, IL13, and RAD50

Variants near the *IL13* and *IL4* genes were first identified by Cargill and confirmed in subsequent larger GWAS studies [8, 32]. The most statistically significant signals for these variants lie closest to *IL4* and *IL13*, and near the *RAD50* gene, a locus that regulates transcription of *IL4, IL5,* and *IL13*. The *IL4, IL5,* and *IL13* genes encode cytokines involved in Th2 immunity, which is central to allergic, asthmatic, and extracellular pathogen responses. IL-4 and IL-13 inhibit the development of naïve (Th0) cells to Th17, but have been shown to paradoxically increase IL-12 production in dendritic cells isolated from mice exposed to Leishmania [36]. It is, therefore, plausible that these genetic variants influence the balance of several cytokines in the Th1, Th2, and Th17 pathways leading to increased psoriasis susceptibility.

TNFAIP3 and TNIP1

Variants near the TNFAIP3 and TNIP1 genes were initially identified by Nair et al. [8] The proteins encoded by these genes (A20 and ABIN1, respectively) are key regulators of NF-kB and TNF-α signaling. Therefore, it is most likely that these variants influence psoriasis susceptibility via dysregulation of the inflammatory response.

One problem of GWAS is that the most significantly associated SNP in each locus (i.e. the index variant) is not typically the causal variant that functionally confers disease susceptibility. Therefore, when an index variant is between genes, it is difficult to determine which gene is causing the disease. This has been seen for the loci *STAT2/IL23A*, *RPS6KA4/PRDX5*, *UBE2L3/YDJC*, *STAT3/STAT5A/STAT5B*, and *MBD2/POL1/STARD6*. Efforts to identify the causal variants within protein-coding regions are lim-

ited and inconclusive [33, 37]. Given that most of the SNPs are common variants with a modest effect on the risk of the disease, it is reasonable to hypothesize that the causal variants are likely non-coding and may alter the expression of causal genes. Fortunately, large-scale targeted sequencing and high-density SNP genotyping array is more affordable. The affordability and increasing availability of new technologies will likely help unravel this issue in the coming years.

"Missing Heritability" of Psoriasis

While linkage analyses and GWAS have successfully identified a number of psoriasis susceptibility loci, about 50 % of the total heritability remains unexplained. *HLA-Cw6* constitutes the largest portion of the explained heritability of psoriasis (Fig. 10.1) as evidenced by its high

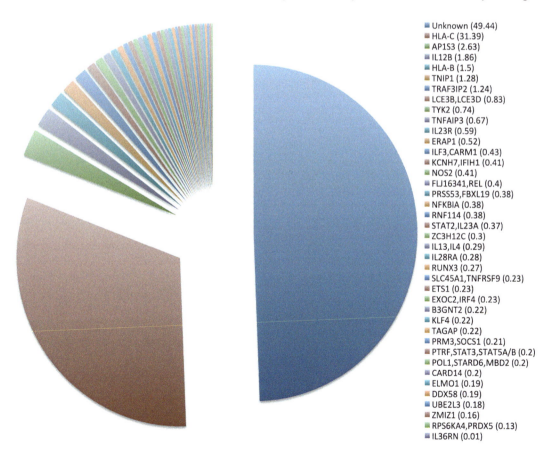

- Unknown (49.44)
- HLA-C (31.39)
- AP1S3 (2.63)
- IL12B (1.86)
- HLA-B (1.5)
- TNIP1 (1.28)
- TRAF3IP2 (1.24)
- LCE3B,LCE3D (0.83)
- TYK2 (0.74)
- TNFAIP3 (0.67)
- IL23R (0.59)
- ERAP1 (0.52)
- ILF3,CARM1 (0.43)
- KCNH7,IFIH1 (0.41)
- NOS2 (0.41)
- FLJ16341,REL (0.4)
- PRSS53,FBXL19 (0.38)
- NFKBIA (0.38)
- RNF114 (0.38)
- STAT2,IL23A (0.37)
- ZC3H12C (0.3)
- IL13,IL4 (0.29)
- IL28RA (0.28)
- RUNX3 (0.27)
- SLC45A1,TNFRSF9 (0.23)
- ETS1 (0.23)
- EXOC2,IRF4 (0.23)
- B3GNT2 (0.22)
- KLF4 (0.22)
- TAGAP (0.22)
- PRM3,SOCS1 (0.21)
- PTRF,STAT3,STAT5A/B (0.2)
- POL1,STARD6,MBD2 (0.2)
- CARD14 (0.2)
- ELMO1 (0.19)
- DDX58 (0.19)
- UBE2L3 (0.18)
- ZMIZ1 (0.16)
- RPS6KA4,PRDX5 (0.13)
- IL36RN (0.01)

Fig. 10.1 List of psoriasis-associated susceptibility loci and their relative contribution (percentage) to psoriasis heritability

odds ratio (4.32) and allele frequency (0.09). Aside from *HLA-Cw6*, other loci that contribute a relatively large proportion of inherited susceptibility include *IL12B*, *HLA-B/MICA*, *TNIP1*, and *TRAF3IP3*. The "missing heritability" may be explained by the common variants conferring a very small risk, rare to low-frequency variants with an intermediate effect, structural variants, allelic or gene-gene interactions, epigenetic inheritance, and/or underestimation of the risk conferred by the GWAS hits.

Pustular Psoriasis Phenotypes and *IL-36RN*

The variants of pustular psoriasis include generalized pustular psoriasis (GPP), pediatric-onset generalized pustular psoriasis (PGPP), adult-onset generalized pustular psoriasis (AGPP), palmoplantar pustulosis (PPP), and acrodermatitis continua of Hallopeau (ACH). These variants have historically been included within the broad spectrum of psoriasis due to its co-occurrence with psoriasis vulgaris, shared histologic features, and common immune cell mediators and inflammatory cytokines. Landry and Muller suggested a heritable basis for this condition when they provided a description of GPP in two Caucasian siblings [38]. However, genetic studies have failed to show consistent MHC or HLA associations between the pustular variants of psoriasis and psoriasis vulgaris [18].

Blumberg et al. [39] published a report suggesting the possible role of the IL-1 family in the pathogenesis of GPP. The IL-1 family is comprised of 11 cytokine proteins, including IL-1-receptor antagonist (IL-1Ra), IL-36α, IL-36β, IL-36γ, and IL-36Ra [40]. IL-1Ra and IL-36Ra are encoded by the *IL-1RN* and *IL-36RN* genes, respectively, and are antagonists of the IL-36α, IL-36β, and IL-36γ cytokines [39]. Blumberg et al. provided the first *in vivo* evidence in transgenic mice for the possible role of *IL-36A*, *IL-36RN*, and other IL-1 family genes in the immunopathogenesis of GPP [39].

Shortly thereafter, Aksentijevich et al. published a report of nine patients with multifocal osteomyelitis, periostitis, failure to thrive, and pustulosis due to a deficiency of *IL-1RN* (now known as deficiency of the interleukin-1 receptor antagonist, or DIRA) [41]. Loss-of-function mutations in *IL-1RN* result in the loss of the IL-1Ra protein and, thus, uninhibited proinflammatory cytokine signaling from IL-1α, and IL-1β, and IL-1γ [41]. Similarly, Marrakchi et al. studied 9 Tunisian families with GPP and found that affected individuals had homozygous germ-line mutations in *IL-36RN* (now known as deficiency of interleukin-36 receptor antagonist, or DITRA) [40, 42]. The *IL-36RN* mutations are analogous to the *IL-1RN* loss-of-function mutations but without the associated skeletal anomalies [43]. Importantly, there are several reports of patients with DIRA and DITRA rapidly responding to treatment with Anakinra, a recombinant human IL-1Ra [41, 44–46].

To date, there are 14 reported *IL-36RN* mutations associated with GPP [47]. While pedigree analyses reveal an inheritance pattern that is primarily autosomal recessive, the genotype-phenotype relationship between *IL-36RN* mutations and pustular psoriasis phenotypes is not entirely understood. The association between pathogenic *IL-36RN* mutations and symptom onset is highly variable and age dependent, suggesting that *IL-36RN* mutations in the absence of specific environmental triggers are not sufficient to cause disease. Additionally, while the majority of GPP patients with no prior history of psoriasis vulgaris harbor *IL-36RN* mutations, these recessive mutations are rarely found in psoriasis vulgaris alone or GPP with a prior history of psoriasis vulgaris [48–50].

CARD14

Caspase recruitment domain family, member 14 (*CARD14*), is another keratinocyte-related protein demonstrated to confer susceptibility to GPP in the European and Japanese populations [50]. *CARD14* encodes a protein that activates NF-κB and inhibits apoptosis. Rare gain-of-function mutations in this gene result in enhanced NF-κB signaling and up-regulation of inflammatory cytokines predisposing affected individuals to GPP, as well as psoriasis vulagris, psoriatic arthritis, and pityriasis rubra pilaris [51–53]. In studied pedigrees, *CARD14* mutations segregated in an autosomal dominant pattern and were highly penetrant [53]. In contrast to *IL-36RN* mutations, gain-of-function mutations in *CARD14* appear to be more strongly associated with GPP patients with a prior history of psoriasis vulgaris as opposed to psoriasis vulgaris alone or GPP without a prior history of psoriasis vulgaris [54].

From GWAS and Epidemiologic Genetic Studies to Molecular and Epigenetic Studies

Evidence is rapidly accumulating for the role of epigenetic changes in the pathogenesis of psoriasis and other chronic inflammatory conditions. In order to improve our understanding of the interaction between psoriasis-related genes and the environment, it is crucial that ongoing studies also evaluate novel mechanisms of epigenetic regulation of gene expression. Epigenetics refers to the study of heritable changes to an individual's genetic material without altering the actual DNA sequence, and includes gene methylation, histone modification, microRNAs (miRNAs), and small interfering RNAs (siRNAs). As one of the most abundant class of regulators in the human genome, miRNAs play an essential role in the post-transcriptional modification of mRNA and are key mediators of the immune system [55]. miRNAs and other non-coding RNAs represent more than 70 % of the human genome and could harbor heritable changes that may contribute to psoriasis susceptibility [56, 57].

One interesting report demonstrates the interplay between miR-148a and cell surface expression of HLA-C [58]. miR-148a binding to the 3'UTR of HLA-C mRNA directly affects cell surface expression of HLA-C and influenced HIV control and Crohn's disease susceptibility [58]. These findings provide a mechanism whereby miRNAs interact with psoriasis susceptibility loci to ultimately impact disease phenotype. In this way, polymorphisms in specific miRNAs and/or their interaction with susceptibility genes may provide insights into the issue of "missing heritability" in psoriasis and other complex, multigenic diseases. The use of *in vivo* animal models of psoriasis will also greatly facilitate our study of the molecular mechanisms and epigenetic alterations contributing to the immunopathogenesis of psoriasis.

Future Directions

GWAS and epidemiologic genetic studies have been fundamental to the identification of psoriasis-associated susceptibility loci. Identifying the major molecular pathways and cell types perturbed by these genetic variants has offered important insights into the pathogenesis of psoriasis. Nevertheless, significant research gaps exist and many individuals with psoriasis do not have any identifiable genetic mutations. Additionally, having a known psoriasis-associated gene variant does not guarantee that the affected individual will go on to develop the disease. These observations highlight the need for continued research intended to better understand the correlation between psoriasis-associated gene variants, phenotype, and environmental triggers. The decreasing cost and rapid advancements in gene sequencing technologies in combination with the formation of multi-institutional patient and tissue registries should make future phenotype-genotype studies more feasible.

References

1. Gudjonsson JE, Elder JT. Psoriasis: epidemiology. Clin Dermatol. 2007;25:535–46.
2. Brandrup F, Holm N, Grunnet N, et al. Psoriasis in monozygotic twins: variations in expression in individuals with identical genetic constitution. Acta Derm Venereol. 1982;62:229–36.
3. Farber EM, Nall ML, Watson W. Natural history of psoriasis in 61 twin pairs. Arch Dermatol. 1974;109: 207–11.
4. Lonnberg AS, Skov L, Skytthe A, et al. Heritability of psoriasis in a large twin sample. Br J Dermatol. 2013;169:412–6.

5. Grjibovski AM, Olsen AO, Magnus P, et al. Psoriasis in Norwegian twins: contribution of genetic and environmental effects. J Eur Acad Dermatol Venereol. 2007;21:1337–43.

6. Russell TJ, Schultes LM, Kuban DJ. Histocompatibility (HL-A) antigens associated with psoriasis. N Engl J Med. 1972;287:738–40.

7. Tiilikainen A, Lassus A, Karvonen J, et al. Psoriasis and HLA-Cw6. Br J Dermatol. 1980;102:179–84.

8. Nair RP, Duffin KC, Helms C, et al. Genome-wide scan reveals association of psoriasis with IL-23 and NF-kappaB pathways. Nat Genet. 2009;41:199–204.

9. Clop A, Bertoni A, Spain SL, et al. An in-depth characterization of the major psoriasis susceptibility locus identifies candidate susceptibility alleles within an HLA-C enhancer element. PLoS One. 2013;8:e71690.

10. Varla-Leftherioti M. The significance of the women's repertoire of natural killer cell receptors in the maintenance of pregnancy. Chem Immunol Allergy. 2005;89:84–95.

11. Uhrberg M, Valiante NM, Shum BP, et al. Human diversity in killer cell inhibitory receptor genes. Immunity. 1997;7:753–63.

12. Hubbard T, Barker D, Birney E, et al. The Ensembl genome database project. Nucleic Acids Res. 2002;30:38–41.

13. Luszczek W, Manczak M, Cislo M, et al. Gene for the activating natural killer cell receptor, KIR2DS1, is associated with susceptibility to psoriasis vulgaris. Hum Immunol. 2004;65:758–66.

14. Martin MP, Gao X, Lee JH, et al. Epistatic interaction between KIR3DS1 and HLA-B delays the progression to AIDS. Nat Genet. 2002;31:429–34.

15. Nelson GW, Martin MP, Gladman D, et al. Cutting edge: heterozygote advantage in autoimmune disease: hierarchy of protection/susceptibility conferred by HLA and killer Ig-like receptor combinations in psoriatic arthritis. J Immunol. 2004;173:4273–6.

16. Gudjonsson JE, Karason A, Antonsdottir A, et al. Psoriasis patients who are homozygous for the HLA-Cw*0602 allele have a 2.5-fold increased risk of developing psoriasis compared with Cw6 heterozygotes. Br J Dermatol. 2003;148:233–5.

17. Lysell J, Tessma M, Nikamo P, et al. Clinical Characterisation at Onset of Childhood Psoriasis – A Cross Sectional Study in Sweden. Acta Derm Venereol. 2015;95:457–61.

18. Asumalahti K, Ameen M, Suomela S, et al. Genetic analysis of PSORS1 distinguishes guttate psoriasis and palmoplantar pustulosis. J Invest Dermatol. 2003;120:627–32.

19. Mallon E, Bunce M, Savoie H, et al. HLA-C and guttate psoriasis. Br J Dermatol. 2000;143:1177–82.

20. Mallbris L, Wolk K, Sanchez F, et al. HLA-Cw*0602 associates with a twofold higher prevalence of positive streptococcal throat swab at the onset of psoriasis: a case control study. BMC Dermatol. 2009;9:5.

21. Fry L, Powles AV, Corcoran S, et al. HLA Cw*06 is not essential for streptococcal-induced psoriasis. Br J Dermatol. 2006;154:850–3.

22. Ozawa A, Miyahara M, Sugai J, et al. HLA class I and II alleles and susceptibility to generalized pustular psoriasis: significant associations with HLA-Cw1 and HLA-DQB1*0303. J Dermatol. 1998;25:573–81.

23. Gonzalez S, Martinez-Borra J, Del Rio JS, et al. The OTF3 gene polymorphism confers susceptibility to psoriasis independent of the association of HLA-Cw*0602. J Invest Dermatol. 2000;115:824–8.

24. Holm SJ, Carlen LM, Mallbris L, et al. Polymorphisms in the SEEK1 and SPR1 genes on 6p21.3 associate with psoriasis in the Swedish population. Exp Dermatol. 2003;12:435–44.

25. Feng BJ, Sun LD, Soltani-Arabshahi R, et al. Multiple Loci within the major histocompatibility complex confer risk of psoriasis. PLoS Genet. 2009;5: e1000606.

26. Knight J, Spain SL, Capon F, et al. Conditional analysis identifies three novel major histocompatibility complex loci associated with psoriasis. Hum Mol Genet. 2012;21:5185–92.

27. Okada Y, Han B, Tsoi LC, et al. Fine mapping major histocompatibility complex associations in psoriasis and its clinical subtypes. Am J Hum Genet. 2014;95:162–72.

28. Matthews D, Fry L, Powles A, et al. Evidence that a locus for familial psoriasis maps to chromosome 4q. Nat Genet. 1996;14:231–3.

29. Tomfohrde J, Silverman A, Barnes R, et al. Gene for familial psoriasis susceptibility mapped to the distal end of human chromosome 17q. Science. 1994;264: 1141–5.

30. Nair RP, Henseler T, Jenisch S, et al. Evidence for two psoriasis susceptibility loci (HLA and 17q) and two novel candidate regions (16q and 20p) by genome-wide scan. Hum Mol Genet. 1997;6:1349–56.

31. International Psoriasis Genetics Consortium. The International Psoriasis Genetics Study: assessing linkage to 14 candidate susceptibility loci in a cohort of 942 affected sib pairs. Am J Hum Genet. 2003;73: 430–7.

32. Cargill M, Schrodi SJ, Chang M, et al. A large-scale genetic association study confirms IL12B and leads to the identification of IL23R as psoriasis-risk genes. Am J Hum Genet. 2007;80:273–90.

33. Tsoi LC, Spain SL, Knight J, et al. Identification of 15 new psoriasis susceptibility loci highlights the role of innate immunity. Nat Genet. 2012;44:1341–8.

34. Xu L, Li Y, Zhang X, et al. Deletion of LCE3C and LCE3B genes is associated with psoriasis in a northern Chinese population. Br J Dermatol. 2011;165: 882–7.

35. Capon F, Di Meglio P, Szaub J, et al. Sequence variants in the genes for the interleukin-23 receptor (IL23R) and its ligand (IL12B) confer protection against psoriasis. Hum Genet. 2007;122:201–6.

36. Hurdayal R, Nieuwenhuizen NE, Revaz-Breton M, et al. Deletion of IL-4 receptor alpha on dendritic cells renders BALB/c mice hypersusceptible to Leishmania major infection. PLoS Pathog. 2013;9:e1003699.

37. Das S, Stuart PE, Ding J, et al. Fine mapping of eight psoriasis susceptibility loci. Eur J Hum Genet. 2015;23:844–53.

38. Landry M, Muller SA. Generalized pustular psoriasis. Observations on the course of the disease in a familial occurrence. Arch Dermatol. 1972;105:711–6.

39. Blumberg H, Dinh H, Trueblood ES, et al. Opposing activities of two novel members of the IL-1 ligand family regulate skin inflammation. J Exp Med. 2007;204:2603–14.

40. Marrakchi S, Guigue P, Renshaw BR, et al. Interleukin-36-receptor antagonist deficiency and generalized pustular psoriasis. N Engl J Med. 2011;365:620–8.

41. Aksentijevich I, Masters SL, Ferguson PJ, et al. An autoinflammatory disease with deficiency of the interleukin-1-receptor antagonist. N Engl J Med. 2009;360:2426–37.

42. Cowen EW, Goldbach-Mansky R. DIRA, DITRA, and new insights into pathways of skin inflammation: what's in a name? Arch Dermatol. 2012;148:381–4.

43. Carapito R, Isidor B, Guerouaz N, et al. Homozygous IL36RN mutation and NSD1 duplication in a patient with severe pustular psoriasis and symptoms unrelated to deficiency of interleukin-36 receptor antagonist. Br J Dermatol. 2015;172:302–5.

44. Brau-Javier CN, Gonzales-Chavez J, Toro JR. Chronic cutaneous pustulosis due to a 175-kb deletion on chromosome 2q13: excellent response to anakinra. Arch Dermatol. 2012;148:301–4.

45. Huffmeier U, Watzold M, Mohr J, et al. Successful therapy with anakinra in a patient with generalized pustular psoriasis carrying IL36RN mutations. Br J Dermatol. 2014;170:202–4.

46. Rossi-Semerano L, Piram M, Chiaverini C, et al. First clinical description of an infant with interleukin-36-receptor antagonist deficiency successfully treated with anakinra. Pediatrics. 2013;132:e1043–7.

47. Li X, Chen M, Fu X, et al. Mutation analysis of the IL36RN gene in Chinese patients with generalized pustular psoriasis with/without psoriasis vulgaris. J Dermatol Sci. 2014;76:132–8.

48. Berki DM, Mahil SK, Burden AD, et al. Loss of IL36RN function does not confer susceptibility to psoriasis vulgaris. J Invest Dermatol. 2014;134:271–3.

49. Li M, Han J, Lu Z, et al. Prevalent and rare mutations in IL-36RN gene in Chinese patients with generalized pustular psoriasis and psoriasis vulgaris. J Invest Dermatol. 2013;133:2637–9.

50. Sugiura K, Muto M, Akiyama M. CARD14 c.526G > C (p.Asp176His) is a significant risk factor for generalized pustular psoriasis with psoriasis vulgaris in the Japanese cohort. J Invest Dermatol. 2014;134:1755–7.

51. Fuchs-Telem D, Sarig O, van Steensel MA, et al. Familial pityriasis rubra pilaris is caused by mutations in CARD14. Am J Hum Genet. 2012;91:163–70.

52. Jordan CT, Cao L, Roberson ED, et al. Rare and common variants in CARD14, encoding an epidermal regulator of NF-kappaB, in psoriasis. Am J Hum Genet. 2012;90:796–808.

53. Jordan CT, Cao L, Roberson ED, et al. PSORS2 is due to mutations in CARD14. Am J Hum Genet. 2012;90:784–95.

54. Sugiura K. The genetic background of generalized pustular psoriasis: IL36RN mutations and CARD14 gain-of-function variants. J Dermatol Sci. 2014;74:187–92.

55. O'Connell RM, Rao DS, Baltimore D. microRNA regulation of inflammatory responses. Annu Rev Immunol. 2012;30:295–312.

56. Esteller M. Non-coding RNAs in human disease. Nat Rev Genet. 2011;12:861–74.

57. Pivarcsi A, Stahle M, Sonkoly E. Genetic polymorphisms altering microRNA activity in psoriasis – a key to solve the puzzle of missing heritability? Exp Dermatol. 2014;23:620–4.

58. Kulkarni S, Qi Y, O'HUigin C, et al. Genetic interplay between HLA-C and MIR148A in HIV control and Crohn disease. Proc Natl Acad Sci U S A. 2013;110:20705–10.

Update on the Genetics of Psoriatic Arthritis

Darren D. O'Rielly, Lihi Eder, and Proton Rahman

Abstract

Psoriatic arthritis (PsA) is a common disease arising from a complex interplay between genetic, environmental and immune related factors. PsA exhibits one of the largest known recurrence risks among first degree relatives in a complex rheumatic disease. While there is substantive evidence supporting a strong genetic component of PsA, it has been difficult to elucidate genes specific to PsA pathogenesis. Investigating the genetic etiology of PsA is inherently challenging given the existence of gene-gene interactions, gene-environment interactions as well as a potential contribution of copy number variants (CNVs) and epigenetic factors. This chapter will provide an overview of the genetics basis of PsA focusing on candidate gene studies, genome-wide linkage and association-based studies, in addition to highlighting the genetics related to PsA pharmacotherapy (i.e., pharmacogenetics).

Keywords

Genetics • Human Leukocyte Antigen (HLA) • Major Histocompatibility Region (MHC) • Candidate gene studies • Genome Wide Association Scans (GWAS) • Pharmacogenetics • Copy Number Variants • Gene-Gene Interactions • Gene-environment interactions

D.D. O'Rielly, PhD, FCCMG
Faculty of Medicine, Memorial University,
St. John's, NL, Canada

L. Eder, MD, PhD
Department of Medicine,
Centre for Prognosis Studies in the Rheumatic Diseases,
Toronto Western Hospital,
Toronto, ON, Canada

P. Rahman, MD, MSc (✉)
Department of Medicine, Memorial University,
St. John's, NL, Canada
e-mail: prahman@mun.ca

Introduction

Psoriatic arthritis (PsA) is a common disease arising from a complex interplay between genetic, environmental and immune related factors. While there is substantive evidence supporting a strong genetic component of PsA, it has been difficult to elucidate genes specific to PsA pathogenesis. This difficulty is likely attributed

© Springer International Publishing Switzerland 2016
A. Adebajo et al. (eds.), *Psoriatic Arthritis and Psoriasis: Pathology and Clinical Aspects*,
DOI 10.1007/978-3-319-19530-8_11

to the modest sample size of PsA cohorts being investigated, small effect sizes of the individual genes, and complexities inherent to multifactorial disease such as gene-gene interactions, gene-environment interactions as well as a potential contribution of copy number variants (CNVs) and epigenetic factors. This chapter will provide an overview of the genetics basis of PsA and will highlight recent developments in this field.

Population-based familial aggregation studies suggest that the heritability of PsA is greater than for psoriasis vulgaris (PsV). In fact, with the exception of ankylosing spondylitis (AS), PsA exhibits one of the largest known recurrence risks among first degree relatives in a complex rheumatic disease with a recurrence risk between 30 and 48 [1, 2]. However, in the absence of large PsA twin studies, heritability estimates in PsA cannot be validated using alternate methodologies.

Candidate Gene Studies: HLA Region

Similar to psoriasis, GWAS studies suggest that the Major Histocompatibility Complex (MHC) region contributes the greatest risk of developing PsA, which is estimated to be about one third of the entire genetic contribution. The MHC region is located on the short arm of chromosome 6 and contains numerous genes that are relevant to immune system function. Within this region, the multi-allele HLA class I genes bear the strongest association with psoriasis and PsA. In general, *HLA-C* alleles are more strongly associated with psoriasis while *HLA-B* alleles are associated with PsA. *HLA-C*0602* allele is the strongest and most consistently reported genetic susceptibility marker for psoriasis [3–5]. The presence of this allele is associated with sub-phenotypes of psoriasis including early-onset disease, severe psoriasis and guttate psoriasis [6, 7]. In addition, gene-gene interactions between endoplasmic reticulum aminopeptidase 1 (*ERAP1*) gene and *HLA-C*0602* plays a role in the susceptibility of psoriasis [8]. Although the *HLA-C*0602* allele is also associated with PsA [9–13], this link is more complex. While the prevalence of *HLA-C*0602* is higher in

PsA patients compared to the general population, this association is stronger with psoriasis itself than with PsA [14, 15]. The frequency of *HLA-C*0602* allele is significantly lower in patients with PsA compared to those with psoriasis alone and while this allele is associated with an early onset of psoriasis, its presence is also associated with a longer psoriasis-arthritis interval and with a milder form of arthritis [13, 14, 16]. *HLA-C*0602* is also inversely associated with psoriatic nail lesions, a clinical marker for PsA, in patients with psoriasis [7]. Collectively, these findings suggest a higher penetration of *HLA-C*0602* for the skin disease compared to the joint manifestations.

In contrast, *HLA-B*27*, one of the features of spondyloarthritis, is consistently associated with PsA but not with psoriasis, and consequently, it can be considered as an independent genetic marker for PsA [13, 15, 17]. The presence of this allele is also associated with a more severe sub-phenotype of PsA, including axial involvement, earlier onset of arthritis and progression of joint damage [18–21]. However, in contrast to the high prevalence of this allele in ankylosing spondylitis, its prevalence in PsA is only approximately 20 %. Therefore, its use in clinical practice for classification of PsA may be limited. Several recent studies that compared patients with PsA to those with psoriasis alone identified additional independent HLA markers for PsA. The frequency of *HLA-B*38, HLA-B*08* and *B*39* was higher in patients with PsA, suggesting that these alleles can be regarded as specific genetic markers of PsA in psoriasis patients [13, 15]. These findings are consistent with a recent fine mapping of the MHC region that found that the presence of glutamine in position 45 of the *HLA-B* antigen confers the strongest risk for PsA. This polymorphism was stronger than any of the classic HLA antigens including *HLA-B*27*. This polymorphic site is located in the binding groove of HLA-B and can influence the binding of a peptide to the HLA molecule. Interestingly, *HLA-B*27, B*39* and *B*38*, that have been identified as "PsA-specific" HLA alleles encode proteins that contain Glu at position 45 [22]. Overall, these data highlight the importance of antigen processing and presentation in the pathogenesis of PsA.

Candidate Gene Studies: Non-HLA Region

Numerous small studies have reported non-*HLA* genes within the MHC region to be associated with psoriasis [(e.g., OTF3, SPR1, SEEK1 and corneodesmosin (CDSN))] as previously reviewed [23]. However, replication studies have been inconsistent and it appears that these genes are in strong LD with known *HLA-B* and *HLA-C* alleles. Likewise, similar issues exist for PsA studies within this region.

Because of their potential biological significance, the two most studied non-*HLA* genes within this region are *TNFα* and *MICA*. The marked clinical response of *TNFα* inhibition in PsA has further reinforced numerous molecular and immunological studies that suggest this pro-inflammatory cytokine, plays a critical role in the pathogenesis of PsA. A recent meta-analysis by Zhu et al. [24] provides the most comprehensive evidence to date for SNP association within the promoter gene of *TNFα* and PsA. Overall, 26 studies involving 2159 PsV and 2360 PsA patients were included in that meta-analysis. Among eight pooled studies which included one Asian cohort that had assessed *TNFα* -238A/G, a significant association was noted between the variant genotypes of *TNFα* -238A/G (AA + AG vs GG) and PsA (OR = 2.242, 95 % CI, 1.710–2.941). The alleles were also correlated with PsA susceptibility to *TNFα* -238A/G (A vs G). There was also a significant association between genotypes of *TNFα* -857 T/C (TT + TC vs CC) and PsA (OR = 1.419, 95 % CI, 1.214–1.658) and for the alleles of *TNFα* -857 T/C (T vs C). Meanwhile *TNFα* -308A/G the variant genotype (AA + AG vs GG) and the allele (A vs G) was not associated with susceptibility to PsA. Also, no association was noted between *TNFα* -1031C/T and -863A/C polymorphism and PsA.

Given the proximity of the *MICA* gene to the *HLA-B* locus and its potential function as an activator of natural killer cells, several association studies in independent cohorts have been performed. In a Spanish cohort, the trinucleotide repeat polymorphism, *MICA-A9,* that corresponds to *MICA*002* was reported to be associated with PsA independent of *HLA Cw6*, *MICB* or *TNF* [25]. However, further studies from the Toronto PsA clinic [26] and a large multinational fine mapping of the MHC region in PsA by Okada et al. [22] failed to validate this association.

Multiple *IL-23R* and *IL-12B* variants have been consistently reported in psoriasis GWAS studies. These cytokines have clear links to the pathogenesis of PsA. Meta-analysis of 13 studies has revealed the minor alleles of rs11209026 to be significantly associated with PsA (OR = 0.630, 95 % CI 0.524–0.757) [27]. Likewise, minor allele of rs7530511 was also associated with PsA (OR = 0.875, 95 % CI 0.766–1.000) [27]. A separate meta-analysis by the same group for *IL-12B* SNPs has been published based on 11 studies [28]. For the *IL-12B*, the odds ratio for rs3212227 and rs6887695 in PsA was 0.707 (95 % CI 0.628–0.797) and 0.677 (95 % CI 0.599–0.767), respectively [28].

Another group of proteins that interact with class I HLA antigens are the killer-cell immunoglobulin-like receptors (KIR). KIRs are encoded by a highly polygenic and polymorphic locus on chromosome 19q13.4 and located on NK cells [29]. The interaction between KIRs and HLA-class I molecules affects NK cell activity. Several *KIR* genes were found to be associated with PsA. The frequency of *KIR2DS2* is elevated in PsA compared with healthy controls. Moreover, the risk of PsA is higher when *KIR2DS2* is present with the HLA-C ligands (C group 1) for the corresponding inhibitory KIRs, and is highest when *KIR2DS2* is present in the absence of HLA-C ligands for homologous inhibitor KIRs, compared with the state when *KIR2DS2* is absent. The association with PsA remained when comparing PsA to patients with psoriasis without arthritis and hence the association between *KIR2DS2* and PsA may likely be specific to arthritis [30].

Case–control association studies suggest that signal-transducer and activator of transcription protein 3 (*STAT3*) and *RUNX3* gene are associated with PsA [31, 32]. These genes have potential functional consequences in PsA as *STAT3* encodes a transducer and transcription factor for cell growth, apoptosis and immune response, while RUNX3 is a transcription factor that promotes the differentiation of T cells to CD8+ cells. In a cohort of 335 PsA patients and 1844 ethnically matched controls, the G allele of SNP rs744166 was significantly associated with PsA (p = 1.36×10^{-3}, OR = 1.35) [31]. In a larger German study, an association with *RUNX3* variant (SNP rs4649038) was noted with an odds ratio of 1.24 (95 % CI 1.15–1.33) [32].

Genome-Wide Association Studies in PsA

Genome-wide association-based studies are comprised of genome-wide linkage studies and genome-wide SNP association studies (GWAS). Linkage studies were the first methods used for the identification of susceptibility determinants across the entire genome in many diseases including PsA. The initial advantage of linkage studies was the ability to identify novel genes. In 2003, the first and only genome-wide linkage study in PsA was completed in Iceland. A suggestive linkage was noted on chromosome 16q and a significant logarithm of odds (LOD) score was achieved when the linkage analysis was conditioned on paternal transmission [33].

Although genome-wide linkage studies have the potential to identify novel genes in psoriatic diseases, such studies have traditionally been underpowered due to sparse marker coverage, relatively small sample sizes, and very few loci identified by linkage studies have been independently replicated. Consequently, a shift occurred in 2007 with the advent of SNP-based GWAS, which compared SNP allele frequencies between cases and controls; circumventing the limitations of family-based linage analysis. In fact, GWAS have revolutionized the identification of genomic regions associated with psoriatic diseases by identifying more candidate genes compared with linkage-based studies or candidate gene association studies.

Compared with psoriasis, a disease closely related to PsA, relatively small GWAS have been completed in PsA cohorts (Table 11.1) [34]. Non-HLA genes identified by GWAS in PsA include *IL-12B, IL-23R, TRAF3IP2, FBXL19, TNIP1,* and *REL* (Table 11.2) [35–39]. *TYK2* has also reached a genome-wide level of significance in GWAS; a finding not yet published (Elder JT, personnel communication, 2014). Genetic variants reaching a genome-wide level of significance identified by psoriasis GWAS that were also associated with PsA but failed to reach GWAS level of significance include *IL-23A, STAT3, IL-2/IL-21, TNFAIP3, NFkBIA,* and *NOS2* (Table 11.2) [35–39]. The relative lack of genome-wide significant genes in PsA compared with PsV can be attributed to a relatively small number of GWAS in PsA and the greater clinical heterogeneity of PsA. The candidate genes identified in PsA have highlighted pathways of critical importance to disease pathogenesis including distinct signaling pathways comprising NFkB signaling, the IL-23/IL-17 axis, and Th-17 signaling.

Activation of the innate immune response represents the initial physiological trigger, which sets in motion an inflammatory cascade initiating PsA pathogenesis. Interferons (IFNs) and TNFα trigger the innate immune response in PsA via the immediate-early response transcription factor, nuclear factor kappa-light-chain-enhancer of activated B cells (NFkB), which represents one of the most important transcriptional regulators of the

Table 11.1 Cohort size and markers genotyped via genome-wide association studies (GWAS) in psoriatic arthritis (PsA)

Group	Year	Markers	Ethnic ancestry	No. of patients
Liu et al.	2008	311,398	European	91
Nair et al.	2009	438,670	European	438
Huffmeier et al.	2010	1,585,307	European	609
Ellinghaus et al.	2010	2,339,118	European	1922
Ellinghaus et al.[a]	2012	1,160,703	European	535
Total				**3595**

[a]Indicates a meta-analysis

Table 11.2 Genetic associations identified in psoriatic arthritis (PsA) reaching or approaching a genome-wide level of significance

Gene/locus	Chromosome	Ethnic ancestry	Signaling pathway affected
IL-23R	1p31.3	European	Th-17 signaling
REL	2p13-p12	European	NFkB activation and signaling
IL-2/IL-21	4q27	European	Th-17 signaling
IL-12β	5q31.1-q33.1	European	Th-17 signaling
TNIP1	5q32-q33.1	European	NFkB activation and signaling
TRAF3IP2	6q21	European	Th-17 signaling
TNFAIP3	6q23	European	NFkB activation and signaling
IL-23A	12q13.3	European	Th-17 signaling
NFkBIA	14q13	European	NFkB activation and signaling
FBXL19	16p11.2	European	NFkB activation and signaling
NOS2	17q11.2-q12	European	NFkB activation and signaling
STAT3	17q21.31	European	Th-17 signaling
TYK2	19p13.2	European	NFkB activation and signaling

Bold represents genetic loci that reached a genome-wide level of significance (5×10^{-8}).

Gene/locus	Chr.	Ethnic ancestry	PsV	PsA	Signaling pathways affected
Th-17 cell differentiation					
IL-12β	5q31.1-q33.1	European	X	X	IL-23 pathway
IL-23A	12q13.3	European	X	X	IL-23 pathway
IL-23R	1p31.3	European	X	X	IL-23 pathway
TYK2	19p13.2	European	X		IL-23 pathway
STAT3	17q21.31	European	X	X	IL-23 pathway
Th-17 effector signaling					
IL-2/IL-21	4q27	European	X	X	IL-21 pathway
Crosstalk with innate immune response (TNF-α & NFkB)					
TNF-α	6p21.3	European	X	X	TNF-induced NFkB-dependent gene expression
TNIP1	5q32-q33.1	European	X	X	TNF-induced NFkB-dependent gene expression
REL	2p13-p12	European	X	X	Essential part of NFkB complex
FBXL19	16p11.2	European	X	X	Inhibits NFkB signaling

Bold represents genetic loci that reached a genome-wide level of significance

innate immune response. Several genetic loci involved in NFkB signaling have reached genome-wide significance (i.e., *TNIP1, FBXL19, REL*, and *TYK2*) or approaching genome-wide significance (i.e., *NFkBIA, NOS2*) in PsA [35–39]. *TNFAIP3* encodes the TNF-induced protein 3 (TNFAIP3) and its ubiquitination in response to NFkB activation prevents subsequent NFκB activation [40].

The product of *TNIP1* interacts with TNFAIP3 to inhibit TNF-induced NFkB-dependent gene expression [41]. The product of *FBXL19* reversibly inhibits NFkB signaling, and the expression of *FBXL19* is significantly elevated in psoriatic compared with normal skin [37]. *REL* genes encode a subunit of the NFkB complex that is essential for proper signaling and the product of *NFkBIA* interferes with nuclear localization signals by inhibiting the activity of dimeric NFkB-REL complexes [42]. *NOS2* encodes an inducible form of nitric oxide synthase which is a known effector of the innate immune system, and whose transcription be induced by NFkB [43]. Whereas, *TYK2* encodes a tyrosine kinase involved in the initiation of IFN-a signaling and NFkB activation [44]. Collectively, the genetic loci revealed by GWAS strongly support a role of NFkB in the pathogenesis of PsA. That the NFkB activation induces expression of the receptor activator of nuclear factor κB (RANK), which is required for the receptor activator of nuclear factor κB ligand (RANKL) to activate osteoclasts, emphasizes the critical role of NFkB signaling in PsA pathogenesis. Moreover, activated osteoclasts which are up-regulated in psoriatic synovial tissues causes bone resorption leading to bone erosion; a feature common in PsA patients [45].

That the IL-23/IL-17 axis play a prominent role in adaptive immunity and forms a complex interplay with TNFα and NFkB [46], suggests that disruption of which by genetic variation can contribute to PsA pathogenesis. Several genetic loci involved in Th-17 signaling have reached genome-wide significance (i.e., *IL-12B*, *IL-23R*, *TYK2*, and *TRAF3IP2*) or approaching genome-wide significance (i.e., *IL-23A*, *STAT3*, and *IL-2/IL-21*) in PsA [35–39]. IL-23 is a heterodimeric cytokine (composed of a p19 subunit and a p40 subunit), which binds IL-23R and IL-12Rβ1; the latter being shared with IL-12 [47, 48]. IL-23 promotes the expansion and survival of Th-17 cells through its receptor and signaling pathway [49], can induce the production of several pro-inflammatory cytokines (e.g., IL-17, TNFα, IL-21, and IL-22) [50, 51], and the binding of IL-23 to its receptor triggers NFkB activation via the degradation of IkB kinase [52]. *TRAF3IP2*

encodes TRAF3 interacting protein 2 or NFkB activator 1 (Act1), which is essential for Th-17 cell-mediated inflammatory responses, and its dysregulation may affect both IL-17 and NFkB signaling cascades [53]. Act1 is also a cytoplasmic adaptor protein that activates NFkB [54]. Indeed, a study of the *TRAF3IP2* variant associated with PsA revealed near complete loss of ability of the protein to activate NFkB signaling [36]. The binding of IL-17 to its receptor also triggers Act1 or the CCAAT-enhancer-binding protein (C/EBP) cascade [53, 55] secondary to Act1 associating with inducible IkB kinase, IKKi [56]. Therefore, both IL-23/IL-17 axis influences the activation of the NFkB pathway in multiple ways and in a synergistic manner [57].

TYK2 encodes Tyk2, which binds directly to IL-12Rβ1 and is essential for IL-23-mediated signaling and Th-17 cell differentiation. *STAT3*, which encodes for STAT3, is also required for the differentiation of Th-17 cells [41]. Specifically, STAT3 is known to induce RAR-related orphan receptor gamma (RORg) and RORa, both of which are encoded by RORC (the master regulator of Th-17 differentiation) to establish Th-17 cell differentiation [48, 58, 59]. IL-21 is a potent immunomodulatory cytokine which plays a key role in Th-17 effector signaling, leading to increased IL-17 production and IL-23R expression [60–62]. A GWAS reported four variants (all in strong LD) within the IL-2/IL-21 region that were associated with PsA [35].

Pharmacogenetics and PsA

Systemic therapies to treat moderate-to-severe PsA include DMARDs, used alone or in combination, or biologic agents, primarily TNFα inhibitors. Given that disease severity varies from patient to patient, treatment requires personalization where the choice of treatment depends on the extent of disease, relative effectiveness of the therapy, and existing comorbidities [63]. Patient preferences for mode and frequency of treatment administration, potential adverse events, and cost are all important factors, as patient compliance is one of the greatest barriers to effective treatment.

In this section, we focus on traditional DMARDs and biologic agents, as these systemic drugs are associated with frequent and often severe adverse events.

Although methotrexate is an inexpensive oral systemic agent that is often highly effective in controlling moderate-to-severe PsA [64], its use is discontinued in approximately 30 % of patients, primarily attributed to hepatotoxicity [65]. Currently, the dose required for clinical efficacy and the ability to accurately identify which patients will develop adverse events is not possible. Only a single study has investigated the pharmacogenetics of methotrexate for PsA patients. Data from 281 patients from the University of Toronto PsA Clinic revealed an association of the A allele of DHFR at +35,289 with response to methotrexate whereas homozygosity for the minor allele of MTHFR 677C>T (genotype 677TT) was associated with increased liver toxicity [66]. Although these results require confirmation in larger prospective cohorts, they do suggest that potential candidate polymorphisms might substantially influence response to methotrexate in patients with PsA.

Biologic agents are increasingly used to treat moderate-to-severe PsA in patients refractory to traditional therapy. TNFα inhibitors represent a major advancement in the symptomatic relief of inflammatory conditions. However, adequate response to treatment is still variable with 20–40 % of patients experiencing an inadequate response. It has been proposed that genetic factors contribute substantially to clinical responses to TNF inhibitors. In a study involving 57 Caucasian PsA patients and 155 healthy matched controls, the TNFα +489A allele showed a trend of association with the response to PsA treatment with etanercept, although there is as yet no evidence for a causal relationship [67]. In a pooled study of AS and PsA patients, PsA patients with the *TNFα* -308 GG genotype respond better to TNFα inhibitors than those with the AA or AG genotypes [68]. The *TNFRSF10A* CC genotype (rs20575) was associated with EULAR response to infliximab at 6 months, whereas the *TNFR1A* AA genotype (rs767455) in was associated with a better EULAR response at 3 months in PsA

patients [69]. This is consistent with evidence that *TNFRSF10A* is expressed in PsA patients, where it can induce cell-cycle arrest of proinflammatory cells and apoptosis in arthritic synovium [70, 71]. In a study of 103 patients with PsA, more patients with high-affinity *FCGR2A* (p.H131R) genotypes (homozygous wild-type or heterozygous combinations) achieved a EULAR response at 6 months compared with patients with the low-affinity genotype (homozygous mutant) [72]. While these results require confirmation in larger prospective cohorts, they do suggest that variants affecting genes involved in general immunity and the TNFα signaling pathway might functionality affect the response to TNFα inhibitors.

Conclusion

Understanding the genetic risk factors for PsA could lead to the development of more effective screening strategies and therapy. Although GWAS have highlighted genes that contribute to the PsA pathogenesis, replication in larger cohorts, fine mapping, resequencing, and functional studies are warranted to better understand susceptibility to and progression of the disease. General agreement has been reached that searching solely for common variants by GWAS will identify only a fraction of the entire genetic burden of disease. Consequently, searching for highly penetrant but rare disease alleles in families with PsA, using next-generation sequencing (e.g., *IL-36RN* and *CARD14* in psoriasis) and through epigenetic investigations, along with structural variations such as CNVs (e.g., *DEFB4* copy number in psoriasis) should also be carefully evaluated. Once genes are identified, investigation of gene-gene (e.g., *ERAP1* and *HLA-B27* in ankylosing spondyloarthritis) and gene-environment (e.g., smoking in psoriasis and PsA) interactions should be performed.

No clinically actionable information can be gleaned by a single variants because of the very low odds ratio for the individual variants identified from GWAS in PsA; a finding consistent with the lack of predictive power in such studies.

Consequently, a global genotype relative risk score that includes clinical, biochemical and genetic markers should be developed for disease susceptibility, expression, and prognosis in PsA.

References

1. Moll JM, Wright V. Familial occurrence of psoriatic arthritis. Ann Rheum Dis. 1973;32:181–201.
2. Chandran V, Schentag CT, Brockbank JE, Pellett FJ, Shanmugarajah S, Toloza SM, et al. Familial aggregation of psoriatic arthritis. Ann Rheum Dis. 2009;68: 664–7.
3. Henseler T, Christophers E. Psoriasis of early and late onset: characterization of two types of psoriasis vulgaris. J Am Acad Dermatol. 1985;13:450–6.
4. Russell TJ, Schultes LM, Kuban DJ. Histocompatibility (HL-A) antigens associated with psoriasis. N Engl J Med. 1972;287:738–40.
5. Feng BJ, Sun LD, Soltani-Arabshahi R, Bowcock AM, Nair RP, Stuart P, et al. Multiple Loci within the major histocompatibility complex confer risk of psoriasis. PLoS Genet. 2009;5:e1000606.
6. Enerback C, Martinsson T, Inerot A, Wahlstrom J, Enlund F, Yhr M, et al. Evidence that HLA-Cw6 determines early onset of psoriasis, obtained using sequence-specific primers (PCR-SSP). Acta Derm Venereol. 1997;77:273–6.
7. Gudjonsson JE, Karason A, Runarsdottir EH, Antonsdottir AA, Hauksson VB, Jónsson HH, et al. Distinct clinical differences between HLA-Cw*0602 positive and negative psoriasis patients – an analysis of 1019 HLA-C- and HLA-B-typed patients. J Invest Dermatol. 2006;126:740–5.
8. Genetic Analysis of Psoriasis Consortium & the Wellcome Trust Case Control Consortium 2, Strange A, Capon F, Spencer CC, Knight J, Weale ME, Allen MH, et al. A genome-wide association study identifies new psoriasis susceptibility loci and an interaction between HLA-C and ERAP1. Nat Genet. 2010;42: 985–90.
9. Espinoza LR, Vasey FB, Gaylord SW, Dietz C, Bergen L, Bridgeford P, et al. Histocompatibility typing in the seronegative spondyloarthropathies: a survey. Semin Arthritis Rheum. 1982;11:375–81.
10. Lopez-Larrea C, Torre Alonso JC, Rodriguez Perez A, Coto E. HLA antigens in psoriatic arthritis subtypes of a Spanish population. Ann Rheum Dis. 1990;49:318–9.
11. McHugh NJ, Laurent MR, Treadwell BL, Tweed JM, Dagger J. Psoriatic arthritis: clinical subgroups and histocompatibility antigens. Ann Rheum Dis. 1987;46:184–8.
12. Chandran V, Bull SB, Pellett FJ, Ayearst R, Rahman P, Gladman DD. Human leukocyte antigen alleles and susceptibility to psoriatic arthritis. Hum Immunol. 2013;74:1333–8.
13. Winchester R, Minevich G, Steshenko V, Kirby B, Kane D, Greenberg DA, et al. HLA associations reveal genetic heterogeneity in psoriatic arthritis and in the psoriasis phenotype. Arthritis Rheum. 2012;64:1134–44.
14. Ho PY, Barton A, Worthington J, Plant D, Griffiths CE, Young HS, et al. Investigating the role of the HLA-Cw*06 and HLA-DRB1 genes in susceptibility to psoriatic arthritis: comparison with psoriasis and undifferentiated inflammatory arthritis. Ann Rheum Dis. 2008;67:677–82.
15. Eder L, Chandran V, Pellet F, Shanmugarajah S, Rosen CF, Bull SB, et al. Human leucocyte antigen risk alleles for psoriatic arthritis among patients with psoriasis. Ann Rheum Dis. 2012;71:50–5.
16. Queiro R, Gonzalez S, Lopez-Larrea C, Alperi M, Sarasqueta C, Riestra JL, et al. HLA-C locus alleles may modulate the clinical expression of psoriatic arthritis. Arthritis Res Ther. 2006;8:R185.
17. Eder L, Chandran V, Pellett F, Shanmugarajah S, Rosen CF, Bull SB, et al. Differential human leucocyte allele association between psoriasis and psoriatic arthritis: a family-based association study. Ann Rheum Dis. 2012;71:1361–5.
18. Chandran V, Tolusso DC, Cook RJ, Gladman DD. Risk factors for axial inflammatory arthritis in patients with psoriatic arthritis. J Rheumatol. 2010;37:809–15.
19. Queiro R, Torre JC, Gonzalez S, Lopez-Larrea C, Tinture T, Lopez-Lagunas I. HLA antigens may influence the age of onset of psoriasis and psoriatic arthritis. J Rheumatol. 2003;30:505–7.
20. Gladman DD, Farewell VT. The role of HLA antigens as indicators of disease progression in psoriatic arthritis. Multivariate relative risk model. Arthritis Rheum. 1995;38:845–50.
21. Haroon M, Winchester R, Giles JT, Heffernan E, FitzGerald O. Certain class I HLA alleles and haplotypes implicated in susceptibility play a role in determining specific features of the psoriatic arthritis phenotype. Ann Rheum Dis. 2014. pii: annrheumdis-2014-205461. doi: 10.1136/annrheumdis-2014-205461. [Epub ahead of print]
22. Okada Y, Han B, Tsoi LC, Stuart PE, Ellinghaus E, Tejasvi T, et al. Fine mapping major histocompatibility complex associations in psoriasis and its clinical subtypes. Am J Hum Genet. 2014;95:162–72.
23. Chandran V, Rahman P. Update on the genetics of spondyloarthritis – ankylosing spondylitis and psoriatic arthritis. Best Pract Res Clin Rheumatol. 2010;24:579–88.
24. Zhu J, Qu H, Chen X, Wang H, Li J. Single nucleotide polymorphisms in the tumor necrosis factor-alpha gene promoter region alter the risk of psoriasis vulgaris and psoriatic arthritis: a meta-analysis. PLoS One. 2013;8:e64376.
25. Gonzalez S, Martinez-Borra J, Torre-Alonso JC, Gonzalez-Roces S, Sanchez del Río J, Rodriguez Pérez A, et al. The MICA-A9 triplet repeat polymorphism in the transmembrane region confers additional susceptibility to the development of psoriatic arthritis and is independent of the association of Cw*0602 in psoriasis. Arthritis Rheum. 1999;42:1010–6.

26. Eder L, Chandran V, Gladman DD. What have we learned about genetic susceptibility in psoriasis and psoriatic arthritis? Curr Opin Rheumatol. 2015;27:91–8.

27. Zhu KJ, Zhu CY, Shi G, Fan YM. Association of IL23R polymorphisms with psoriasis and psoriatic arthritis: a meta-analysis. Inflamm Res. 2012;61: 1149–54.

28. Zhu KJ, Zhu CY, Shi G, Fan YM. Meta-analysis of IL12B polymorphisms (rs3212227, rs6887695) with psoriasis and psoriatic arthritis. Rheumatol Int. 2013;33:1785–90.

29. Lanier LL. NK cell recognition. Annu Rev Immunol. 2005;23:225–74.

30. Chandran V, Bull SB, Pellett FJ, et al. Killer-cell immunoglobulin-like receptor gene polymorphisms and susceptibility to psoriatic arthritis. Rheumatology. 2014;53:233–9.

31. Cénit MC, Ortego-Centeno N, Raya E, Callejas JL, García-Hernandez FJ, Castillo-Palma MJ, et al. Influence of the STAT3 genetic variants in the susceptibility to psoriatic arthritis and Behcet's disease. Hum Immunol. 2013;74:230–3.

32. Apel M, Uebe S, Bowes J, Giardina E, Korendowych E, Juneblad K, et al. Variants in RUNX3 contribute to susceptibility to psoriatic arthritis, exhibiting further common ground with ankylosing spondylitis. Arthritis Rheum. 2013;65:1224–31.

33. Karason A, Gudjonsson JE, Upmanyu R, Antonsdottir AA, Hauksson VB, Runasdottir EH, et al. A susceptibility gene for psoriatic arthritis maps to chromosome 16q: evidence for imprinting. Am J Hum Genet. 2003;72:125–31.

34. Bowes J, Orozco G, Flynn E, Ho P, Brier R, Marzo-Ortega H, et al. Confirmation of TNIP1 and IL23A as susceptibility loci for psoriatic arthritis. Ann Rheum Dis. 2011;70:1641–4.

35. Liu Y, Helms C, Liao W, Zaba LC, Duan S, Gardner J, et al. A genome-wide association study of psoriasis and psoriatic arthritis identifies new disease loci. PLoS Genet. 2008;4:e1000041.

36. Hüffmeier U, Uebe S, Ekici AB, Bowes J, Giardina E, Korendowych E, et al. Common variants at TRAF3IP2 are associated with susceptibility to psoriatic arthritis and psoriasis. Nat Genet. 2010;42:996–9.

37. Stuart PE, Nair RP, Ellinghaus E, Ding J, Tejasvi T, Gudjonsson JE, et al. Genome-wide association analysis identifies three psoriasis susceptibility loci. Nat Genet. 2010;42:1000–4.

38. Ellinghaus E, Ellinghaus D, Stuart PE, Nair RP, Debrus S, Raelson JV, et al. Genome-wide association study identifies a psoriasis susceptibility locus at TRAF3IP2. Nat Genet. 2010;42:991–5.

39. Ellinghaus E, Stuart PE, Ellinghaus D, Nair RP, Debrus S, Raelson JV, et al. Genome-wide meta-analysis of psoriatic arthritis identifies susceptibility locus at REL. J Invest Dermatol. 2012;132:1133–40.

40. Vereecke L, Beyaert R, van Loo G. The ubiquitin-editing enzyme A20 (TNFAIP3) is a central regulator of immunopathology. Trends Immunol. 2009;30: 383–91.

41. Verstrepen L, Carpentier I, Verhelst K, Beyaert R. ABINs: A20 binding inhibitors of NF-kappa B and apoptosis signaling. Biochem Pharmacol. 2009;78: 105–14.

42. De Molfetta GA, Lucíola Zanette D, Alexandre Panepucci R, Dos Santos AR, da Silva Jr WA, Antonio Zago M. Role of NFKB2 on the early myeloid differentiation of CD34+ hematopoietic stem/progenitor cells. Differentiation. 2010;80:195–203.

43. Lowenstein CJ, Padalko E. iNOS (NOS2) at a glance. J Cell Sci. 2004;117:2865–7.

44. Strobl B, Stoiber D, Sexl V, Mueller M. Tyrosine kinase 2 (TYK2) in cytokine signaling and host immunity. Front Biosci. 2011;16:3214–32.

45. Ritchlin CT, Haas-Smith SA, Li P, Hicks DG, Schwarz EM. Mechanisms of TNFalpha- and RANKL-mediated osteoclastogenesis and bone resorption in psoriatic arthritis. J Clin Invest. 2003;111:821–31.

46. Miossec P. IL-17 and Th17 cells in human inflammatory diseases. Microbes Infect. 2009;11:625–30.

47. Oppmann B, Lesley R, Blom B, Timans JC, Xu Y, Hunte B, et al. Novel p19 protein engages IL-12p40 to form a cytokine, IL-23, with biological activities similar as well as distinct from IL-12. Immunity. 2000;13:715–25.

48. Parham C, Chirica M, Timans J, Vaisberg E, Travis M, Cheung J, et al. A receptor for the heterodimeric cytokine IL-23 is composed of IL-12Rbeta1 and a novel cytokine receptor subunit, IL-23R. J Immunol. 2002;168:5699–708.

49. Langrish CL, Chen Y, Blumenschein WM, Mattson J, Basham B, Sedgwick JD, et al. IL-23 drives a pathogenic T cell population that induces autoimmune inflammation. J Exp Med. 2005;201:233–40.

50. Pappu R, Ramirez-Carrozzi V, Sambandam A. The interleukin-17 cytokine family: critical players in host defence and inflammatory diseases. Immunology. 2011;134:8–16.

51. McGeachy MJ, Cua DJ. The link between IL-23 and Th17 cell-mediated immune pathologies. Semin Immunol. 2007;19:372–6.

52. Cheung PF, Wong CK, Lam CW. Molecular mechanisms of cytokine and chemokine release from eosinophils activated by IL-17A, IL-17F, and IL-23: implication for Th17 lymphocytes-mediated allergic inflammation. J Immunol. 2008;180:5625–35.

53. Sønder SU, Saret S, Tang W, Sturdevant DE, Porcella SF, Siebenlist U. IL-17-induced NF-kappaB activation via CIKS/Act1: physiologic significance and signaling mechanisms. J Biol Chem. 2011;286: 12881–90.

54. Li X, Commane M, Nie H, Hua X, Chatterjee-Kishore M, Wald D, et al. Act1, an NF-kappa B-activating protein. Proc Natl Acad Sci U S A. 2000;97:10489–93.

55. Fujioka S, Niu J, Schmidt C, Sclabas GM, Peng B, Uwagawa T, et al. NF-kappaB and AP-1 connection: mechanism of NF-kappaB-dependent regulation of AP-1 activity. Mol Cell Biol. 2004;24:7806–19.

56. Bulek K, Liu C, Swaidani S, Wang L, Page RC, Gulen MF, et al. The inducible kinase IKKi is required for

IL-17-dependent signaling associated with neutrophilia and pulmonary inflammation. Nat Immunol. 2011;12:844–52.

57. Chiricozzi A, Guttman-Yassky E, Suarez-Farinas M, Nograles KE, Tian S, Cardinale I, et al. Integrative responses to IL-17 and TNF-a in human keratinocytes account for key inflammatory pathogenic circuits in psoriasis. J Invest Dermatol. 2011;131:677–87.

58. Ivanov II, McKenzie BS, Zhou L, Tadokoro CE, Lepelley A, Lafaille JJ, et al. The orphan nuclear receptor RORgammat directs the differentiation program of proinflammatory IL-17+ T helper cells. Cell. 2006;126:1121–33.

59. Yang XO, Pappu BP, Nurieva R, Akimzhanov A, Kang HS, Chung Y, et al. T helper 17 lineage differentiation is programmed by orphan nuclear receptors ROR alpha and ROR gamma. Immunity. 2008;28:29–39.

60. Hoeve MA, Savage ND, de Boer T, Langenberg DM, de Waal Malefyt R, Ottenhoff TH, et al. Divergent effects of IL-12 and IL-23 on the production of IL-17 by human T cells. Eur J Immunol. 2006;36:661–70.

61. Korn T, Bettelli E, Gao W, Awasthi A, Jäger A, Strom TB, et al. IL-21 initiates an alternative pathway to induce proinflammatory T(H)17 cells. Nature. 2007;448:484–7.

62. Nurieva R, Yang XO, Martinez G, Zhang Y, Panopoulos AD, Ma L, et al. Essential autocrine regulation by IL-21 in the generation of inflammatory T cells. Nature. 2007;448:480–3.

63. Chen H, Poon A, Yeung C, Helms C, Pons J, Bowcock AM, et al. A genetic risk score combining ten psoriasis risk loci improves disease prediction. PLoS One. 2011;6:e19454.

64. Cronstein BN. Low-dose methotrexate: a mainstay in the treatment of rheumatoid arthritis. Pharmacol Rev. 2005;57:163–72.

65. Zachariae H, Sogaard H. Liver biopsy in psoriasis. A controlled study. Dermatologica. 1973;146:149–55.

66. Chandran V, Siannis F, Rahman P, Pellett FJ, Farewell VT, Gladman DD. Folate pathway enzyme gene polymorphisms and the efficacy and toxicity of methotrexate in psoriatic arthritis. J Rheumatol. 2010;37:1508–12.

67. Murdaca G, Gulli R, Spanò F, Lantieri F, Burlando M, Parodi A, et al. TNF-α gene polymorphisms: association with disease susceptibility and response to anti-TNF-α treatment in psoriatic arthritis. J Invest Dermatol. 2014;134:2503–9.

68. Seitz M, Wirthmüller U, Möller B, Villiger PM. The −308 tumour necrosis factor-alpha gene polymorphism predicts therapeutic response to TNFalpha-blockers in rheumatoid arthritis and spondyloarthritis patients. Rheumatology (Oxford). 2007;46:93–6.

69. Morales-Lara MJ, Cañete JD, Torres-Moreno D, Hernández MV, Pedrero F, Celis R, et al. Effects of polymorphisms in TRAILR1 and TNFR1A on the response to anti-TNF therapies in patients with rheumatoid and psoriatic arthritis. Joint Bone Spine. 2012;79:591–6.

70. Pundt N, Peters MA, Wunrau C, Strietholt S, Fehrmann C, Neugebauer K, et al. Susceptibility of rheumatoid arthritis synovial fibroblasts to FasL- and TRAIL-induced apoptosis is cell cycle-dependent. Arthritis Res Ther. 2009;11:R16.

71. Hofbauer LC, Schoppet M, Christ M, Teichmann J, Lange U. Tumour necrosis factor-related apoptosis-inducing ligand and osteoprotegerin serum levels in psoriatic arthritis. Rheumatology (Oxford). 2006;45:1218–22.

72. Ramírez J, Fernández-Sueiro JL, López-Mejías R, Montilla C, Arias M, Moll C, et al. FCGR2A/CD32A and FCGR3A/CD16A variants and EULAR response to tumor necrosis factor-α blockers in psoriatic arthritis: a longitudinal study with 6 months of followup. J Rheumatol. 2012;39:1035–41.

Animal Models of Psoriasis and Psoriatic Arthritis

12

Rik J. Lories and Barbara Neerinckx

Abstract

Animal models are important tools in biomedical research. However, the development of animal models that mimic psoriatic disease is a challenge as the characteristic skin and joint manifestations appear unique for humans. For skin disease different models have been developed mostly by tissue-specific overexpression or loss of function approaches. Important translational insights have come from patient skin transplantation models. The development of specific models for psoriatic arthritis appears even more challenging, in particular given the diverse disease manifestation seen in man. Nevertheless, models such as the spontaneous ankylosing enthesitis model in DBA/1 mice, the beta-glucan driven arthritis and spondylitis in SKG mice and the recent use of minicircle-driven IL-23 overexpression have all contributed to our understanding of joint disease.

Keywords

Psoriasis • Psoriatic arthritis • Animal models • Translational research • Pathogenesis

Introduction

Animal models are essential tools in modern biomedical research to understand mechanisms of disease and to pre-clinically evaluate novel therapeutic strategies. Mouse models in particular have already greatly contributed to our understanding of human diseases as mouse genes can be targeted to generate transgenic animals, resulting in either deletion or overexpression of specific genes [1]. The last decade has seen an unprecedented evolution in genome editing technologies now allowing cell-specific and inducible gene targeting. In addition, international collaborative consortia have generated thousands of knockout mice or mice carrying modified alleles that are available to individual research laboratories thereby enormously increasing the access to novel animal models while also reducing the associated cost. As a consequence, mouse models

R.J. Lories, MD, PhD (✉) • B. Neerinckx, MD
Laboratory of Tissue Homeostasis and Disease,
Skeletal Biology and Engineering
Research Center, KU Leuven, Herestraat 49,
BOX 813, Leuven 3000, Belgium
e-mail: Rik.Lories@uz.kuleuven.be

© Springer International Publishing Switzerland 2016
A. Adebajo et al. (eds.), *Psoriatic Arthritis and Psoriasis: Pathology and Clinical Aspects*,
DOI 10.1007/978-3-319-19530-8_12

will further contribute to our understanding of development, health and disease.

Animal models have also important limitations. With the exception of monogenic disorders, it is rarely seen that an animal model exactly mimics human disease. This is particularly true for complex diseases such as psoriasis and psoriatic arthritis in which environmental and genetic factors interact, and that are both characterized by a heterogeneous clinical presentation.

The use of animal models for biomedical research is also a matter of debate in society as ethical concerns are strongly voiced. From the patient perspective, an animal model is likely to be considered useful and acceptable if it directly contributes to a better understanding of the disease and at least indirectly to the potential development of treatments. Therefore animal models of psoriasis and psoriatic arthritis should be specifically considered in this context. In this chapter we discuss the challenges faced to introduce such models for psoriasis and psoriatic arthritis, give an overview of the models that are currently used including an assessment of their strong points and eventual weaknesses, and further shortly reflect on the lessons that can be learned from decades of intense research and progress in both skin and joint disease.

The Heterogeneity of Psoriatic Disease Is a Challenge for the Development of Disease Models

There is increasing evidence and growing consensus that Psoriasis, Psoriatic arthritis and associated co-morbidity are best considered under the umbrella of the "psoriatic disease" concept [2, 3]. This unifying view is based on the overlap in clinical symptoms, the common genetic susceptibility factors, the shared successes in targeted therapies and the global impact of comorbidity. Nevertheless the relationship between skin, nail and joint disease remains hard to define. Only a limited percentage of psoriasis patients also suffer from chronic arthritis. There is no good correlation between severity or flares of joint and skin disease and each primary disease

manifestation can occur simultaneously with, before or completely without the other.

Both Psoriasis and Psoriatic arthritis have strong differences in clinical manifestations within the disease entity. For Psoriasis, *psoriasis vulgaris* or plaque psoriasis is the most common disease type but other types such as *psoriasis guttata, inversa, pustulosa, erythroderma* and *palmo-plantaris* are also regularly seen [4, 5]. For Psoriatic arthritis, Moll and Wright defined five different types of disease: distal interphalangeal joint disease, *oligoarthritis, polyarthritis, arthritis mutilans*, and *spondylitis* [6]. This diversity in clinical manifestations is difficult to match in a mouse model.

Psoriatic disease appears to be unique for our species. There is no known naturally occurring disorder in other species that shows all the cardinal features of Psoriasis and that responds to the same therapies [7]. From this perspective, any animal model will have some limitations.

Specific Translational Challenges for Psoriasis Models

The skin of a mouse is different in many ways from that of humans [8]. From the structural point of view only sparse hair follicles and large interfollicular zones are found on the human skin as opposed to the densely packed hair follicles in mice. The mouse epidermis is thinner than its human counterpart and shows faster epidermal cell turnover. Mouse skin also regenerates more effectively than human skin, mostly without scarring. In addition, the mouse skin contains a number of immune cell types that are not found in humans and vice versa [8, 9]. This is an important observation as the skin can be considered a specialized immunological tissue in which the cellular immune players form the skin-associated lymphoid tissue (SALT) [10]. Hence, differences in cellular composition between species may result in distinct types of inflammatory reactions complicating translational insights and the evaluation of therapeutic strategies.

A second major challenge for the development of psoriasis models is the intrinsic nature of the disease. Many of the mechanisms that have been defined agree with the intriguing concept that the immune pathways that become activated in Psoriasis represent an amplification of background immune circuits that are essential for the skin's barrier role [7]. Thus in the experimental setting of a mouse model it has become clear that strongly similar inflammation and hyperproliferation in the mouse skin can be induced by many approaches including gene overexpression and knockout models. This suggests that the chronic inflammatory skin disease reported in different models represents a relative non-specific form of chronic cutaneous inflammation resulting from various primary disturbances of skin homeostasis.

This is further illustrated by the observation that psoriasis-like disease in mouse skin can be triggered by targeting genes in both the keratinocytes or in the dermal layer (in particular immunity associated genes) [7–9]. Strong shifts in cellular and molecular signaling in one skin compartment seem sufficient to spark complex disease. On the other hand, the intrinsic disease heterogeneity of psoriasis, with a number of manifestations that are distinct from classic *psoriasis vulgaris,* makes it unlikely that a single gene approach will lead to the development of the full clinical picture, including these alternative manifestations.

Finally, the world of the laboratory mouse is vastly different from the complex environmental exposure of psoriasis patients. Psoriasis is a disease that develops specifically in a tissue that acts as an interface and a battleground of host defense. Many laboratory animals are raised in a (semi)-sterile environment and small changes in the circumstances or in mouse strain used can strongly affect the phenotype of the model. Many genetic mouse models are developed in specific backgrounds and may not be reproducible in other strains. This highlights the great impact of modifier genes on such model systems [7].

Models of Psoriasis

Research groups currently use different models of psoriasis. These include some mouse strains with spontaneous development of a psoriasis-like disease, a large number of genetically modified

Table 12.1 Overview of psoriasis models

Spontaneous disease models
These animals show epidermal thickening and vascular changes but do not have an epidermal T cell infiltrate
Flaky skin – (Ttc7$^{fsn/fsn}$ mice), Chronic proliferative dermatitis -(Sharpin$^{cpdm/cpdm}$ mice), Homozygous asebia – *Scd1*$^{ab/ab}$ mice
Mutated animals
Overexpression in the basal epidermal layer: promoter keratin-5 (K5) and 14 (K14)
K5-latent-TGFb1, K5-STAT3C, K5-Tie2, K5-PPARb/g, K14-TGFa, K14-IL-6, K14-KGF, K14-IL-1a, K14-p40, K14-IL-20, K14-VEGF, K14-amphiregulin, K14-TNF, K14-Raf1
Overexpression in the supradermal epidermal layer: promoter keratin-10 (K10) and involucrin (invol)
K10-BMP6, Invol-integrina2,5 – b1, Invol-amphiregulin, Invol-IFNg, Invol-MEK1
Many of the overexpression models show epidermal thickening but also features unlike psoriasis such as alopecia and early lethality
Knockout and conditional knockout animals
Systemic gene targeting
Hypomorphic CD18, IRF-2, Integrin aE, IL-1RA
Cell-specific gene targeting
K5-SRF, K14-IKKb, K5-Ick-IkBa, K5-JunB/c-Jun
Phenotypes are often mixed with many non-psoriatic features. The K5-JunB/c-jun conditional knockout also shows joint involvement
Transplantation models
Skin transplantation in immune deficient mice (affected and non-affected skin)
Human T cell transfer
Direct induction
Injection of cytokines: IL-17, IL-23, IL-12
Chemically drive: Imiquimod

More details about the models can be found in Ref. [8, 9]

mice, induced models of psoriasis and human skin or immune cell transplantation models (Table 12.1).

Spontaneous Models of Psoriasis-Like Skin Disease in Mice

Spontaneous mutations occur in laboratory mouse strains. Psoriasiform lesions have been recognized in mice that are homozygous for the mutated asebia allele in the stearoyl-CoA desaturase 1 gene (*Scd1*$^{ab/ab}$ mice) [11], for the chronic proliferative dermatitis allele in the Sharpin gene (*Sharpin^{cpdm/cpdm}* mice) [12] and for the flaky skin mutation in the tetratricopeptide repeat domain 7 gene (*Ttc7^{fsn/fsn}* mice) [13]. However, T cells, essential players in the human disease, are mostly absent in these models and their translational potential, in particular their response to therapy, appears limited [9, 14].

Transgenic Approaches: Gain and Loss of Function

The availability of well-characterized promoters for genes that are specifically expressed in the basal epidermal layer (e.g. keratin-5 and 14), and for genes associated with the suprabasal epidermal layer (e.g. involucrin and keratin-10) has defined a great toolbox to study tissue-specific overexpression of target genes. Effectively, a large number of growth factors, cytokines and intracellular signaling molecules have been overexpressed in this way resulting mostly in hyperkeratosis, and also often in epidermal inflammation [8, 9]. The relative drawback of this type of model is that the local dosing of the gene of interest is difficult to control and that therefore a causal effect in the human disease for that gene is difficult to ascertain.

Knockout or other loss of function approaches (such as mutated alleles resulting in partial loss of function) may come closer to the physiological situation but still lead to potentially major shifts in gene networks. Full or conditional knockout models targeting integrins, NFkappaB signaling and cytokine antagonists (e.g. IL-1RA) have demonstrated development of psoriasiform lesions [8, 9]. Of note, inducible epidermal specific deletion of c-Jun and JunB not only leads to skin symptoms but has also been associated with changes in the joint [15].

Induced Models of Psoriasis

Direct evidence for a role of cytokines interleukin (IL)-21 and IL-23 has been found by injection of these molecules into the skin [16, 17]. An alternative approach that may come close to the events associated with initiation of disease in psoriasis is the topical application of imiquimod, that activates toll-like receptor 7 [18]. This relatively cheap and straightforward model has potential for pre-clinical treatment evaluation, in particular as it has been associated with activation of the IL-23/IL-17 axis [18].

Humanized Models

The transfer of lesional and pre-lesional patient skin compared to skin biopsies of normal donors onto immune deficient mice is an attractive translational model although technically challenging [8, 9, 19]. The combined transfer of the epidermis and the SALT in the biopsy allows the study of interactions in an *in vivo* setting. These models have not only demonstrated the importance of T cells in psoriasis but again have strong translational potential as drugs can be tested in a pre-clinical setting (see for instance [20]). Additional evidence that T cells play a critical role in psoriasis has come from T cell transfer experiments onto immune deficient mice [21].

Specific Challenges Associated with Models of Psoriatic Arthritis

The nature of psoriatic arthritis is not well understood. Although the clinical skills and experience of the trained rheumatologist aid greatly in making a correct diagnosis in a majority of patients, it remains difficult to precisely define psoriatic arthritis as one disease. Most easily classified as a chronic inflammatory skeletal disease it is characterized by an enormous heterogeneity in clinical manifestations and severity, perhaps even more than the related skin disorder. The different subtypes of the disease, as originally described by Moll and Wright, are for sure not found in one specific mouse model [6].

The intrinsic differences in clinical manifestations are further emphasized by the different types of structural damage that occur in the joint.

Joint damage in psoriatic arthritis can be characterized by cartilage loss, by bone erosion and by new bone formation with progression towards ankylosis. Up till now, there is no mouse model that covers all the essential features of psoriatic arthritis: distal joints, axial joints, skin, nail disease, bone destruction and bone remodeling. Therefore, taking into account a translational perspective and an instrumental view on animal models to improve either diagnosis or therapy, animal model data of interest for psoriatic arthritis can come from different approaches and some may overlap with models of rheumatoid arthritis or have originally been defined as models of spondyloarthritis.

Specific Models of Psoriatic Arthritis (Table 12.2)

Spontaneous Models of Psoriatic Arthritis

Aging male DBA/1 mice from different litters that are caged together spontaneously develop arthritis of the hind paws, in particular the interphalangeal and ankle joints [22, 23]. The DBA/1 strain is considered immunologically normal. Microscopic studies demonstrated that the clinically apparent arthritis is caused by enthesitis and mild synovitis, progressively leading to joint remodeling with new cartilage and bone formation, eventually leading to ankylosis. Other remarkable features of the model include occasional nail lesions associated with distal phalanx destruction and dactylitis [22]. This model helped to identify the role of growth factors, in particular bone morphogenetic proteins, in ankylosis [24].

Nail and toe lesions have also been described in mice lacking endogenous major histocompatibility class II genes [25]. Other models of ankylosis include the ANKENT phenotype in C57/Bl6 mice albeit with a low penetrance as compared to DBA/1 mice [26, 27]. Incidence of disease appeared to increase however in the presence of the spondyloarthritis associated HLA-27 gene [26].

Table 12.2 Overview of psoriatic arthritis models

Spontaneous disease models
Spontaneous arthritis in aging male DBA/1 mice
Characterized by ankylosing enthesitis, no skin features, sometime nail disease and dactylitis
ANKENT mice
Ankylosing enthesitis of the ankle
Mice without endogenous MHC genes
Erosive toe and nail disease
Transgenic animals (overexpression and knockout)
Conditional knockout of JunB and c-Jun in the epidermis
Primarily skin phenotype but also arthritis associated with new bone formation has been described
Overexpression of amphiregulin in the epidermis
Mild signs of arthritis reported
Induced models
Minicircle overexpression of IL-23
Enthesitis, arthritis, destruction and new bone formation
Beta-glucan treatment in SKG mice
Arthritis, enthesitis, spondylitis

Transgenic Approaches towards Psoriatic Arthritis Models

As already mentioned above, specific epidermal deletion of JunB and c-Jun not only resulted in psoriasiform skin lesions but also in signs of arthritis and the presence of periosteal new bone formation [15]. Additional experiments targeting tumor necrosis factor (TNF) suggest that this type of arthritis is TNF dependent. Overexpression of amphiregulin in the suprabasal epidermis also leads to mild arthritis in mice [28]. Together these models suggest that primary disease manifestations in the skin may also trigger symptoms in the joint, at least in mouse models.

Induced Models of Psoriatic Arthritis

Interesting observations in induced models support the view that the IL23-IL17 axis plays an important role, not only in Psoriasis but also in psoriatic arthritis. Systemic overexpression of IL-23 using minicircle technology results in enthesitis and remodeling arthritis [29]. Early signs of disease are specifically found in the enthesis. Within these tendon and ligament insertion sites, a novel population of RoRγT and IL-23 receptor positive T cells was found. Entheseal tissue exposed to IL-23 showed increased production of IL-17, TNF and IL-22 as well as of growth factors such as BMPs. In contrast to the data obtained in the *JunB/c-Jun* knockout mice, there is no evidence of crosstalk between joints and skin.

Another model pointing towards a critical role for the IL23/IL17 axis was described after beta-glucan treatment of SKG mice [30]. The SKG mice are a known model of rheumatoid arthritis and carry a mutation in the *Zap-70* gene affecting selection in the thymus and leading to overt auto-immunity [31]. However, the fungal beta-glucan administration strongly influenced the clinical signs of disease with arthritis, spondylitis and dactylitis developing. The underlying mechanisms are incompletely understood but a relationship with increased auto-reactivity of T cells primed by the gut flora has been proposed.

In addition, mechanisms of joint remodeling can also be studied in mice with transient destructive arthritis such as collagen-induced arthritis, collagen antibody induced arthritis [32] and the KP/N serum transfer model [33]. As inflammation subsides in the late phase of disease, new bone formation can be spectacular in these models and used to get better insights into mechanisms of disease and evaluation of therapeutic targets.

Lessons Learned and Future Perspectives

Psoriatic disease is unique for humans and none of the animal models exactly mimics it. Nevertheless, animal models that highlight specific aspects of skin and joint disease have been instrumental in shaping our concepts of psoriatic disease. Taken together, investigators using such models identified tissues, cells and molecules that play an active role in the disease. Such models have also allowed researchers to provide proof-of-principle for treatment approaches. In particular for psoriasis induced models or xeno-tissue-transfer setups remain of great interest. Transgenic and knockout approaches will likely further contribute to define the role of new genes and cells that are hypothesized to play a role in the disease e.g. based on genetic studies or tissue analysis. Such models are currently still missing for psoriatic arthritis and represent an enormous challenge due to the striking heterogeneity of the disease in all aspects. However, clever use of existing models, e.g. bone remodeling models and cytokine overexpression models, should further contribute to improve our understanding of psoriatic arthritis and most in particular to identify what makes this form of arthritis unique among chronic inflammatory joint diseases.

References

1. Nguyen D, Xu T. The expanding role of mouse genetics for understanding human biology and disease. Dis Model Mech. 2008;1(1):56–66.
2. Olivieri I, D'Angelo S, Palazzi C, Padula A. Advances in the management of psoriatic arthritis. Nat Rev Rheumatol. 2014;10:531–42.
3. Scarpa R. New insights into the concept of psoriatic disease. J Rheumatol Suppl. 2012;89:4–6.
4. Perera GK, Di Meglio P, Nestle FO. Psoriasis. Annu Rev Pathol. 2012;7:385–422.
5. Nestle FO, Kaplan DH, Barker J. Psoriasis. N Engl J Med. 2009;361(5):496–509.
6. Moll JM, Wright V. Psoriatic arthritis. Semin Arthritis Rheum. 1973;3(1):55–78.
7. Schon MP. Animal models of psoriasis: a critical appraisal. Exp Dermatol. 2008;17(8):703–12.
8. Gudjonsson JE, Johnston A, Dyson M, Valdimarsson H, Elder JT. Mouse models of psoriasis. J Invest Dermatol. 2007;127(6):1292–308.
9. Wagner EF, Schonthaler HB, Guinea-Viniegra J, Tschachler E. Psoriasis: what we have learned from mouse models. Nat Rev Rheumatol. 2010;6(12):704–14.
10. Lowes MA, Suarez-Farinas M, Krueger JG. Immunology of psoriasis. Annu Rev Immunol. 2014;32:227–55.
11. Brown WR, Hardy MH. A hypothesis on the cause of chronic epidermal hyperproliferation in asebia mice. Clin Exp Dermatol. 1988;13(2):74–7.
12. HogenEsch H, Gijbels MJ, Offerman E, van Hooft J, van Bekkum DW, Zurcher C. A spontaneous mutation characterized by chronic proliferative dermatitis in C57BL mice. Am J Pathol. 1993;143(3):972–82.

13. Sundberg JP, France M, Boggess D, Sundberg BA, Jenson AB, Beamer WG, et al. Development and progression of psoriasiform dermatitis and systemic lesions in the flaky skin (fsn) mouse mutant. Pathobiology. 1997;65(5):271–86.

14. Gijbels MJ, Elliott GR, HogenEsch H, Zurcher C, van den Hoven A, Bruijnzeel PL. Therapeutic interventions in mice with chronic proliferative dermatitis (cpdm/cpdm). Exp Dermatol. 2000;9(5):351–8.

15. Zenz R, Eferl R, Kenner L, Florin L, Hummerich L, Mehic D, et al. Psoriasis-like skin disease and arthritis caused by inducible epidermal deletion of Jun proteins. Nature. 2005;437(7057):369–75.

16. Zheng Y, Danilenko DM, Valdez P, Kasman I, Eastham-Anderson J, Wu J, et al. Interleukin-22, a T(H)17 cytokine, mediates IL-23-induced dermal inflammation and acanthosis. Nature. 2007;445(7128): 648–51.

17. Chan JR, Blumenschein W, Murphy E, Diveu C, Wiekowski M, Abbondanzo S, et al. IL-23 stimulates epidermal hyperplasia via TNF and IL-20R2-dependent mechanisms with implications for psoriasis pathogenesis. J Exp Med. 2006;203(12): 2577–87.

18. van der Fits L, Mourits S, Voerman JS, Kant M, Boon L, Laman JD, et al. Imiquimod-induced psoriasis-like skin inflammation in mice is mediated via the IL-23/IL-17 axis. J Immunol. 2009;182(9):5836–45.

19. Krueger GG, Manning DD, Malouf J, Ogden B. Long-term maintenance of psoriatic human skin on congenitally athymic (nude) mice. J Invest Dermatol. 1975;64(5):307–12.

20. Schafer PH, Parton A, Gandhi AK, Capone L, Adams M, Wu L, et al. Apremilast, a cAMP phosphodiesterase-4 inhibitor, demonstrates anti-inflammatory activity in vitro and in a model of psoriasis. Br J Pharmacol. 2010;159(4):842–55.

21. Schon MP, Detmar M, Parker CM. Murine psoriasis-like disorder induced by naive CD4+ T cells. Nat Med. 1997;3(2):183–8.

22. Lories RJ, Matthys P, de Vlam K, Derese I, Luyten FP. Ankylosing enthesitis, dactylitis, and onychoperiostitis in male DBA/1 mice: a model of psoriatic arthritis. Ann Rheum Dis. 2004;63(5):595–8.

23. Braem K, Carter S, Lories RJ. Spontaneous arthritis and ankylosis in male DBA/1 mice: further evidence for a role of behavioral factors in "stress-induced arthritis". Biol Proced online. 2012;14(1):10.

24. Lories RJ, Derese I, Luyten FP. Modulation of bone morphogenetic protein signaling inhibits the onset and progression of ankylosing enthesitis. J Clin Invest. 2005;115(6):1571–9.

25. Bardos T, Zhang J, Mikecz K, David CS, Glant TT. Mice lacking endogenous major histocompatibility complex class II develop arthritis resembling psoriatic arthritis at an advanced age. Arthritis Rheum. 2002;46(9):2465–75.

26. Capkova J, Ivanyi P. H-2 influence on ankylosing enthesopathy of the ankle (ANKENT). Folia Biol. 1992;38(3–4):258–62.

27. Capkova J, Stepankova R, Hudcovic T, Sinkora J, Rehakova Z. Experimental colitis does not increase the prevalence of ANKENT, a spontaneous joint disease in mice. Folia Microbiol. 2004;49(6):745–50.

28. Cook PW, Pittelkow MR, Piepkorn M. Overexpression of amphiregulin in the epidermis of transgenic mice induces a psoriasis-like cutaneous phenotype. J Invest Dermatol. 1999;113(5):860.

29. Sherlock JP, Joyce-Shaikh B, Turner SP, Chao CC, Sathe M, Grein J, et al. IL-23 induces spondyloarthropathy by acting on ROR-gammat(+) CD3(+) CD4(−)CD8(−) entheseal resident T cells. Nat Med. 2012;18(7):1069–76.

30. Ruutu M, Thomas G, Steck R, Degli-Esposti MA, Zinkernagel MS, Alexander K, et al. beta-glucan triggers spondylarthritis and Crohn's disease-like ileitis in SKG mice. Arthritis Rheum. 2012;64(7): 2211–22.

31. Sakaguchi N, Takahashi T, Hata H, Nomura T, Tagami T, Yamazaki S, et al. Altered thymic T-cell selection due to a mutation of the ZAP-70 gene causes autoimmune arthritis in mice. Nature. 2003;426(6965): 454–60.

32. Jacques P, Lambrecht S, Verheugen E, Pauwels E, Kollias G, Armaka M, et al. Proof of concept: enthesitis and new bone formation in spondyloarthritis are driven by mechanical strain and stromal cells. Ann Rheum Dis. 2014;73(2):437–45.

33. Ruiz-Heiland G, Horn A, Zerr P, Hofstetter W, Baum W, Stock M, et al. Blockade of the hedgehog pathway inhibits osteophyte formation in arthritis. Ann Rheum Dis. 2012;71(3):400–7.

Mechanisms of Bone Remodelling in Psoriatic Arthritis

13

Nigil Haroon and Christopher Ritchlin

Abstract

Psoriatic arthritis (PsA) is characterized by chronic inflammatory arthritis associated with skin and/or nail changes of psoriasis. PsA manifests in the peripheral joints with both bone destruction and new bone formation while in the spine there is aberrant bone formation and vertebral fusion. The pathogenic basis for the co-existence of bone loss and paradoxical bone formation has not been explained. Several exciting discoveries in this area has improved our understanding of bone homeostatic abnormalities in PsA and these will be explored in this chapter.

Keywords

Psoriasis • Inflammatory arthritis • Spondyloarthritis • Osteoblast • Osteoclast

Introduction

Psoriatic arthritis (PsA) is a chronic inflammatory arthritis with varied joint manifestations and association with psoriasis of the skin and/or nail. The peripheral arthritis associated with PsA can range from relatively mild oligoarticular, nonerosive joint inflammation to polyarticular erosive and severely deforming arthritis. Inflammation in the spinal joints resembling other forms of axial spondyloarthritis (AxSpA) is seen as well. A characteristic and striking feature that distinguishes PsA in all its different forms, is altered bone remodeling phenotypes. These striking manifestations, viewed on plain radiographs, arise by reciprocal osteoblastic (bone formation) and osteoclastic (bone resorption) activities. While bone formation is also a characteristic feature in axial spondyloarthritis (SpA), PsA is distinct because complete bony fusion and the presence of enthesophytes often arises in the appendicular skeleton, even in the absence of contiguous bone erosion.

N. Haroon MD, PhD (✉)
Department of Medicine and Rheumatology,
Toronto Western Hospital, University Health
Network, University of Toronto, 1 East-wing-425,
399 Bathurst St., Toronto, ON M5T 2S8, Canada
e-mail: Nigil.Haroon@uhn.ca

C. Ritchlin, MD, MPH
Immunology and Rheumatology Division, University
of Rochester Medical Center, Rochester, NY, USA

© Springer International Publishing Switzerland 2016
A. Adebajo et al. (eds.), *Psoriatic Arthritis and Psoriasis: Pathology and Clinical Aspects*,
DOI 10.1007/978-3-319-19530-8_13

Although we still lack a detailed understanding of the events that underlie altered bone remodeling, significant advances over the past decade are beginning to complete the puzzle. Insights regarding the cell lineages that promote bone resorption and formation to maintain homeostasis in the normal skeleton cleared the way for working models to explain the pathologic state in SpA and in particular, PsA. The recent discovery of the IL-23/Th17 pathway opened new avenues of investigation that directly address the events in psoriatic bone. In this chapter we will review the recent advances in our understanding of bone homeostasis and abnormalities in the involved biological pathways.

Bone Remodeling across the Spectrum of Psoriatic Arthritis

As discussed in previous chapters, the clinical spectrum of PsA is broad. Patients may present with typical spondyloarthritis manifestations including monoarthritis or oligoarthritis and/or

spinal arthritis. Spinal arthritis can result in new bone formation manifesting as syndesmophytes and ankylosis (Fig. 13.1a). Polyarthritis mimicking rheumatoid arthritis may be the presenting manifestation or the result of cumulative joint involvement over years. Severe destruction of joints can lead to arthritis mutilans, a striking form of the disease characterized by tuft and digit resorption with flail digits in the hands and feet. Radiographically, this form of arthritis can be viewed as complete or partial digit loss and the pencil-in-cup deformity in which the distal tuft is whittled down to a point and the distal end of the middle phalanx is significantly widened [1]. Extra-articular manifestations including enthesitis, tenosynovitis and dactylitis are often seen in PsA. Depending on the clinical presentation, the bone remodeling pathways involved may have differential regulation. Most importantly, bone erosion (Fig. 13.1b) is a prevalent finding in PsA; almost half of patients show bone damage on radiographs with 2 years of disease onset [2]. Moreover, a proportion of these patients show evidence of new bone formation (Fig. 13.1b) in

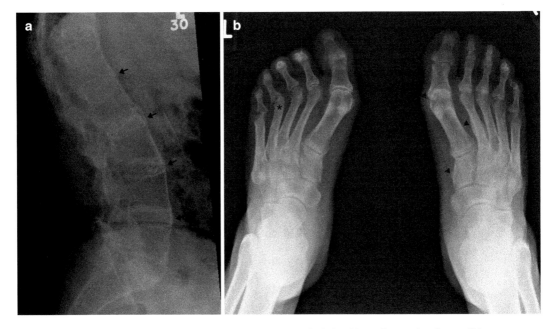

Fig. 13.1 Radiographic changes of psoriatic arthritis. (**a**) Spinal new bone formation manifesting as bridging syndesmophytes (*arrows*) resulting in bamboo spine appearance. (**b**) Typical peripheral joint radiographic changes

seen in PsA with erosions and early pencil in cup appearance (*asterisk*) and periosteal new bone formation (*arrow heads*)

the periosteal and periarticular regions that may progress to peripheral ankylosis. Similarly patients with enthesitis can manifest erosions and new bone formation in the affected area. Generally the erosive peripheral arthritis patients have intra articular erosions while new bone formation is evident in the juxta-articular areas raising the possibility of altered inflammatory or cytokine milieu driving these divergent presentations.

Differentiation of PsA from RA and osteoarthritis on plain radiographs can be challenging at times but high-resolution micro-CT scanning of MCP joints has provided unique insights. First, the number of erosions in PsA and RA were similar but those in RA take on a U-shape while those in PsA tend to be smaller in size and depth and show a tubular or omega (Ω) appearance, likely a reflection of reparative bone formation in the periosteum [3]. Second, large osteophytes lining the circumference of the bone, were more typical of PsA. Third, the osteophytes in OA were more palmar and dorsal compared to PsA which were more commonly located on the radial side and more likely to be at enthesial insertion sites to the bone. Lastly, enthesiophytes were significantly increased in number and size in psoriasis patients without arthritis compared to controls. These data underscore the unique bone formation processes in PsA which appear to begin in psoriasis patients without musculoskeletal symptoms.

Pathways Linking Psoriasis and Arthritis

Psoriasis and PsA are closely associated clinical features and in the majority of cases, development of plaques precedes the onset of arthritis by about 10 years. Thus, it is reasonable to postulate that events that culminate in joint inflammation and damage originate in an aberrant immune profile that arises in the skin. Raised, erythematous plaques with silvery scale with predilection for the scalp and extensor surfaces are defining features of psoriasis. The current model, based on data from animal models and human tissues indicate that the early events are promoted by release

of DNA by stressed keratinocytes which binds to the antibacterial peptide cathelicidin LL-37 [4]. The DNA-LL37 complex binds Toll-like receptor 9 (TLR-9) on plasmacytoid dendritic cells and triggers interferon (IFN)-α release. Activation of dermal dendritic cells by IFN-α is followed by migration of these cells to the draining lymph node.

Within the lymph node, DCs that originated in the plaque, stimulate differentiation of naïve T cells into the Th1 and Th17 cells. These T cells migrate back to the skin in the vasculature. Once in the dermis, Th1 cells release IFN-γ and TNF-α while the Th17 cells produce TNF-α, IL-1, IL-17 and IL-22. Other immune cells also produce IL-17 including CD8+ lymphocytes, innate lymphocytes, γ-δ and NK-T cells and neutrophils. Th17 cells invading the dermis release IL-1, IL-6, and TNF-α as well as chemokines and most importantly IL-22 that promote keratinocyte proliferation. Dermal dendritic cells synthesize IL-23 which leads to further proliferation and survival of Th17 cells. A combination of IL-17A, IL-22, and TNF-α to lead to the stimulate cutaneous IL-19 synthesis and release. IL-19 induces production of anti-bacterial proteins in keratinocytes including S100A7, S100A8, S100A9. Cytokines IL-1β, IL-20, CXCL-8, and matrix metalloproteinase-1 are increased in the presence of IL-19. IL-36 γ, which is stimulated by LL-37 and found in abundance in psoriatic plaques, leads to production of neutrophil-attracting IL-8 and CXCL1 [5]. Neutrophil collections, termed Munro's abscesses, are formed which develop into psoriatic plaques.

Nail Involvement and Distal Arthritis

Nail disease (pits, erosions, oncycholysis) are commonly observed in psoriasis and are even more prevalent in PsA. Clinical observations also noted the close relationship between DIP arthritis and nail disease in PsA. McGonagle et al. postulated an important link between the nail bed and joint damage in distal joints. His group demonstrated that the extensor tendon enthesis fuses with the nail root providing a direct link between the DIP joint and the nail [6]. Thus inflammation in the nail may promote inflammation in the neighboring distal joint. Another potential link between psoriatic nail disease and joint inflammation was the finding in a psoriasiform murine model, nocioceptors activated in the skin promoted accumulation of dermal dendritic cells adjacent to the nerve fibers that released IL-23 [7]. As will be discussed below, IL-23 is a critical cytokine that may direct aberrant bone remodeling thus linking psoriatic nail disease and joint damage.

Enthesitis

The enthesis is the attachment site of the joint capsule, tendon or ligament to bone. Enthesitis is a common manifestation in PsA, presenting as plantar fasciitis, Achilles tendonitis, lateral or medial epicondylitis to name a few [8]. Enthesitis is of great interest because it is a cardinal element in SpA and PsA. Recent efforts were directed to better understand the structure and function of the enthesis in order to define its role in psoriatic disease and SpA. MRI imaging studies in PsA revealed widespread bone marrow edema along with tendon, synovium and bursal inflammation at enthesial attachement sites. The term "enthesis organ" was advanced based on a collection of tissues comprised of sesamoid and periosteal cartilage along with collagen fibers, bursae and lining synovial tissue that serves to dissipate stress [9]. More recently, the term synovial-enthesial complex was proposed to describe this integrated set of tissues [10]. Under normal conditions, the enthesis lacks vasculature or cells. However, during times of shear stress or enthesial damage, danger signals lead to cytokine production by lymphocytes and monocytes found in the adjacent synovial tissues [11]. Thus, in psoriatic arthritis it is hypothesized that the enthesis is the site of origin for the inflammatory response, which is in contrast to rheumatoid arthritis where the inflammatory site is believed to be the synovium [12]. This view has been challenged and at this time definitive support for this model awaits

future study. Mechanical trauma has been proposed as an inciting factor for the development of enthesitis and has been shown in mouse models. In the TNF Δ ARE mouse model, unloading of the hind limbs results in a decrease in inflammation of the Achilles tendon supporting this hypothesis [13].

Dactylitis

Initial MRI studies of dactylitic joints were interpreted as a form of flexor tenosynovitis but subsequent studies indicate widespread inflammation that can involve soft tissues, bone and cartilage [14, 15]. The pathophysiologic events responsible for the diffuse swelling of a digit or dactylitis but animal studies discussed below suggest a role for the IL-23/Th17 pathway [16, 17]. It is important to note that erosions, not commonly observed in dactylitis digits, were reported mainly in tender vs. non-tender digits [15]. One possibility is that the diffuse tissue inflammation begins at the attachment of the capsule onto the phalanx and represents a form of enthesitis accompanied by aberrant bone remodeling [18].

Synovitis

Histologic analysis of psoriatic synovial tissue demonstrates findings remarkably similar to RA in appearance, with lining-layer hyperplasia and a subsynovial infiltrate of T cells, B cells, and monocytes. Digital image analysis of biopsy tissues revealed that PsA tissues had a lower number of infiltrating T and plasma cells but the expression of TNF-α, IL-β, IL6, and IL18 protein expression was similar in the two diseases. Activated T cells have been identified in the skin and joints in PsA patients; T cells in the epidermis joint fluid are predominately CD8$^+$ although more recent studies have uncovered a prominent Th17 response in the psoriatic plaque [19, 20]. Most interestingly, CD8+IL-17+ cells were identified in the synovial fluid of PsA but not RA joints. Th17 cells were identified in the psoriatic synovium and mast cells in the joint tissue were also noted to express IL-17 [21, 22]. Subsequent unpublished studies suggest that mast cells do not synthesize IL-17 but take up this cytokine from the surrounding microenvironment.

Pathologic Bone Resorption in PsA

Bone homeostasis is maintained by a coordinated interaction between osteoclasts and osteoblasts. Osteoclasts are the only cells capable of resorbing the inorganic matrix of bone while osteoblasts synthesize osteoid required for bone formation [23]. Osteoclasts are multinucleated cells that possess a ruffled border that seals them off from the surrounding microenviroment to release enzymes (H$^+$ ions, cathpesin K and others) that degrade bone (Fig. 13.2). During inflammation, the fraction of circulating CD14+ monocytes rise and these cells enter joint spaces where under the right cytokine stimulation, they differentiate into osteoclasts. The cytokines M-CSF and RANKL are critical for the differentiation of monocytes into osteoclasts, a process termed osteoclastogenesis. TNF-α, a pro-inflammatory cytokine, can induce osteoclast-associated receptor (OSCAR) on monocytes [24] and potentiates the actions of RANKL. Binding of OSCAR by denatured activates the receptor and provides a second signal to activate osteoclast promoting genes. This requirement for dual

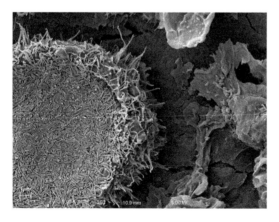

Fig. 13.2 Osteoclast with ruffled membrane. Scanning electron microscopic image of an osteoclast on a bone wafer, surrounded by monocytes

activation of RANK and OSCAR or TREM 2 another receptor that can deliver a second signal is analogous to the two-step process required for T cell activation [25]. An array of cytokines including TNF-α, IL-1, IL-6, IL-17 and VEGF induce RANK-L expression. Engagement of RANK on pre-osteoclasts triggers NFκB and AP-1 signaling, that fosters cell fusion and the formation of the polykaryon followed by terminal differentiation of the resorption organelles.

In psoriatic joint tissues, marked upregulation of RANKL protein and low expression of its antagonist OPG were identified in the adjacent synovial lining [26]. RANK-L is inhibited when it is bound by osteoprotegerin (OPG). Thus, the ratio of high RANK-L to OPG favors an osteoclastogenic environment. OPG is secreted by osteocytes, osteoblasts and osteogenic stromal stem cells, protecting the body from excessive bone resorption. Osteoclasts were also noted in cutting cones traversing the subchondral bone, supporting bidirectional attack on bone. In addition, osteoclast precursors (OCPs) derived from circulating CD14+ monocytes were markedly elevated in the peripheral blood of PsA patients and a fourth of psoriasis patients without arthritis compared with healthy controls. Treatment of PsA patients with anti-TNF agents significantly decreased the level of circulating OCP, thus supporting a central effect of TNF in the generation of precursor formation.

It is now well established that RANK-L expressed on the surface of Th17 cells can also cause osteoclast cells to switch from a non-resorptive to resorptive phenotype [27]. Th17 cells are capable of directly producing RANK ligand as well as indirectly through the action of IL-17 on synovial fibroblasts, which can induce RANK ligand expression. In contrast, Th1 and Th2 cells were did not induce osteoclastogenesis in co-culture experiments with monocytes [28]. In preclinical models, IL-23 and IL-17 knock out mice exhibit significantly inflammatory bone destruction than wild-type mice. These experiments support a pathway were IL-23 induced differentiation of naïve lymphocytes to the Th17 subset strongly favors a resorptive phenotype characteristic of pathologic bone destruction

[28]. These studies outlined above support the concept that both TNF and Th17 cells strongly induce osteoclastogenesis through both direct and indirect mechanisms.

Additional evidence for the importance of TNF in pathways that promote bone damage was provided in clinical translational studies. In particular, anti-TNF therapy resulted in decreased numbers of circulating osteoclast precursors in the peripheral blood of PsA patients [29]. Blocking TNF has direct effects on bone metabolism, but also modulates trafficking of T lymphocytes. In the collagen-induced arthritis (CIA) mouse model, anti-TNF therapy was associated with a decrease in number of Th17 cells within the joints, but increased numbers within the draining lymph nodes [30]. While anti-TNF therapy has effects on bone erosion, TNF blockade does not influence the formation of osteophytes or syndesmophytes as discussed in detail below [31].

Pathways of Aberrant New Bone Formation in PsA

Wnt Signaling Pathway

The Wnt Signaling Pathway can be considered a 'pluripotent' pathway by virtue of the numerous cellular processes it could affect. The Wnt pathway is known to play a role in cell proliferation, polarity and embryogenesis. The term 'Wnt' is derived from the names of two genes *Wingless* (*Wg*) and *Integration1* (*Int1*). *Wingless1* mutations were initially reported to cause abnormal embryogenesis and wing formation in Drosophila [32] while *Int1* was found to be activated in mouse mammary carcinomas [33]. It was later discovered that both genes are homologous. Wnt signaling pathway is critical in the regulation of cell growth, differentiation and death [32, 34–36] and it has been linked to limb development, antero-posterior axial patterning and eye formation [32, 34, 36]. The Wnt pathway has been found to play a significant role in bone homeostasis.

Decreased Dkk-1 and increased nuclear localization of β-catenin, implying activation of the Wnt-signalling pathway, has been reported in the lesional psoriasis skin [37, 38]. Wnt proteins signal (Fig. 13.3) through its receptor Frizzled and co-receptors LDL-receptor like protein (LRP) -5 and 6. β-catenin, the key transcription factor mediating the Wnt signaling, is trapped in a complex and programmed for ubiquitination and degradation when the pathway is inactive. Upon activation, the inhibitory complex around β-catenin breaks down permitting its nuclear translocation. Dishevelled is activated which inhibits Glycogen Synthase Kinase-3β (GSK-3β) and Axin moves out of the complex. This pathway is activated in committed osteoblasts while deficiency of β-catenin in osteoblast precursor cells results in reduced bone deposition [39]. The synthesis of chondrogenic and osteoblastic factors results from the nuclear translocation of β-catenin and binding to transcription factor T cell Factor 4 (TCF). Excess Wnt signaling can stimulate bone formation and Wnt signalling abnormalities have been linked to osteoporosis, RA, AS, osteoarthritis, and Paget's disease [40–47]. *LRP5* mutations are associated with Osteoporosis and Pseudoglioma (OPPG) syndrome in humans [48].

BMP Pathway

BMPs belong to the TGF-β superfamily and acts through the dimerization of BMP receptors I and II (Fig. 13.3) that results in activation of SMAD signaling [49]. Conflicting reports on the role of BMP in axial SpA and boned formation have been published. BMP2, BMP4 and BMP7 were reported in AS patients to correlate with the degree of radiographic fusion [50]. In another study while BMP7 did correlate with radiographic damage, BMP2 levels correlated with BASDAI and not radiographic damage by BASRI [51]. Interestingly in the same study showed elevated BMP2 and BMP7 levels in RA patients where erosive arthritis, rather than new bone formation is seen [51]. Hence it remains to be seen if studies on blood levels of BMPs are indeed reflective of pathogenesis or simply detecting changes secondary to inflammation.

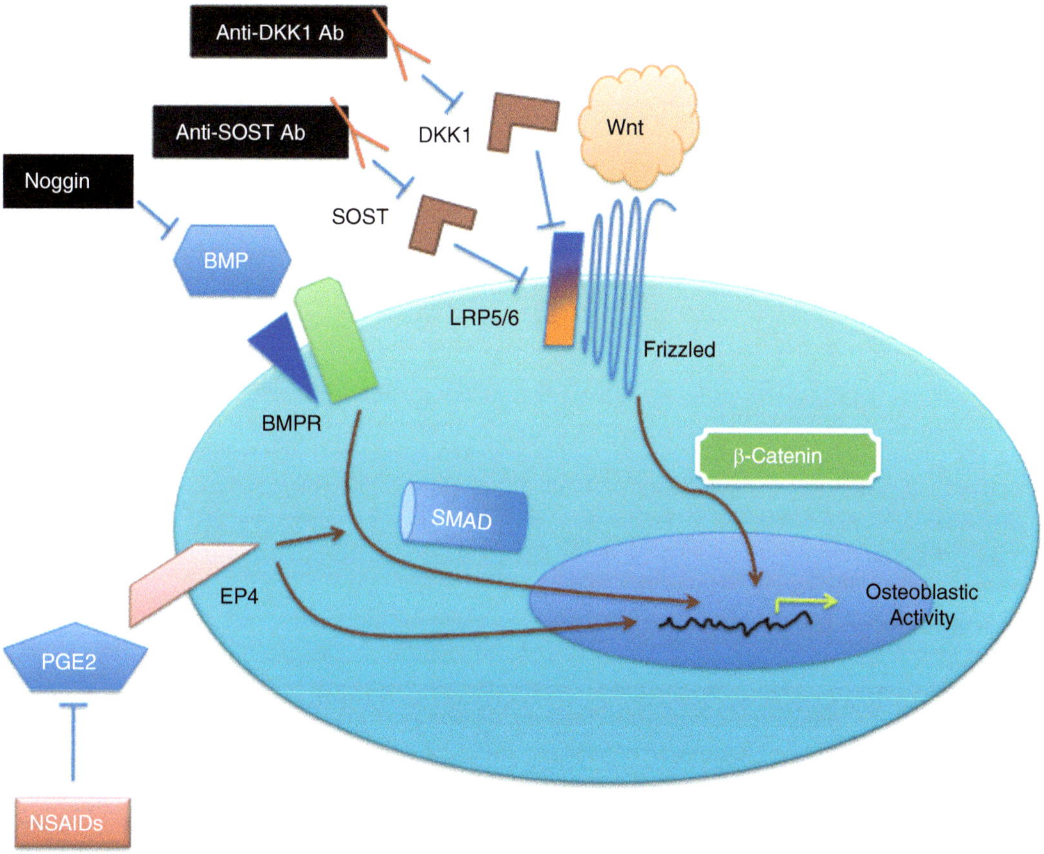

Fig. 13.3 Cartoon showing three major pathways currently associated with bone homeostasis in spondyloarthritis. *Arrows* indicate positive signaling through BMP, Wnt and PGE2. SOST, DKK1, Noggin and NSAIDs are inhibitors of these pathways. Antibodies against DKK1 and SOST can result in activation of osteoblastic pathways by inhibiting the inhibitors DDK1 and SOST respectively. *NSAIDs* Nonsteroidal anti-inflammatory drugs, *PGE2* Prostaglandin E2, EP4: PGE2 receptor type 4, *BMP* bone morphogenic protein, *BMPR* BMP receptor, *SOST* Sclerostin, DKK1: Dickopff 1, *LRP* low density lipoprotein receptor-related protein

BMPs are important for endochondral bone formation and have been demonstrated in hypertrophic cartilage [52, 53]. In a spontaneous model of peripheral ankylosing enthesitis, dactylitis and nail changes similar to PsA, BMP2, BMP6 and BMP7 were detected in different stages of chondrocyte hypertrophy and ankylosing enthesitis [54]. Blocking BMP signaling with noggin prevented the spontaneous arthritis in mice [54]. In addition active BMP signaling was demonstrated in entheseal sites of patients with spondyloarthritis [54]. Recently BMP6 polymorphisms were found to be associated with radiographic severity in Korean AS patients [55]. Thus there is increasing evidence for BMP signaling in the pathogenesis of new bone formation in spondyloarthritis.

Mechanical Stress

A major clinical feature of PsA is enthesitis. Associated with entheseal inflammation, there can be significant new bone formation. The special anatomical organization of the entheseal sites have been well described. Severe enthesitis has been reported in the TNFΔAIRE mice, where TNF overexpression occurs due to deletion of a TNF regulatory region [13]. Unloading of the hind paws by tail suspension resulted in protection from arthritis and enthesitis in this animal model [13]. A distant parallel in human studies is rather correlational with AS patients engaged in more physically demanding jobs having greater radiographic damage [56]. AS patients with bending, twisting, stretching and exposure to vibration at work were more likely to have poor radiographic and functional outcomes [56]. Definitive studies looking at this aspect, though difficult to design, are important to formulate our exercise recommendations for patients with AS.

Spinal Arthritis and Fusion

New bone formation in the form of syndesmophytes eventually leading to spinal fusion and possible bamboo spine is the hallmark of spondyloarthritis. A proportion of PsA patients will develop spinal fusion. Due to the relative inaccessibility of human spinal tissue the pathogenesis of spinal new bone formation is not well understood. There is a strong association of SpA with HLA-B27 which is a class-I Major Histocompatibility Complex molecule that presents antigens to CD8+ T cells. Interestingly, CD8+T cells have been shown to produce wnt10b, a wnt family protein that can stimulate osteoblastic activity [57].

Advanced forms of spinal involvement in PsA may be indistinguishable from AS. In fact patients with significant sacroiliitis in X-rays and having back pain satisfy the criteria for AS, with or without psoriasis. Lessons from the pathogenesis of AS could give us clues on the mechanisms of bone remodeling especially new bone formation seen. It seems logical that spinal inflammation is followed by new bone formation but the evidence for this is scanty. In a study including 39 AS patients followed over 2 years, significantly ($p<0.01$) higher proportion of corners with (6.5 %) than without (2.0 %) inflammation developed syndesmophytes [58]. However, using a different model for analysis and considering all syndesmophytes at follow up, a greater proportion of syndesmophytes developed from corners that had no baseline inflammation (62 % vs. 38 %; P=0.03). It is possible that basal inflammation in corners that developed syndesophytes indeed had inflammation but was missed due to

either sensitivity or timing of MRI. The 'TNF-brake hypothesis' was proposed based on another study on AS patients with a similar design [59]. In this study as well syndesmophytes developed more frequently in vertebral corners with baseline inflammation than in those without (20 % vs. 5.1 %). However syndesmophytes developed more frequently at the corners in which inflammation resolved (14.3 %) than at those where inflammation persisted (2.9 %) suggesting that resolution of inflammation ('TNF-Brake') may drive new bone formation. As outlined above, to date there is no evidence of increased spinal fusion resulting from TNFi therapy. The TNF-transgenic mouse develops sacroiliitis that is controlled by TNF blockade with no evidence of new bone formation [60]. DKK1 blockade however promoted sacroiliac joint ankylosis [60].

There are contradictory reports on Wnt signalling abnormalities in AS. DKK-1 is a circulating inhibitor of the Wnt-signaling pathway. In AS, DKK-1 levels are low, resulting in excess osteoblastic activity [40]. This is not exclusive to AS and has been reported in Diffuse Idiopathic Skeletal Hyperostosis (DISH) where excess bone formation is seen in the spine [61]. These results have been replicated in another AS cohort [44] and when tested in a Jurkat T-cell model, was found to be dysfunctional in AS patients at activating the Wnt pathway [62]. Thus not only is DKK-1 lower in AS, it is also less effective in activating the Wnt signalling pathway.

Lessons from Animal Models

The study of psoriatic arthritis has been hampered by the difficulty in obtaining patient tissues from involved joints. Many animal models share some features with psoriatic arthritis patients (Table 13.1) but the complete phenotype has proven elusive. Inducible deletion of transcription factors JunB and c-Jun within keratinocytes produce skin disease and erosive arthritis with periostitis. Although initially interpreted as a model of joint disease in PsA subsequent evaluation did not support this initial view.

Table 13.1 Animal models of psoriatic arthritis

Species	Manipulation	Skin or nail	Joint	Enthesitis	Dactylitis	Author
Baboon	Spontaneous		+			Rothschild [63]
Mouse	Act1-D10N transgenic	+				Wang et al. [64]
Mouse	Amphiregulin expression under control of INF-AR	+	+			Cook et al. [65]
Mouse	IL-23 Minicircle		+	+		Sherlock et al. [66]
Mouse	Inducible epidermal deletion of JunB and c-Jun	+	+		+	Zenz et al. [67]
Mouse	Lacks endogenous MHC class II molecules	+				Bardos et al. [68]
Mouse	ZAP 70/curdlan		+	+	+	Benham et al. [16, 69], Rehaume et al. [16, 69]
Mouse	K749 KI **Cross with K5.Stat.3C**	+	+	+	+	Ruutu et al. [17]
Mouse	B10Q Mannan injection	+	+	+	+	Khmaladze et al. [70]
Mouse	Doxycycline inducible TNF	+	+	+	+	Retser et al. [71]

Nonetheless, this model demonstrated that deletion of a keratinocyte transcription factor could result in musculoskeletal inflammation that required a functional acquired immune response [67]. In another important model, male DBA/1 mice housed under crowded conditions, which induced fighting and trauma, developed distal arthritis, dactylitis, and ankylosing enthesitis. This phenotype was not observed in germ-free environments and was less severe when male mice were housed in larger cages with filter tops that prevented exposure to the scent from neighboring mice [72, 73]. Transgenic mice lacking endogenous MHC class II develop resorption of the distal phalanx, nail pitting, and hyperkeratosis [74]. In another model. mice lacking β2 microglobulin exhibit paw swelling, joint ankyloses, and nail changes [74].

Introduction HLA-B27/β2 microglobulin transgenes in the rat caused psoriaform skin lesions, nail changes, peripheral non-erosive arthritis, and gut lesions [75]. The arthritis did not develop under germfree conditions. Overexpression of human amphiregulin in the epidermis of transgenic mice produced skin lesions and knee synovitis [65]. K5.Stat3C transgenic mice, who have with constitutively active Stat3 signaling in their keratinocytes, when crossed with F759, who have amplified IL-6 signaling due to impaired SOCS3-negative

feedback, develop a scaling skin disease similar to psoriasis and go on to develop enthesitis, nail deformities, paw swelling and bone erosions [76]. Up to 30 % of baboons may exhibit spondyloarthropy, but psoriasiform lesions have not been identified [63].

The most compelling models of PsA illustrate the potential importance of the IL-23/Th17 pathway in musculoskeletal pathology. In 2 different models, passive induction of collagen-induced arthritis and administration of IL-23 mini circles in B10.R111 mice, Sherlock et al. demonstrated that overexpression of IL-23 produced a mouse model with all the hallmarks of psoriatic arthritis: paw swelling, sacroiliitis and peripheral arthritis, axial enthesitis, and skin psoriasis. This model also had aortic wall and aortic valve inflammation [66]. Of direct relevance to the bone, was the finding of both pathologic bone resorption and new periosteal bone formation. The enthesial interface of tendon and bones in both axial and peripheral joints contain cells which express IL-23 receptor. These IL-23R expressing cells were further characterized in mice as double negative T lymphocytes (CD3+ CD4- CD8-RoRγt+) [66]. Furthermore, the phenotype persisted when CD4+ cells were depleted a finding that underscored the central importance of a non-T helper cell population. This population was found only at the interface of the tendon and bone and not in the belly of the tendon. In response to IL-23, IL-17A, IL-22, and Bmp7 genes were upregulated. Additional experiments in this mice with IL-22 minicircles suggested that IL-22 induced genes associated with inflammation and bone formation while IL-23 promoted gene activation profiles consistent with inflammation and bone resorption. Additional support for the importance of IL-23 in the development of psoriasiform lesions, enthesitis, dactylitis and arthritis was demonstrated in the SKG mice with a Zap 70 mutation that alters T cell receptor signaling. When exposed to curdlan or other fungal products, these mice demonstrate the features outlined above which are IL-23 dependent [16, 17, 69].

Lessons from Genetic Studies

With the advent of genome wide association studies (GWAS) several new genetic loci associated with PsA have been identified. No clear links with bone homeostasis however are evident from the GWAS hits. A large proportion of loci are related to cytokine expression including *TNF*, IL1, IL17, IL22, IL23, NFkB, and *TNFAIP3*. *TNFAIP3* encodes for Act1 that activates NFκB signalling by inhibiting the inhibitor of NFκB Kinase (IKKγ) [77]. Interestingly, the deficiency of Act1 in osteoblasts has limits osteoclastogenesis and this could be an important molecule maintaining bone homeostasis [78].

Genetic studies in PsA have not shown strong links with bone related genes. This could be due to analysis with pooled data from patients with varying phenotypes ranging from severe peripheral erosive arthritis to spinal fusion. Clues from recent genetic studies in AS may be informative in understanding bone homeostasis abnormalities in PsA. The genetic association of *HLA-B27* with PsA is not as strongly as seen in AS but there is a link to spinal involvement in PsA. Despite the strong link to susceptibility, HLA-B27 has not been found to be associated with radiographic progression in prospective studies of AS [79]. However recent literature suggests that HLA-B27 positive individuals, especially men, have higher spinal radiographic damage than HLA-B27 negative individuals [80]. Other MHC loci have been linked to spinal damage in some studies in AS [81, 82]. The short duration of follow up in radiographic progression studies, diagnostic delays and the relative low number of HLA-B27 negative individuals may have decreased the power for detecting B27 influences in prospective studies.

In the initial GWAS studies, two genes *ANTXR2* (codes for Anthrax Toxin Receptor 2) and *PTGER4* (codes for EP4, the Prostaglandin E Receptor 4) that could have an impact on bone homeostasis were identified in the Caucasian population [83–86]. ANTXR2 interacts functionally with LRP6 and thus could impact the Wnt signaling pathway [87]. However, no evidence to date directly links ANTXR2 and bone abnormalities. Prostaglandin E2 (PGE2), through interactions with EP4, can induce mineralized bone formation [88]. The PGE2-EP4 action can be direct or through modification of the BMP signaling pathway (Fig. 13.3). Regular use of high dose non-steroidal anti-inflammatory drugs (NSAIDs) have been reported to slow radiographic progression in a couple of studies [89, 90]. Thus the link between *PTGER4* and AS could have therapeutic implications.

Three other bone related genes were recently associated with AS in Han Chinese [91]. The chloride channel Anoctamin 6 (ANO6 or TMEM16F), coded by *ANO6,* is a transmembrane protein responding to intracellular calcium concentration exposure and aiding the cell surface exposure of phosphatidylserine [92]. TMEM16F is expressed in osteoblasts and deficiency can lead to skeletal abnormalities [93].

The link proteins help stabilize cartilage by linking aggrecan and hyaluronan. Mice lacking the linker protein have abnormalities in cartilage development and bone formation [94]. The linker protein Hyaluronan and proteoglycan link protein 1 (HAPLN1), coded by *HAPLN1*, is an interesting molecule to study in SpA [91]. Antibodies against HAPLN1 have been reported in multiple diseases including PsA [95]. *HAPLN1* is associated with AS in Han Chinese population and with spinal osteophyte formation in the Japanese [91, 96].

The GWAS study on Han Chinese population referred to above also reported an association with *EDIL3* [91]. *EDIL3* codes for EGF-like repeats and discoidin I-like domains 3 also known as Del1. Del1 is an integrin receptor with prominent roles in angiogenesis and prevention of the neutrophil adhesion [97]. Del1 can modulate the Wnt and BMP pathways and could be important in bone homeostasis and pathology seen in PsA [98]. Interestingly bone loss and increased IL-17 production have been reported in mice deficient in Del1 [99]. This may be of therapeutic importance in PsA as local Del1 therapy in this mouse model prevented IL17 overexpression and bone loss [99].

Other interesting genes that have been explored in AS studies are *LMP2, ERAP1, RANK* and *PTGS1* [79, 100]. LMP2 is an immunoproteosome and *LMP2* has been reported to be associated with uveitis [101]. It was found to be associated with radiographic progression in a prospective cohort of AS patients while the aminopeptidase gene *ERAP1* was associated with baseline radiographic severity. In a recent large study on spinal radiographic damage in AS, associations were reported with two genes *RANK* (Receptor Activator of Nuclear Factor kB) and *PTGS1* (Prostaglandin Endoperoxide Synthase 1). RANK, a receptor in osteoclast development and PTGS1, the cyclogenase enzyme involved in the prostaglandin pathway are interesting candidate molecules involved in bone homeostasis SpA.

Treatment Effects on Bone Remodeling

The most compelling findings to support the seminal importance of TNF and the IL-23/Th17 pathway in psoriatic bone damage arise from clinical trials with these agents. Phase III trials with etanercept, adalimumab, golimumab, infliximab and certolizumab demonstrate inhibition of radiographic progression not observed in patients on placebo [102–104]. In addition, ustekinumab, a monoclonal antibody to the p40 subunit present in both IL-12 and IL-23, also limited radiographic progression in phase III trials [105]. Additionally, secukinumab, an agent that blocks

IL-17A resulted in a decline in radiographic progression [106]. In contrast, both methotrexate and anti-TNF agents do not inhibit progression of hand osteophytes in PsA illustrating that bone anabolic pathways are distinct and not tightly bound to bone resorption in the peripheral skeleton [3].

Disease modification in axial spondyloarthritis is being actively explored in recent years. Contrary to previous reports, recent evidence suggests that disease modification is a reasonable treatment target in axial spondyloarthritis. Initial evidence of disease modification in AS with NSAID use and then with TNFi have been demonstrated. The first randomized controlled trial looked at the role of regular celecoxib dosing in comparison to PRN basis celecoxib on reducing spinal radiographic progression in AS patients [89]. There was significantly lower progression of spinal x-rays as assessed by the modified Stoke's AS spine score (mSASSS) by 2 years in patients randomized to receive regular celecoxib [89]. In a follow up secondary analysis of this data, the NSAID effect was present only in patients with elevated baseline CRP [107]. In a small subset of patients from the German GESPIC cohort with baseline syndesmophytes and elevated CRP, a similar effect was seen with high dose NSAIDs [90]. Thus it appears that NSAIDs could potentially slow the progression of syndesmophytes in patients who have risk factors for progression (elevated CRP and damage at baseline). NSAIDs have been implicated in the past to impair fracture healing and surgical spinal fusion, which may indicate a true biological effect on slowing bone formation [108–110].

TNFi are very effective suppressors of inflammation in axial spondyloarthritis. Initial studies however failed to show a disease modifying effect of TNFi in AS [111–114]. Subsequent studies did show suppression of radiographic progression in AS patients especially when started early in the disease course [115, 116]. The earlier we start and the more sustained the treatment with TNFi, the higher the likelihood of seeing a disease modifying effect [115]. Thus earlier studies that included patients with long disease duration and followed for 4 years or less were not able to show this effect. Large studies with long follow up are required to validate these results. In addition, all patients included in these studies started TNFi therapy for symptoms of AS and it is unclear if TNFi can provide additional disease modifying effect in patients who are well controlled on NSAIDs. On the other hand, patients who are well controlled on TNFi often stop their NSAIDs. Does this have an impact on spinal radiographic progression? Several questions remain unanswered.

Conclusion

Recent studies have led to significant improvement in our understanding of the pathogenesis of SpA. Animal models of psoriatic arthritis and genetic studies have led to the unraveling of novel pathways in pathogenesis. More studies on bone homeostasis and pathways triggering new bone formation in SpA are warranted.

References

1. Jacobson JA, Girish G, Jiang Y, Resnick D. Radiographic evaluation of arthritis: inflammatory conditions. Radiology. 2008;248:378–89.
2. Kane D, Stafford L, Bresnihan B, FitzGerald O. A prospective, clinical and radiological study of early psoriatic arthritis: an early synovitis clinic experience. Rheumatology. 2003;42:1460–8.
3. Finzel S, Kraus S, Schmidt S, et al. Bone anabolic changes progress in psoriatic arthritis patients despite treatment with methotrexate or tumour necrosis factor inhibitors. Ann Rheum Dis. 2013;72:1176–81.
4. Lowes MA, Kikuchi T, Fuentes-Duculan J, et al. Psoriasis vulgaris lesions contain discrete populations of Th1 and Th17 T cells. J Invest Dermatol. 2008;128:1207–11.
5. Li N, Yamasaki K, Saito R, et al. Alarmin function of cathelicidin antimicrobial peptide LL37 through IL-36gamma induction in human epidermal keratinocytes. J Immunol. 2014;193:5140–8.
6. Tan AL, Benjamin M, Toumi H, et al. The relationship between the extensor tendon enthesis and the nail in distal interphalangeal joint disease in psoriatic arthritis–a high-resolution MRI and histological study. Rheumatology. 2007;46:253–6.
7. Riol-Blanco L, Ordovas-Montanes J, Perro M, et al. Nociceptive sensory neurons drive interleukin-23-mediated psoriasiform skin inflammation. Nature. 2014;510:157–61.
8. Siegel EL, Orbai AM, Ritchlin CT. Targeting extra-articular manifestations in PsA: a closer look at enthesitis and dactylitis. Curr Opin Rheumatol. 2015;27:111–7.
9. Benjamin M, Moriggl B, Brenner E, Emery P, McGonagle D, Redman S. The "enthesis organ" concept: why enthesopathies may not present as focal insertional disorders. Arthritis Rheum. 2004;50: 3306–13.
10. Benjamin M, McGonagle D. Histopathologic changes at "synovio-entheseal complexes" suggesting a novel mechanism for synovitis in osteoarthritis and spondylarthritis. Arthritis Rheum. 2007;56:3601–9.
11. Benjamin M, McGonagle D. The enthesis organ concept and its relevance to the spondyloarthropathies. Adv Exp Med Biol. 2009;649:57–70.
12. McGonagle D. Imaging the joint and enthesis: insights into pathogenesis of psoriatic arthritis. Ann Rheum Dis. 2005;(64 Suppl 2):ii58–60.
13. Jacques P, Lambrecht S, Verheugen E, et al. Proof of concept: enthesitis and new bone formation in spondyloarthritis are driven by mechanical strain and stromal cells. Ann Rheum Dis. 2014;73:437–45.
14. Healy PJ, Helliwell PS. Dactylitis: pathogenesis and clinical considerations. Curr Rheumatol Rep. 2006;8: 338–41.
15. Healy PJ, Groves C, Chandramohan M, Helliwell PS. MRI changes in psoriatic dactylitis–extent of pathology, relationship to tenderness and correlation with clinical indices. Rheumatology. 2008;47: 92–5.
16. Benham H, Rehaume LM, Hasnain SZ, et al. Interleukin-23 mediates the intestinal response to microbial beta-1,3-glucan and the development of spondyloarthritis pathology in SKG mice. Arthritis Rheumatol. 2014;66:1755–67.
17. Ruutu M, Thomas G, Steck R, et al. beta-glucan triggers spondylarthritis and Crohn's disease-like ileitis in SKG mice. Arthritis Rheum. 2012;64:2211–22.
18. Tan AL, Fukuba E, Halliday NA, Tanner SF, Emery P, McGonagle D. High-resolution MRI assessment of dactylitis in psoriatic arthritis shows flexor tendon pulley and sheath-related enthesitis. Ann Rheum Dis. 2015;74:185–9.
19. Lowes MA, Suarez-Farinas M, Krueger JG. Immunology of psoriasis. Annu Rev Immunol. 2014; 32:227–55.
20. Menon B, Gullick NJ, Walter GJ, et al. Interleukin-17+CD8+ T cells are enriched in the joints of patients with psoriatic arthritis and correlate with disease activity and joint damage progression. Arthritis & Rheumatol. 2014;66:1272–81.
21. Noordenbos T, Yeremenko N, Gofita I, et al. Interleukin-17-positive mast cells contribute to synovial inflammation in spondylarthritis. Arthritis Rheum. 2012;64:99–109.
22. Raychaudhuri SP. Role of IL-17 in psoriasis and psoriatic arthritis. Clin Rev Allergy Immunol. 2013;44: 183–93.
23. Boyce BF. Advances in osteoclast biology reveal potential new drug targets and new roles for osteoclasts. J Bone Miner Res. 2013;28:711–22.

24. Herman S, Muller RB, Kronke G, et al. Induction of osteoclast-associated receptor, a key osteoclast costimulation molecule, in rheumatoid arthritis. Arthritis Rheum. 2008;58:3041–50.

25. Nakashima T, Takayanagi H. Osteoimmunology: crosstalk between the immune and bone systems. J Clin Immunol. 2009;29:555–67.

26. Ritchlin CT, Haas-Smith SA, Li P, Hicks DG, Schwarz EM. Mechanisms of TNF-alpha- and RANKL-mediated osteoclastogenesis and bone resorption in psoriatic arthritis. J Clin Invest. 2003;111:821–31.

27. Kikuta J, Wada Y, Kowada T, et al. Dynamic visualization of RANKL and Th17-mediated osteoclast function. J Clin Invest. 2013;123:866–73.

28. Sato K, Suematsu A, Okamoto K, et al. Th17 functions as an osteoclastogenic helper T cell subset that links T cell activation and bone destruction. J Exp Med. 2006;203:2673–82.

29. Anandarajah AP, Schwarz EM, Totterman S, et al. The effect of etanercept on osteoclast precursor frequency and enhancing bone marrow oedema in patients with psoriatic arthritis. Ann Rheum Dis. 2008;67:296–301.

30. Notley CA, Inglis JJ, Alzabin S, McCann FE, McNamee KE, Williams RO. Blockade of tumor necrosis factor in collagen-induced arthritis reveals a novel immunoregulatory pathway for Th1 and Th17 cells. J Exp Med. 2008;205:2491–7.

31. Sieper J, Appel H, Braun J, Rudwaleit M. Critical appraisal of assessment of structural damage in ankylosing spondylitis: implications for treatment outcomes. Arthritis Rheum. 2008;58:649–56.

32. Klaus A, Birchmeier W. Wnt signalling and its impact on development and cancer. Nat Rev Cancer. 2008;8:387–98.

33. Nusse R, van Ooyen A, Cox D, Fung YK, Varmus H. Mode of proviral activation of a putative mammary oncogene (int-1) on mouse chromosome 15. Nature. 1984;307:131–6.

34. Pinzone JJ, Hall BM, Thudi NK, et al. The role of Dickkopf-1 in bone development, homeostasis, and disease. Blood. 2009;113:517–25.

35. Mikheev AM, Mikheeva SA, Rostomily R, Zarbl H. Dickkopf-1 activates cell death in MDA-MB435 melanoma cells. Biochem Biophys Res Commun. 2007;352:675–80.

36. Niehrs C. Function and biological roles of the Dickkopf family of Wnt modulators. Oncogene. 2006;25:7469–81.

37. Hampton PJ, Ross OK, Reynolds NJ. Increased nuclear beta-catenin in suprabasal involved psoriatic epidermis. Br J Dermatol. 2007;157:1168–77.

38. Seifert O, Soderman J, Skarstedt M, Dienus O, Matussek A. Increased expression of the Wnt signalling inhibitor Dkk-1 in Non-lesional skin and peripheral blood mononuclear cells of patients with plaque psoriasis. Acta Derm Venereol. 2014;95(4): 407–10.

39. Kim KA, Wagle M, Tran K, et al. R-Spondin family members regulate the Wnt pathway by a common mechanism. Mol Biol Cell. 2008;19:2588–96.

40. Diarra D, Stolina M, Polzer K, et al. Dickkopf-1 is a master regulator of joint remodeling. Nat Med. 2007;13:156–63.

41. Marshall MJ, Evans SF, Sharp CA, Powell DE, McCarthy HS, Davie MW. Increased circulating Dickkopf-1 in Paget's disease of bone. Clin Biochem. 2009;42:965–9.

42. Rawadi G, Roman-Roman S. Wnt signalling pathway: a new target for the treatment of osteoporosis. Expert Opin Ther Targets. 2005;9:1063–77.

43. Hopwood B, Tsykin A, Findlay DM, Fazzalari NL. Microarray gene expression profiling of osteoarthritic bone suggests altered bone remodelling. WNT and transforming growth factor-beta/bone morphogenic protein signalling. Arthritis Res Ther. 2007;9:R100.

44. Kwon SR, Lim MJ, Suh CH, et al. Dickkopf-1 level is lower in patients with ankylosing spondylitis than in healthy people and is not influenced by anti-tumor necrosis factor therapy. Rheumatol Int. 2012;32(8): 2523–7.

45. Honsawek S, Tanavalee A, Yuktanandana P, Ngarmukos S, Saetan N, Tantavisut S. Dickkopf-1 (Dkk-1) in plasma and synovial fluid is inversely correlated with radiographic severity of knee osteoarthritis patients. BMC Musculoskelet Disord. 2010;11:257.

46. Daoussis D, Andonopoulos AP. The emerging role of dickkopf-1 in bone biology: is it the main switch controlling bone and joint remodeling? Semin Arthritis Rheum. 2011;41(2):170–7.

47. Garnero P, Tabassi NC, Voorzanger-Rousselot N. Circulating dickkopf-1 and radiological progression in patients with early rheumatoid arthritis treated with etanercept. J Rheumatol. 2008;35:2313–5.

48. Yavropoulou MP, Yovos JG. The role of the Wnt signaling pathway in osteoblast commitment and differentiation. Hormones (Athens). 2007;6:279–94.

49. Massague J. How cells read TGF-beta signals. Nat Rev Mol Cell Biol. 2000;1:169–78.

50. Chen HA, Chen CH, Lin YJ, et al. Association of bone morphogenetic proteins with spinal fusion in ankylosing spondylitis. J Rheumatol. 2010;37: 2126–32.

51. Park MC, Chung SJ, Park YB, Lee SK. Bone and cartilage turnover markers, bone mineral density, and radiographic damage in men with ankylosing spondylitis. Yonsei Med J. 2008;49:288–94.

52. Gitelman SE, Kobrin MS, Ye JQ, Lopez AR, Lee A, Derynck R. Recombinant Vgr-1/BMP-6-expressing tumors induce fibrosis and endochondral bone formation in vivo. J Cell Biol. 1994;126:1595–609.

53. Lories RJ, Luyten FP, de Vlam K. Progress in spondylarthritis. Mechanisms of new bone formation in spondyloarthritis. Arthritis Res Ther. 2009;11:221.

54. Lories RJ, Derese I, Luyten FP. Modulation of bone morphogenetic protein signaling inhibits the onset and progression of ankylosing enthesitis. J Clin Invest. 2005;115:1571–9.

55. Joo YB, Bang SY, Kim TH, et al. Bone morphogenetic protein 6 polymorphisms are associated with radiographic progression in ankylosing spondylitis. PLoS One. 2014;9:e104966.

56. Ward MM, Reveille JD, Learch TJ, Davis Jr JC, Weisman MH. Occupational physical activities and long-term functional and radiographic outcomes in patients with ankylosing spondylitis. Arthritis Rheum. 2008;59:822–32.

57. Terauchi M, Li JY, Bedi B, et al. T lymphocytes amplify the anabolic activity of parathyroid hormone through Wnt10b signaling. Cell Metab. 2009;10: 229–40.

58. Baraliakos X, Listing J, Rudwaleit M, Sieper J, Braun J. The relationship between inflammation and new bone formation in patients with ankylosing spondylitis. Arthritis Res Ther. 2008;10:R104.

59. Maksymowych WP, Chiowchanwisawakit P, Clare T, Pedersen SJ, Ostergaard M, Lambert RG. Inflammatory lesions of the spine on magnetic resonance imaging predict the development of new syndesmophytes in ankylosing spondylitis: evidence of a relationship between inflammation and new bone formation. Arthritis Rheum. 2009;60:93–102.

60. Uderhardt S, Diarra D, Katzenbeisser J, et al. Blockade of Dickkopf (DKK)-1 induces fusion of sacroiliac joints. Ann Rheum Dis. 2010;69:592–7.

61. Senolt L, Hulejova H, Krystufkova O, et al. Low circulating Dickkopf-1 and its link with severity of spinal involvement in diffuse idiopathic skeletal hyperostosis. Ann Rheum Dis. 2012;71(1):71–4.

62. Daoussis D, Liossis SN, Solomou EE, et al. Evidence that Dkk-1 is dysfunctional in ankylosing spondylitis. Arthritis Rheum. 2010;62:150–8.

63. Rothschild BM. Primate spondyloarthropathy. Curr Rheumatol Rep. 2005;7:173–81.

64. Wang Y, Chen J, Zhao Y, Geng L, Song F, Chen HD. Psoriasis is associated with increased levels of serum leptin. Br J Dermatol. 2008;158:1134–5.

65. Cook PW, Brown JR, Cornell KA, Pittelkow MR. Suprabasal expression of human amphiregulin in the epidermis of transgenic mice induces a severe, early-onset, psoriasis-like skin pathology: expression of amphiregulin in the basal epidermis is also associated with synovitis. Exp Dermatol. 2004;13:347–56.

66. Sherlock JP, Joyce-Shaikh B, Turner SP, et al. IL-23 induces spondyloarthropathy by acting on ROR-gammat+CD3+CD4-CD8- entheseal resident T cells. Nat Med. 2012;18:1069–76.

67. Zenz R, Eferl R, Kenner L, et al. Psoriasis-like skin disease and arthritis caused by inducible epidermal deletion of Jun proteins. Nature. 2005;437:369–75.

68. Bardos T, Zhang J, Mikecz K, David CS, Glant TT. Mice lacking endogenous major histocompatibility complex class II develop arthritis resembling psoriatic arthritis at an advanced age. Arthritis Rheum. 2002;46:2465–75.

69. Rehaume LM, Mondot S, Aguirre de Carcer D, et al. ZAP-70 genotype disrupts the relationship between microbiota and host, leading to spondyloarthritis and ileitis in SKG mice. Arthritis Rheumatol. 2014;66: 2780–92.

70. Khmaladze I, Kelkka T, Guerard S, et al. Mannan induces ROS-regulated, IL-17A-dependent psoriasis arthritis-like disease in mice. Proc Natl Acad Sci U S A. 2014;111:E3669–78.

71. Retser E, Schied T, Skryabin BV, et al. Doxycycline-induced expression of transgenic human tumor necrosis factor alpha in adult mice results in psoriasis-like arthritis. Arthritis Rheum. 2013;65:2290–300.

72. Lories RJ, Matthys P, de Vlam K, Derese I, Luyten FP. Ankylosing enthesitis, dactylitis, and onychoperiostitis in male DBA/1 mice: a model of psoriatic arthritis. Ann Rheum Dis. 2004;63:595–8.

73. Braem K, Carter S, Lories RJ. Spontaneous arthritis and ankylosis in male DBA/1 mice: further evidence for a role of behavioral factors in "stress-induced arthritis". Biol Proced Online. 2012;14:10.

74. Khare SD, Luthra HS, David CS. Spontaneous inflammatory arthritis in HLA-B27 transgenic mice lacking beta 2-microglobulin: a model of human spondyloarthropathies. J Exp Med. 1995;182: 1153–8.

75. Yanagisawa H, Richardson JA, Taurog JD, Hammer RE. Characterization of psoriasiform and alopecic skin lesions in HLA-B27 transgenic rats. Am J Pathol. 1995;147:955–64.

76. Yamamoto M, Nakajima K, Takaishi M, et al. Psoriatic inflammation facilitates the onset of arthritis in a mouse model. J Invest Dermatol. 2015;135: 445–53.

77. Li X, Commane M, Nie H, et al. Act1, an NF-kappa B-activating protein. Proc Natl Acad Sci U S A. 2000;97:10489–93.

78. DeSelm CJ, Takahata Y, Warren J, et al. IL-17 mediates estrogen-deficient osteoporosis in an Act1-dependent manner. J Cell Biochem. 2012;113: 2895–902.

79. Haroon N, Maksymowych W, Rahman P, Tsui F, O'Shea F, Inman R. Radiographic severity in ankylosing spondylitis is associated with polymorphism in large multifunctional peptidase 2 (LMP2) in the SPARCC cohort. Arthritis Rheum. 2012;64(4): 1119–26.

80. Ramiro S, Stolwijk C, van Tubergen A, et al. Evolution of radiographic damage in ankylosing spondylitis: a 12 year prospective follow-up of the OASIS study. Ann Rheum Dis. 2015;74:52–9.

81. Ward MM, Hendrey MR, Malley JD, et al. Clinical and immunogenetic prognostic factors for radiographic severity in ankylosing spondylitis. Arthritis Rheum. 2009;61:859–66.

82. Bartolome N, Szczypiorska M, Sanchez A, et al. Genetic polymorphisms inside and outside the MHC improve prediction of AS radiographic severity in addition to clinical variables. Rheumatology (Oxford). 2012;51:1471–8.

83. Australo-Anglo-American Spondyloarthritis Consortium (TASC), Reveille JD, Sims AM, et al. Genome-wide association study of ankylosing spondylitis identifies non-MHC susceptibility loci. Nat Genet. 2010;42:123–7.

84. Chen C, Zhang X, Wang Y. ANTXR2 and IL-1R2 polymorphisms are not associated with ankylosing

spondylitis in Chinese Han population. Rheumatol Int. 2012;32:15–9.

85. Guo C, Xia Y, Yang Q, Qiu R, Zhao H, Liu Q. Association of the ANTXR2 gene polymorphism and ankylosing spondylitis in Chinese Han. Scand J Rheumatol. 2012;41:29–32.

86. The Australo-Anglo-American Spondyloarthritis Consortium (TASC), the Wellcome Trust Case Control Consortium 2 (WTCCC2), Evans DM, et al. Interaction between ERAP1 and HLA-B27 in ankylosing spondylitis implicates peptide handling in the mechanism for HLA-B27 in disease susceptibility. Nat Genet. 2011;43:761–7.

87. Wei W, Lu Q, Chaudry GJ, Leppla SH, Cohen SN. The LDL receptor-related protein LRP6 mediates internalization and lethality of anthrax toxin. Cell. 2006;124:1141–54.

88. Minamizaki T, Yoshiko Y, Kozai K, Aubin JE, Maeda N. EP2 and EP4 receptors differentially mediate MAPK pathways underlying anabolic actions of prostaglandin E2 on bone formation in rat calvaria cell cultures. Bone. 2009;44:1177–85.

89. Wanders A, Heijde D, Landewe R, et al. Nonsteroidal antiinflammatory drugs reduce radiographic progression in patients with ankylosing spondylitis: a randomized clinical trial. Arthritis Rheum. 2005;52:1756–65.

90. Poddubnyy D, Rudwaleit M, Haibel H, et al. Effect of non-steroidal anti-inflammatory drugs on radiographic spinal progression in patients with axial spondyloarthritis: results from the German Spondyloarthritis Inception Cohort. Ann Rheum Dis. 2012;71(10):1616–22.

91. Lin Z, Bei JX, Shen M, et al. A genome-wide association study in Han Chinese identifies new susceptibility loci for ankylosing spondylitis. Nat Genet. 2011;44:73–7.

92. Jacobsen KS, Zeeberg K, Sauter DR, Poulsen KA, Hoffmann EK, Schwab A. The role of TMEM16A (ANO1) and TMEM16F (ANO6) in cell migration. Pflugers Arch. 2013;465:1753–62.

93. Ehlen HW, Chinenkova M, Moser M, et al. Inactivation of anoctamin-6/Tmem16f, a regulator of phosphatidylserine scrambling in osteoblasts, leads to decreased mineral deposition in skeletal tissues. J Bone Miner Res. 2013;28:246–59.

94. Watanabe H, Yamada Y. Mice lacking link protein develop dwarfism and craniofacial abnormalities. Nat Genet. 1999;21:225–9.

95. Austin AK, Hobbs RN, Anderson JC, Butler RC, Ashton BA. Humoral immunity to link protein in patients with inflammatory joint disease, osteoarthritis, and in non-arthritic controls. Ann Rheum Dis. 1988;47:886–92.

96. Urano T, Narusawa K, Shiraki M, et al. Single-nucleotide polymorphism in the hyaluronan and proteoglycan link protein 1 (HAPLN1) gene is associated with spinal osteophyte formation and disc degeneration in Japanese women. Eur Spine J. 2011;20:572–7.

97. Choi EY, Chavakis E, Czabanka MA, et al. Del-1, an endogenous leukocyte-endothelial adhesion inhibitor, limits inflammatory cell recruitment. Science. 2008;322:1101–4.

98. Takai A, Inomata H, Arakawa A, Yakura R, Matsuo-Takasaki M, Sasai Y. Anterior neural development requires Del1, a matrix-associated protein that attenuates canonical Wnt signaling via the Ror2 pathway. Development. 2010;137:3293–302.

99. Eskan MA, Jotwani R, Abe T, et al. The leukocyte integrin antagonist Del-1 inhibits IL-17-mediated inflammatory bone loss. Nat Immunol. 2012;13:465–73.

100. Cortes A, Maksymowych WP, Wordsworth BP, et al. Association study of genes related to bone formation and resorption and the extent of radiographic change in ankylosing spondylitis. Ann Rheum Dis. 2015;74(7):1387–93.

101. Maksymowych WP, Adlam N, Lind D, Russell AS. Polymorphism of the LMP2 gene and disease phenotype in ankylosing spondylitis: no association with disease severity. Clin Rheumatol. 1997;16:461–5.

102. Kavanaugh A, McInnes IB, Mease P, et al. Clinical efficacy, radiographic and safety findings through 5 years of subcutaneous golimumab treatment in patients with active psoriatic arthritis: results from a long-term extension of a randomised, placebo-controlled trial (the GO-REVEAL study). Ann Rheum Dis. 2014;73:1689–94.

103. Ritchlin CT, Kavanaugh A, Gladman DD, et al. Treatment recommendations for psoriatic arthritis. Ann Rheum Dis. 2009;68:1387–94.

104. Mease PJ, Fleischmann R, Deodhar AA, et al. Effect of certolizumab pegol on signs and symptoms in patients with psoriatic arthritis: 24-week results of a Phase 3 double-blind randomised placebo-controlled study (RAPID-PsA). Ann Rheum Dis. 2014;73:48–55.

105. Kavanaugh A, Ritchlin C, Rahman P, et al. Ustekinumab, an anti-IL-12/23 p40 monoclonal antibody, inhibits radiographic progression in patients with active psoriatic arthritis: results of an integrated analysis of radiographic data from the phase 3, multicentre, randomised, double-blind, placebo-controlled PSUMMIT-1 and PSUMMIT-2 trials. Ann Rheum Dis. 2014;73:1000–6.

106. Mease PJ, McInnes IB, Kirkham B, et al. Secukinumab, a human anti–interleukin-17A monoclonal antibody, improves active psoriatic arthritis and inhibits radiographic progression: efficacy and safety data from a phase 3 randomized, multicenter, double-blind, placebo-controlled study. Arthritis Rheum. 2014;66:963.

107. Kroon F, Landewe R, Dougados M, van der Heijde D. Continuous NSAID use reverts the effects of inflammation on radiographic progression in patients with ankylosing spondylitis. Ann Rheum Dis. 2012;71(10):1623–9.

108. Spiro AS, Beil FT, Baranowsky A, et al. BMP-7-induced ectopic bone formation and fracture healing is impaired by systemic NSAID application in C57BL/6-mice. J Orthop Res. 2010;28: 785–91.

109. Li Q, Zhang Z, Cai Z. High-dose ketorolac affects adult spinal fusion: a meta-analysis of the effect of perioperative nonsteroidal anti-inflammatory drugs on spinal fusion. Spine (Phila Pa 1976). 2011;36:E461–8.

110. Glassman SD, Rose SM, Dimar JR, Puno RM, Campbell MJ, Johnson JR. The effect of postoperative nonsteroidal anti-inflammatory drug administration on spinal fusion. Spine (Phila Pa 1976). 1998;23:834–8.

111. van der Heijde D, Landewe R, Einstein S, et al. Radiographic progression of ankylosing spondylitis after up to two years of treatment with etanercept. Arthritis Rheum. 2008;58:1324–31.

112. van der Heijde D, Landewe R, Baraliakos X, et al. Radiographic findings following two years of infliximab therapy in patients with ankylosing spondylitis. Arthritis Rheum. 2008;58:3063–70.

113. van der Heijde D, Salonen D, Weissman BN, et al. Assessment of radiographic progression in the spines of patients with ankylosing spondylitis treated with adalimumab for up to 2 years. Arthritis Res Ther. 2009;11:R127.

114. Baraliakos X, Listing J, Brandt J, et al. Radiographic progression in patients with ankylosing spondylitis after 4 yrs of treatment with the anti-TNF-alpha antibody infliximab. Rheumatology (Oxford). 2007;46: 1450–3.

115. Haroon N, Inman RD, Learch TJ, et al. The impact of tumor necrosis factor alpha inhibitors on radiographic progression in ankylosing spondylitis. Arthritis Rheum. 2013;65:2645–54.

116. Baraliakos X, Haibel H, Listing J, Sieper J, Braun J. Continuous long-term anti-TNF therapy does not lead to an increase in the rate of new bone formation over 8 years in patients with ankylosing spondylitis. Ann Rheum Dis. 2014;73(4):710–5.

Part IV

Clinical Aspects

Wolf-Henning Boehncke

Psoriasis

14

Bahar Shafaeddin Schreve
and Wolf-Henning Boehncke

Abstract

Psoriasis is a common, chronic-recurrent inflammatory dermatosis. Its most typical clinical manifestation are well-demarked, erythemato-squamous plaques, namely on the extensor sites of the extremities. In this case, the diagnosis can easily be made clinically. However, this chronic plaque-type manifestation accounts for only around 70 % of cases. There are numerous other clinical manifestations, including inverse psoriasis lacking scales, acute exanthematic as well as localized manifestations, and finally pustular forms, some of which may represent pathogenetically distinct entities. In these cases, biopsies might be necessary to establish the diagnosis and to exclude numerous differential diagnoses.

Clinical assessment of psoriasis comprises both aspects accessible by physicians' observation as well as patient-reported outcomes. The best-known tool to assess chronic plaque-type psoriasis is the Psoriasis Area and Severity Index (PASI), quantifying the involved body surface area along with the extent of redness, infiltration, and scaling. Given its limitations, numerous modifications of the PASI have been proposed. An alternative approach is to assess psoriasis more globally, e.g. by the Physician Global Assessment (PGA). The most widely used tool to document patient-reported outcomes is the Dermatology Life Quality Index (DLQI), a 10-item questionnaire that can also be used to assess other dermatoses.

Keywords

Plaque-type psoriasis • Guttate psoriasis • Pustular psoriasis • Erythroderma • Inverse psoriasis • Palmoplantar psoriasis • Assessment • Psoriasis area and severity index • Physician global assessment • Dermatology life quality index

B. Shafaeddin Schreve, MD (✉)
Faculty of Medicine, University of Geneva,
Rue Gabrielle-Perret-Gentil 4, Geneva 1211,
Switzerland
e-mail: bahar.shafaeddin@gmail.com

W.-H. Boehncke, MD, MA
Service de Dermatologie et Vénéréologie,
Hopitaux Universitaires de Genève, Geneva
Switzerland

© Springer International Publishing Switzerland 2016
A. Adebajo et al. (eds.), *Psoriatic Arthritis and Psoriasis: Pathology and Clinical Aspects*,
DOI 10.1007/978-3-319-19530-8_14

Psoriasis is among the most common skin diseases, with a wide spectrum of clinical manifestations. This inflammatory skin disease is characterized by its chronic- relapsing course and its genetic predisposition. The hallmark of this disease is altered epidermal differentiation and hyperproliferation as well as inflammation. It classically manifests by erythemato-squamous plaques but there are also other manifestations. It is one of the most prevalent inflammatory skin diseases, affecting around 2 % of the Caucasian population (Europe and North America). The disease is rarer in some genetically distinct populations (Native Americans, African Americans, Eskimos).

Based on disease severity, family history, and genetics, two types of plaque-type psoriasis can be differentiated: Type I psoriasis is characterized by an early onset (<40 years), a severe course, positive family history, and an HLA cw6 positive genotype, while type II psoriasis patients have a later onset (>50 years), a milder course, a negative family history, and no association with HLA cw6.

The heredity of the disease is polygenetic, but is triggered by numerous exogenous and endogenous factors. Exogenous factors comprise trauma (Koebner effect), sunburn, irritative topical therapy, and mechanic trauma. Endogenous factors are infections (streptococcal), drugs (beta-blockers, lithium, and chloroquine) and emotional stress. Patients often improve during the summer and worsen in winter, reflecting how the disease is influenced by different environmental factors. The role of mechanical stress on the disease is illustrated by "Koebner's phenomenon" (or isomorphic response) illustrated in Fig. 14.1, where psoriasis skin lesions are triggered by sites of injury or trauma. Drug-induced flaring of psoriasis is not completely understood. Beta-adrenergic blockers may induce epidermal hyperproliferation by decrease of intraepidermal cyclic AMP, lithium may increase proinflammatory cytokines and stimulate leukocyte recruitment, and chloroquine blocks epidermal transglutaminase which is involved in terminal differentiation of keratinocytes. Infections, especially streptococcal infections of the upper respiratory tract, are recognized triggers of psoriasis. There is also

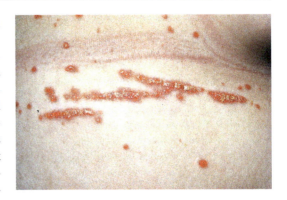

Fig. 14.1 Koebner Phenomenon in plaque-type psoriasis. Typical psoriatic lesions can be triggered through physical trauma such as scratching or cutting (e.g. surgical procedures)

exacerbation or initial manifestation of psoriasis in patients infected by HIV. Alcohol ingestion is also a trigger factor.

Clinical Manifestation

The classic manifestation is **plaque-type psoriasis**, exhibiting well delineated, red, infiltrated plaques covered with silver white scales (Fig. 14.2). Lesions are most active at their edge, sometimes conferring nearly an annular appearance. Scales are easily removed by scratching, and removal results in the appearance of small blood droplets (Auspitz sign) (Fig. 14.3). This is caused by the thinning of the epidermal layer overlying the tips of the dermal papillae which contain dilated and tortuous capillaries, which bleed readily when the scale is removed. Plaques may coalesce into polycyclic or serpiginous patterns, and are usually distributed symmetrically. Predilection sites comprise elbows and knees, the scalp (where they usually do not extend beyond the hairline and may cause non-scarring alopecia; (Fig. 14.4), periumbilical and lumbar regions, but any anatomical site may be affected, including nails. Nail changes are common, and often consist in pitting (best seen under oblique light), oil spots (yellow-brown spots under the nail plate) and dystrophy. Psoriatic arthritis, a seronegative inflammatory arthritis which occurs in the presence of psoriasis may affect up to 30 % of

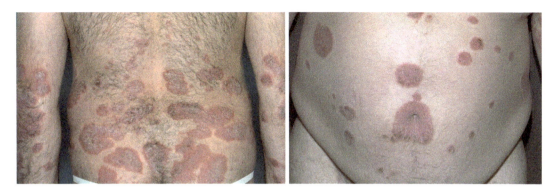

Fig. 14.2 Chronic plaque-type psoriasis in predilection sites, which include the lumbar (*left*) and periumbilical (*right*) areas

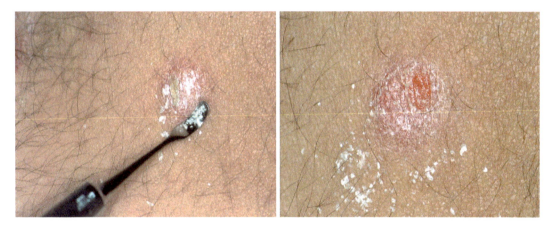

Fig. 14.3 Auspitz phenomenon in chronic plaque-type psoriasis. Scales can easily be removed by gently scratching the lesion, leaving a glossy erythematous area on which blood droplets appear rapidly

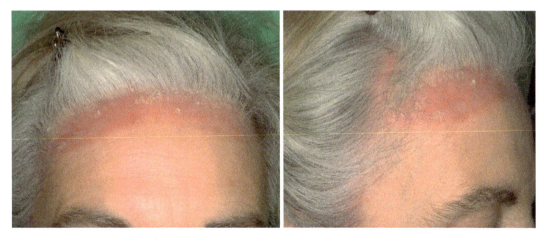

Fig. 14.4 Scalp psoriasis. The scalp is another predilection site. Well-defined erythemato-squamous plaques are often found behind the ears or on the forehead (*above*). Typically, the border of the lesion(s) goes about two fingers wide beyond the scalp

patients (discussed separately). Pruritis is common, especially in scalp and anogenital psoriasis. The morphological variants of psoriasis are illustrated in Table 14.1.

Table 14.1 Clinical classification of psoriasis

Clinical classification of psoriasis
Psoriasis vulgaris
Chronic plaque-type
Acute exanthematic type
Inverse psoriasis
Isolated psoriasis of the nails
Psoriasis pustulosa
Pustular palmoplantar psoriasis (Königsbeck-Berber)
Acrodermatitis continua suppurativa (Hallopeau)
Generalized pustular psoriasis (von Zumbusch)
Impetigo herpetiformis
Pustulous psoriasis of the type of erythema annulare centrifugum
Erythrodermic psoriasis
Psoriatic arthritis

In inverse psoriasis, lesions are located in intertriginous sites such as the groins and axilla, sparing the typical predilection areas. In this type of psoriasis, lesions are sharply defined, dark red moist plaques, and lack the typical scaling (Fig. 14.5) rendering diagnosis difficult. A pustular pattern may be present on the palms and soles.

Acute guttata psoriasis, is an exanthematic inflammatory form of psoriasis (guttata meaning droplet in Latin), and is relatively rare (2 % of all psoriasis). This form is characterized by an eruption of disseminated dark pink or red keratotic papules of 1–2 cm of diameter, with or without scaling, generally appearing on the trunk (but may affect any site of the body), usually sparing the palms and soles (Fig. 14.6). This form occurs often preceded by a beta-hemolytic streptococcal or a viral infection 2–3 weeks prior, especially in children and adolescents. It is a self-limiting disease, resolving within 3–4 months of onset, but its long term prognosis is unknown. Some studies

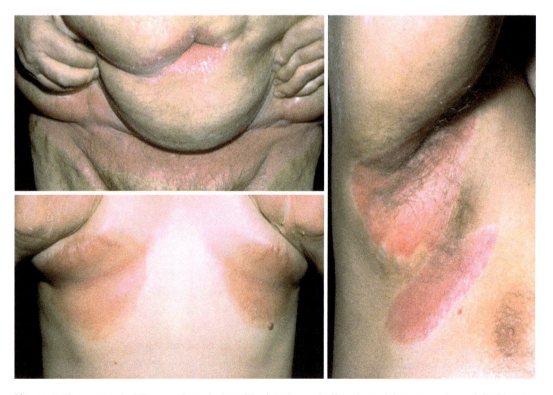

Fig. 14.5 "Inverse psoriasis" spares the typical predilection sites and affects intertriginous areas instead. In this case, the erythema is still sharply demarked, but scaling is usually absent

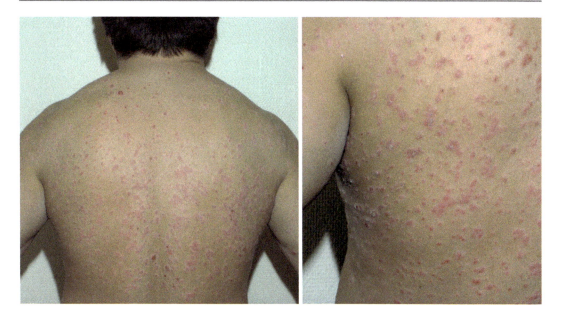

Fig. 14.6 Guttate psoriasis is characterized by the eruptive manifestation of multiple, monomorphic, erythematous keratotic papules, maturing into small plaques

indicated that one third of patients develop into classic chronic plaque disease

Pustular psoriasis must be differentiated from other pustular dermatoses. The pustules are 2–5 mm, deep seated, yellow, develop into reddish macules and crusts, and are present in areas of erythema and scaling and normal skin. The lesions are not associated to hair follicles, and are always sterile. This is a rare form of psoriasis which occurs in adults, and rarely in children. There are known precipitating factors and patients may or may not be known for stable plaque-type psoriasis. Pustular psoriasis is categorized in **localized forms and generalized disease**.

Generalized pustular psoriasis (von Zumbusch) is an acute form of psoriasis with abrupt onset of disseminated small, monomorphic inflammatory sterile pustules in painful inflamed skin. The pustules may evolve into major bullae. Patients often show signs of systemic inflammation such as fever. Triggers of generalized pustular psoriasis are infections, abrupt withdrawal of systemic treatment, and sometimes withdrawal of potent topical corticosteroids. Severe forms of generalized pustular psoriasis may also affect the oral cav-

ity (stomatitis geographica, stomatits areata migrans, lingua geographica). These patients are often seen in an emergency setting due to their acute symptoms. Laboratory examinations show a polymorphonouclear leukocytosis with white blood cells reaching 20,000/μL. Bacterial cultures of tissue show sterile pustules. Blood cultures should be performed because of the risk of superinfection, particularly with S. aureus. Generalized HSV infection must be ruled out with Tzanck tests and viral cultures must be established. Generalized pustular drug eruptions (acute generalized exanthematous pustulosis) may have a similar presentation. The course of this disease is characterized by relapses and remissions over a period of years. It may precede or be followed by psoriasis vulgaris. The prognosis may be dire in the elderly.

Palmoplantar pustular psoriasis consists of yellow-brown sterile pustules located on the palms and soles. a quarter of patients with PP psoriasis also have chronic plaque psoriasis. This form of disease has a different demographic (predominating in women with a 9:1 ratio, more frequent in current or previous smokers (95 %) and a later onset (fourth and fifth decades) and differ-

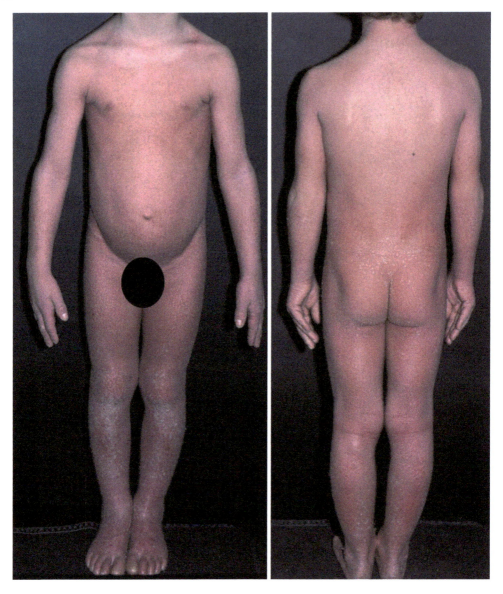

Fig. 14.7 Erythrodermic psoriasis. Psoriasis is one of the dermatoses which can cover the complete skin, resulting in the clinical picture of erythroderma

ent causes. A severe manifestation of localized pustular psoriasis is *acrodermatitis continua suppurativa* affects toes and fingers and confluent pustules, primarily in the area of nails, forming major bullae. This disease is persistent for years and characterized by periods of remission and exacerbations. It may result in loss of finger and/or toe nails.

The differential diagnosis of pustular psoriasis comprises fungal infections, dyshidrotic eczema-

tous dermatitis, irritant or allergic contact dermatitis, herpes simplex virus (HSV) infection (if localized in one site).

Erythrodermic psoriasis is defined as psoriasis affecting the whole body surface (Fig. 14.7). It may arise from any type of psoriasis and may develop progressively or acutely. Factors inducing erythroderma are irritating treatments, sunburns, discontinuation of steroid therapy. This is potentially a life-threatening condition with complications such as protein loss, impaired thermoregulation, electrolyte loss, impaired response, superinfection, and cardiac failure.

Differential Diagnosis

Typical chronic plaque-type psoriasis affecting the classical predilection sites can easily be recognized. The differential diagnosis comprises seborrheic dermatitis, seborrhiasis, and lichen simplex chronicus. Besides, psoriasifrom drug eruptions, caused by drugs such as beta blockers, gold, and methyldopa, are also to be considered. Tinea corporis, often showing much smaller scales, can quickly be excluded with a KOH examination. Mycosis fungoides may sometimes mimick plaque-type psoriasis, as it may present with scaly plaques. Typically plaques in the case of mycosis fungoides are ovally shaped and localized on the trunk Rather than the typical predilection sites of psoriasis.

Acute rashes consisting of erythematosquamous lesions in a patient with positive personal or family history are also easy to diagnose. The presence of an Auspitz phenomenon is also a helpful clue to this diagnosis.

When the lesions are less typical, it may be difficult to diagnose the disease. One must search for subtle history (i.e. medication, recent infections), perform further diagnostic tests (syphilis serology, HIV) and a biopsy may be required. One must always take into account the possibility of drug-induced psoriasis, but in the absence of distinct patient and family history of psoriasis, it may be difficult to distinguish a drug-induced psoriasis from a psoriasiform drug eruption.

The differential diagnosis of acute guttata psoriasis comprises maculopapular drug eruption, secondary syphilis, and pityriasis rosea, while in the case of inverse psoriasis fungal infections, Hailey-Hailey, intertrigo, and extramammary Paget disease should be considered. Glucagonoma syndrome is an important differential as lesions are similar to inverse psoriasis. Nail psoriasis might at times mimick onychomycosis, as it may cause onychodystrophy.

Table 14.2 Differential diagnosis of psoriasis

Manifestations of psoriasis	Differential diagnosis
Psoriasis vulgaris	Bowen's disease Parapsoriasis en plaques Mycosis fungoides Nummular ecznema CDLE Tinea Reiter's disease Seborrhoic dermatitis
Acute exanthematic type	Syphilis II Psoriasiform drug reaction HIV exanthema Pityrisis lichenoides chronica Irritated pityriasis rosea SCLE
Isolated psoriatic plaque	Tinea Eczema CDLE Psoriasiform lupus vulgaris Pagetoid reticulosis Basal cell carcinoma lichen simplex chronicus
Isolated psoriasis of the scalp	Tinea amiantacea Seborrrhiasis
Inverse psoraisis	Intertrigo Candidosis Extramamary Paget's disease
Generalized pustular psoriasis	Acute generalized pustulosa
Pustular palmoplantar psoriasis	Hand –and –feet dermatitis Palmoplantar pustulosis

Table 14.2 summarizes the most important differential diagnoses of psoriasis.

Assessment Tools for Psoriasis

Accurate and reliable assessments tools are important to document the severity of psoriasis and to quantify the effect of the treatment. Historically, the extent of the lesions as well as redness, infiltration, and scaling were assessed, eventually leading to the development of the Psoriasis Area and Severity Index (PASI, see below). The PASI is often used in the context of clinical trials, while many practicing dermatologists find it impractical for use in the daily practice. Thus, alternative measures such as the extent of the lesions in percent of the body surface (Body Surface Affected – BSA), or global assessments (Physician Global Assessment – PGA) are widely used.

In recent years, the importance of the patients' perspective became increasingly acknowledged. Thus, tools to document patient reported outcomes (PROs) were developed, with the Dermatology Life Quality Index (DLQI) being currently the most widely used tool for this purpose in the indication of psoriasis.

In many countries, the combination of PASI, BSA, and DLQI is being used as a reference point to classify psoriasis as being either "mild" or "moderate-to-severe", with the cut-off being a PASI, BSA, or DLQI of 10 ("rule of 10s").

The **PASI** is currently the most widely used assessment tool in the context of clinical trials. Many trials look at a 75 % reduction in this score as the primary end point (PASI75). It takes into account the extent of the lesions, along with redness, infiltration, and scaling. Head, arms, trunk, and legs are being assessed separately.

The body surface area is commonly estimated using the rule of nines: In an adult, the head accounts for 9 % of the body surface area, each arm represents 9 %, the front of the trunk is 18 %, the back is 18 %, and each leg accounts for 18 % of the body surface area. When assessing the percent of affected body surface, the patient' hand can be used as a hint, with the palm corresponding to approximately 1 % of the patient's body surface. Once the percentage of the affected body surface is established for a given anatomic site, the percentage is transformed into a numerical score. The severity of redness, infiltration, and scaling is done based on a scale from "0" to "3", corresponding to "none", "mild", "moderate", and "severe". Finally, the results for the different anatomical sites are "weighted", using a multiplier, the addition of the resulting numbers gives the final absolute PASI. To facilitate the calculation of the PASI, score sheets, calculators, and even aps for smartphones exist.

The PASI shows considerable intra-rater and inter-rater variability, the former often diminishing with experience, while the latter can be reduced through vigorous PASI training. The

Table 14.3 Example of a 6-point static Physician Global Assesment (PGA)

Physician Global Assessment (PGA)	
5 severe	Very marked plaque elevation, scaling, and/or erythema
4 moderate to severe	Marked plaque elevation, scaling, and/or erythema
3 mild to moderate	Moderate plaque elevation, scaling, and/or erythema
2 mild	Slight plaque elevation, scaling, and/or erythema
1 almost clear	Intermediate between mild and clear
0 clear	No signs of psoriasis (postinflammatory hyperpigmentation may be present)

domain usually showing the largest variability is the estimation of the area component. Additional limitations of the PASI include its low power of discrimination in mild psoriasis and its limitation to plaque-type psoriasis. Moreover, affection of different anatomical sites is not weighted with regard to the significance for the patient: Involvement of visible areas such as hands or face is assessed in the same way by the PASI as sites that can easily be covered by clothes (such as the trunk), but the impact on the patient is different.

Given the limitations of the PASI on one hand and the concerns of practicing dermatologists to use the PASI as part of their daily practice on the other hand, different types of **Physician Global Assessment** (PGA) were developed. Principally, static and dynamic scales can be differentiated, the latter aiming at assessing improvement of psoriasis over time. Numerous static PGAs have been developed, where the investigator assigns a single estimate of the patient's overall severity of disease on a 5, 6 or 7 point ordinal rating ranging from clear to very severe psoriasis. Table 14.3 gives an example of a 6-point static PGA. Generally, this method is a more intuitive one and does not integrate plaque morphology or BSA.

The **Lattice System Physicians' Global assessment tool (LS-PGA)** was developed to address deficiencies in other assessments of psoriasis: The PASI can be difficult to use and has no clear clinical frame of reference, while numerous

PGA systems exist in parralel. The LS-PGA addresses these deficiencies by providing a clear method of rating and clinical description of the results in an eight step method. This system has a more quantitative approach to global assessment of disease severity as it integrates the BSA involved and the plaque morphology. It gives more weight to plaque elevation than to scale or redness, which is not the case in the PASI. This is due to the fact that scaling and redness may vary with environmental conditions and other factors (emollients, ambient conditions). Plaque elevation is given more weight as it may be more related to inflammation and proliferation, hallmarks of psoriasis activity.

PASI, PGA, and LS-PGA show high correlations with each other. The LS-PGA has the advantage of having a better reproducibility from one session to the next than the PGA and less variation from one physician to another when compared to the PASI.

None of the above-mentioned assessment tools take into account the patient's perspective. The currently most widely used tool to document the latter is the **Dermatology Life Quality Index** (DLQI). This tool was developed as a simple compact and practical questionnaire and has been shown to be reliable and valid in dermatology clinical settings. It contains ten questions, the answers of the patients yielding between 0 and 3 points. The score ranges from 0 to 30, with 0 being the best score documenting absence of any burden of disease, and 30 documenting the maximum burden of disease. A change of five or more points is considered to be clinically meaningful. It is suggested that a DLQI below five should be a treatment goal in psoriasis. The DLQI is intended for use in dermatology at large and therefore does not specifically focus on psoriasis. Other questionnaires evaluating perception and social and emotional impact of a disease, such as the SF 36 or EuroQOL 5D, can generally be used in all clinical specialties, but their use to assess psoriasis in particular is often limited to clinical studies.

In recent years, several experts have suggested additional tools to document patient reported outcomes, e.g. the Patient Benefit Index (PBI). It will be important to carefully validate and evaluate the new tools, as well as potential new tools attempting to "objectively" measure disease activity and severity in psoriasis. Ideally, this should be done through a rigid, well-defined process. A good example for a comprehensive approach to develop clinical assessment tools is OMERACT in rheumatology. With IDEOM, there is now an initiative aiming at implementing a similar approach in dermatology.

Scalp Psoriasis: Clinical Features and Assessment

15

William Tuong and April W. Armstrong

Abstract

Many patients with psoriasis have scalp lesions as well. Progressive disease may lead to worsening quality of life. Specific clinical features of scalp psoriasis may help differentiate it from other dermatological diseases, such as seborrheic dermatitis. Several clinical assessment tools have been developed to help dermatologist ascertain severity of scalp disease.

Keywords

Scalp • Psoriasis • Clinical features • Clinical assessment • Differential diagnosis

Introduction

Psoriasis may initially present on the scalp in 25–50 % of patients [1–3]. Overall, psoriatic scalp lesions are estimated to affect 40–90 % of patients with psoriasis [1, 2]. Scalp lesions have also been associated with an increased risk for psoriatic arthritis [3]. Progressive disease may significantly lower quality of life, which emphasizes the importance of early diagnosis and treatment [2]. The clinical features and means of assessing scalp psoriasis severity are discussed below.

Clinical Features

Scalp psoriasis may have similar features to psoriatic lesions found elsewhere on the skin [4]. Specifically, the typical lesions of scalp psoriasis are well-demarcated, thick, asymmetric plaques with silver-white scale (Fig. 15.1) [2, 5]. However, mild scalp psoriasis may present with minimal scaling and erythema [4]. An important clinical

W. Tuong, MD
Department of Dermatology, University of California Davis, Sacramento, CA, USA

A.W. Armstrong, MD, MPH (✉)
Department of Dermatology,
University of Colorado Denver,
11801 E. 17th Avenue, Campus Mailbox 8127,
Aurora, CO 80045, USA
e-mail: aprilarmstrong@post.harvard.edu

© Springer International Publishing Switzerland 2016
A. Adebajo et al. (eds.), *Psoriatic Arthritis and Psoriasis: Pathology and Clinical Aspects*,
DOI 10.1007/978-3-319-19530-8_15

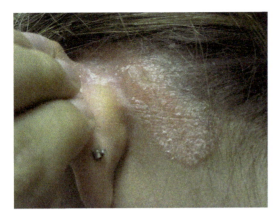

Fig. 15.1 Post auricular well-defined, erythematous plaque with thick silvery scale

feature is the extension of plaques past the hairline to involve the adjacent skin of the face, neck, or post-auricular regions [2, 4]. Pruritus associated with scalp lesions may also be a significant complaint amongst some patients [2].

Although scalp psoriasis does not commonly cause hair loss [4], several reports indicate that this may be an important clinical feature among some patients [6–8]. The largest case series of 47 patients with acute or chronic hair loss and scalp psoriasis found that circumscribed alopecia (75 % of patients) was more common than diffuse alopecia (25 %) [8]. Although most patients showed complete hair regrowth after psoriasis treatment, five patients demonstrated residual scarring [8]. Although several case reports have suggested that scalp psoriasis may cause scarring alopecia, the pathogenesis remains unclear [6, 7].

Clinical Assessment

The Psoriasis Area and Severity Index (PASI) is considered the standard assessment tool for psoriasis. To review, the PASI system grades the severity of erythema, induration, and desquamation present on the head, upper extremities, lower extremities, and trunk with a 5-point scale (0 = absent to 4 = most severe) [9]. These scores are weighted according to the surface area of the evaluated region (head = 0.1, upper extremities = 0.2,

trunk = 0.3, and lower extremities = 0.4) [9]. Weighted scores are multiplied by an integer (0 = 0 % to 6 = 90–100 %) that represents the amount of surface area affected, yielding a final score between zero and 72 [9].

Several scoring systems have modified the PASI to help determine the severity of scalp psoriasis. The Psoriasis Scalp Severity Index (PSSI) [10] and Scalp-modified PASI (S-mPASI) [11] exclusively assess severity of scalp disease along the parameters of erythema, induration, and desquamation. Specifically, the PSSI uses a 5-point scale to grade the three aforementioned clinical parameters [10]. The parameter scores are summed and multiplied by an integer (0–6) that represents the area of affected scalp. The PSSI score ranges from zero to 72 [10]. The S-mPASI uses a similar calculation, but multiplies the disease severity score by a constant integer of 0.1 to yield a score between 0 and 7.2 [11].

Other instruments include the Total Severity Scale (TSS) [12], the Scalp-specific Physician's Global Assessment (S-PGA) [11], and the Global Severity Score (GSS) [12]. The TSS scores the scalp on the three PASI parameters and sums these three values to produce a score that ranges between zero and nine [12]. The S-PGA provides an overall assessment of current scalp disease compared to baseline severity using a 5-point scale (−2 = much worse to 2 = much improvement) [11]. The GSS uses a 6-point scale (0 = none to 5 = very severe) to evaluate overall severity of scalp disease [12].

Differential Diagnosis

Several common diseases should be differentiated from scalp psoriasis during clinical assessment. Seborrheic dermatitis may also present with well-defined, scaly erythematous patches on the scalp. However, the scales of seborrheic dermatitis are typically greasy-appearing and commonly involve other skin sites, such as the nasolabial folds, ears, eyebrows, and chest. Moreover, non-inflammatory tinea capitis usually presents with fine scaling and ovoid patches of alopecia.

References

1. Farber EM, Nall L. Natural history and treatment of scalp psoriasis. Cutis. 1992;49(6):396–400.
2. van de Kerkhof PC, Franssen ME. Psoriasis of the scalp. Diagnosis and management. Am J Clin Dermatol. 2001;2(3):159–65.
3. Wilson FC, Icen M, Crowson CS, McEvoy MT, Gabriel SE, Kremers HM. Incidence and clinical predictors of psoriatic arthritis in patients with psoriasis: a population-based study. Arthritis Rheum. 2009; 61(2):233–9. doi:10.1002/art.24172.
4. Crowley J. Scalp psoriasis: an overview of the disease and available therapies. J Drugs Dermatol. 2010; 9(8):912–8.
5. Wozel G. Psoriasis treatment in difficult locations: scalp, nails, and intertriginous areas. Clin Dermatol. 2008;26(5):448–59. doi:10.1016/j.clindermatol.2007. 10.026.
6. Almeida MC, Romiti R, Doche I, Valente NY, Donati A. Psoriatic scarring alopecia. An Bras Dermatol. 2013;88(6 Suppl 1):29–31. doi:10.1590/abd1806-4841.20132241.
7. Bardazzi F, Fanti PA, Orlandi C, Chieregato C, Misciali C. Psoriatic scarring alopecia: observations in four patients. Int J Dermatol. 1999;38(10):765–8.
8. Runne U, Kroneisen-Wiersma P. Psoriatic alopecia: acute and chronic hair loss in 47 patients with scalp psoriasis. Dermatology. 1992;185(2):82–7.
9. Fredriksson T, Pettersson U. Severe psoriasis – oral therapy with a new retinoid. Dermatologica. 1978; 157(4):238–44.
10. Thaci D, Daiber W, Boehncke WH, Kaufmann R. Calcipotriol solution for the treatment of scalp psoriasis: evaluation of efficacy, safety and acceptance in 3,396 patients. Dermatology. 2001; 203(2):153–6.
11. Krell J, Nelson C, Spencer L, Miller S. An open-label study evaluating the efficacy and tolerability of alefacept for the treatment of scalp psoriasis. J Am Acad Dermatol. 2008;58(4):609–16. doi:10.1016/j.jaad. 2007.12.031.
12. Reygagne P, Mrowietz U, Decroix J, de Waard-van der Spek FB, Acebes LO, Figueiredo A, et al. Clobetasol propionate shampoo 0.05% and calcipotriol solution 0.005%: a randomized comparison of efficacy and safety in subjects with scalp psoriasis. J Dermatolog Treat. 2005;16(1):31–6. doi:10.1080/09546630410024853.

Nail Psoriasis: Clinical Features and Assessment

William Tuong and April W. Armstrong

Abstract

Many patients with psoriasis have involvement of the nails. Nail psoriasis can range from asymptomatic, limited involvement to being physically and functionally debilitating. Psoriatic lesions affecting the nail matrix can lead to pitting, leukonychia, red spots on the lunula, and nail plate crumbling. Moreover, nail bed lesions may result in onycholysis, splinter hemorrhages, oil drop discoloration, or nail bed hyperkeratosis. Clinical assessment of disease severity can be performed through various tools and may help clinicians track progress and response to treatment.

Keywords

Nail • Psoriasis • Clinical features • Clinical assessment • Differential diagnosis

Introduction

Several epidemiological studies indicate that the majority of patients with psoriasis have involvement of the nails as well [1–3]. Specifically, between 80 and 90 % of psoriatic patients are estimated to develop nail psoriasis in their lifetime [4, 5]. Although early stage nail

W. Tuong, MD
Department of Dermatology, University of California Davis, Sacramento, CA, USA

A.W. Armstrong, MD, MPH (✉)
Department of Dermatology, University of Colorado Denver, 11801 E. 17th Avenue, Campus Mailbox 8127, Aurora, CO 80045, USA
e-mail: aprilarmstrong@post.harvard.edu

psoriasis is often asymptomatic, progressive disease can lead to worsening physical and psychological functioning [6]. Moreover, the data regarding the association between nail changes and psoriatic arthritis are mixed. In particular, onycholysis and other nail dystrophies may be associated with developing psoriatic arthritis later in life [7, 8]. However, a separate study found low correlation between severity of nail disease and joint symptoms [9]. Taken together, the data emphasize the complex phenotype of psoriasis and its potential effect on skin, nails, and joints.

The clinical signs of nail psoriasis are attributable to psoriatic lesions that extend to the nail matrix or nail bed. Psoriatic lesions affecting the

© Springer International Publishing Switzerland 2016
A. Adebajo et al. (eds.), *Psoriatic Arthritis and Psoriasis: Pathology and Clinical Aspects*,
DOI 10.1007/978-3-319-19530-8_16

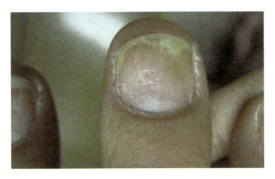

Fig. 16.1 Fingernail with proximal pitting, right-sided oil drop discoloration, distal onycholysis, and distal splinter hemorrhaging

nail matrix can lead to pitting, leukonychia, red spots on the lunula, and nail plate crumbling. Moreover, nail bed lesions may result in onycholysis, splinter hemorrhages, oil drop discoloration, or nail bed hyperkeratosis. These clinical features are discussed further below and several are depicted in Fig. 16.1.

Clinical Features

Nail Matrix Disease

Pitting is a common clinical feature of nail psoriasis [10, 11] and is characterized by superficial depressions in the nail plate [12]. Psoriatic lesions involving the dorsal (proximal) nail matrix lead to shallow punctate depressions [12], whereas deeper pits indicate involvement of the intermediate and ventral nail matrices [13]. Moreover, leukonychia are opaque white lesions in the nail plate caused by inflammation in the intermediate nail matrix [14]. Although it has been traditionally considered a common finding among nail psoriasis patients, several studies indicate that leukonychia lacks specificity and may be less helpful in diagnosing nail psoriasis if found exclusively [15, 16].

Other clinical findings caused by nail matrix disease are red spots in the lunula and nail plate crumbling. Red spots in the lunula are erythematous lesions located within the white crescent-shaped area at the nail base. It is an uncommon

finding [16] that may indicate the presence of dilated vasculature in the nail matrix [17]. Severe inflammation of the nail matrix may lead to compromised keratinization of the nail plate and crumbling [18].

Nail Bed Disease

Onycholysis is common feature of nail psoriasis [2, 16] and refers to the distal separation of the nail bed from the nail plate [12]. Its specificity for nail psoriasis may be higher if the area of detachment is bordered by erythema [12]. Importantly, onycholysis compromises the protective barrier around the nail parenchyma and increases the risk of local infection [5].

Several other clinical features are due to nail bed disease. Splinter hemorrhages are minute, reddish-brown lines from focal rupture of longitudinal vasculature within the nail bed [13]. Although its prevalence is significantly higher among patients with nail psoriasis [16], splinter hemorrhages can also be caused by trauma or indicate systemic disease, such as infective endocarditis [19]. The translucent red-yellow focal discoloration of the nail bed is called the "oil drop" or "salmon-spot" sign [12]. It is considered a specific feature of nail psoriasis that represents accumulation of cellular debris and serum within a focal area of separation between the nail plate and nail bed [13]. Additionally, subungual hyperkeratosis clinically presents as nail plate thickening. Although it is a non-specific feature, subungual hyperkeratosis due to psoriasis can exhibit a white-silvery appearance not commonly seen in other nail diseases [13].

Clinical Assessment

The Psoriasis Area and Severity Index (PASI) is the considered the standard assessment tool for psoriasis involving the skin. However, numerous scoring systems have been proposed for nail psoriasis because the PASI does not include an evaluation of nail involvement.

The Nail Psoriasis Severity Index (NAPSI) is a commonly used scoring system among psoriasis clinical trials [20] that has demonstrated good reproducibility [21] and inter-rater reliability [22]. In this system, the nail is divided into four quadrants and assessed on the presence or absence of nail matrix findings (pitting, leukonychia, red spots in the lunula, and crumbling) or nail bed changes (onycholysis, splinter hemorrhages, oil drop/salmon-spot sign, and subungual hyperkeratosis) [21]. For each quadrant, one point is given if any nail matrix findings are found and one point is given for the presence of any nail bed signs [21]. The nail matrix score and nail bed score are summed to produce a total score for each nail that ranges from 0 to 8 [21]. The total possible score for fingernails ranges from 0 to 80. If the toenails are included, the total score ranges from 0 to 160 [21].

However, the NAPSI may lack adequate sensitivity to capture meaningful clinical improvements [23, 24]. As such, the modified NAPSI (mNAPSI) was created to better account for the severity of certain nail changes [24]. Specifically, pitting, onycholysis and oil-drop discoloration (evaluated together), and crumbling are each graded from 0 to 3 depending on severity [24]. Leukonychia, splinter hemorrhages, hyperkeratosis, and red spots in the lunula are each scored as either present (score of 1) or absent (score of 0) [24]. Therefore, each nail has a possible score of 0–13 or 0–130 if all fingernails are considered [24].

Several other scoring systems have been developed. The Nail Area Severity (NAS) system scores the area of pitting, subungual hyperkeratosis, onycholysis, and oil-drop dyschromia on a 5-point scale (0 = none and 4 = very severe) [25]. Alternatively, the Nijmegen-Nail psoriasis Activity Index tooL (N-NAIL) scores five features of nail psoriasis (onycholysis/oil-drop, pitting, crumbling, Beau's lines, and subungual hyperkeratosis) on a 4-point scale [26].

The scoring systems described in this section are primarily used in clinical trials, and their detailed evaluation of nail changes may not be feasible in outpatient settings. Serial digital photographs may be a more practical means to track the progress of patients with nail psoriasis.

Differential Diagnosis

The differential diagnosis for nail psoriasis includes several diseases, and the most commonly encountered are discussed here. Onychomycosis shares several similar clinical features with nail psoriasis, such as nail thickening, discoloration, and onycholysis. However, onychomycosis is more likely to affect toenails and typically involves fewer digits compared to psoriasis. Additionally, nail pitting is less common in onychomycosis. It may be useful to rule out onychomycosis with a fungal culture or KOH preparation of scrapings. Lichen planus of the nails can be differentiated from nail psoriasis by several clinical features, such as longitudinal splitting, longitudinal melonychia, onychorrhexis, nail plate thinning, and the presence of dorsal pterygium. Although both psoriasis and alopecia areata may cause nail pitting, patchy areas of hair loss is more suggestive of the latter.

References

1. de Jong EM, Seegers BA, Gulinck MK, Boezeman JB, van de Kerkhof PC. Psoriasis of the nails associated with disability in a large number of patients: results of a recent interview with 1,728 patients. Dermatology. 1996;193(4):300–3.
2. Brazzelli V, Carugno A, Alborghetti A, Grasso V, Cananzi R, Fornara L, et al. Prevalence, severity and clinical features of psoriasis in fingernails and toenails in adult patients: Italian experience. J Eur Acad Dermatol Venereol. 2012;26(11):1354–9. doi: 10.1111/j.1468-3083.2011.04289.x.
3. Kyriakou A, Patsatsi A, Sotiriadis D. Detailed analysis of specific nail psoriasis features and their correlations with clinical parameters: a cross-sectional study. Dermatology. 2011;223(3):222–9. doi:10.1159/ 000332974.
4. Baran R. The burden of nail psoriasis: an introduction. Dermatology. 2010;221 Suppl 1:1–5. doi:10.1159/ 000316169.
5. de Berker D. Management of nail psoriasis. Clin Exp Dermatol. 2000;25(5):357–62.

6. Ortonne JP, Baran R, Corvest M, Schmitt C, Voisard JJ, Taieb C. Development and validation of nail psoriasis quality of life scale (NPQ10). J Eur Acad Dermatol Venereol. 2010;24(1):22–7.

7. Love TJ, Gudjonsson JE, Valdimarsson H, Gudbjornsson B. Small joint involvement in psoriatic arthritis is associated with onycholysis: the Reykjavik Psoriatic Arthritis Study. Scand J Rheumatol. 2010;39(4):299–302. doi:10.3109/03009741003604559.

8. Wilson FC, Icen M, Crowson CS, McEvoy MT, Gabriel SE, Kremers HM. Incidence and clinical predictors of psoriatic arthritis in patients with psoriasis: a population-based study. Arthritis Rheum. 2009;61(2):233–9. doi:10.1002/art.24172.

9. Wittkowski KM, Leonardi C, Gottlieb A, Menter A, Krueger GG, Tebbey PW, et al. Clinical symptoms of skin, nails, and joints manifest independently in patients with concomitant psoriasis and psoriatic arthritis. PLoS One. 2011;6(6):e20279. doi:10.1371/journal.pone.0020279.

10. Salomon J, Szepietowski JC, Proniewicz A. Psoriatic nails: a prospective clinical study. J Cutan Med Surg. 2003;7(4):317–21. doi:10.1007/s10227-002-0143-0.

11. Tham SN, Lim JJ, Tay SH, Chiew YF, Chua TN, Tan E, et al. Clinical observations on nail changes in psoriasis. Ann Acad Med Singapore. 1988;17(4):482–5.

12. Tan ES, Chong WS, Tey HL. Nail psoriasis: a review. Am J Clin Dermatol. 2012;13(6):375–88. doi:10.2165/11597000-000000000-00000.

13. Jiaravuthisan MM, Sasseville D, Vender RB, Murphy F, Muhn CY. Psoriasis of the nail: anatomy, pathology, clinical presentation, and a review of the literature on therapy. J Am Acad Dermatol. 2007;57(1):1–27. doi:10.1016/j.jaad.2005.07.073.

14. Sandre MK, Rohekar S. Psoriatic arthritis and nail changes: exploring the relationship. Semin Arthritis Rheum. 2014;44(2):162–9. doi:10.1016/j.semarthrit.2014.05.002.

15. van der Velden HM, Klaassen KM, van de Kerkhof PC, Pasch MC. Fingernail psoriasis reconsidered: a case-control study. J Am Acad Dermatol. 2013;69(2):245–52. doi:10.1016/j.jaad.2013.02.009.

16. Garzitto A, Ricceri F, Tripo L, Pescitelli L, Prignano F. Possible reconsideration of the Nail Psoriasis Severity Index (NAPSI) score. J Am Acad Dermatol. 2013;69(6):1053–4. doi:10.1016/j.jaad.2013.06.051.

17. Morrissey KA, Rubin AI. Histopathology of the red lunula: new histologic features and clinical correlations of a rare type of erythronychia. J Cutan Pathol. 2013;40(11):972–5. doi:10.1111/cup.12218.

18. Omura EF. Histopathology of the nail. Dermatol Clin. 1985;3(3):531–41.

19. Wolff K, Johnson RA, Saavedra AP, Fitzpatrick TB. In: Wolff K, Johnson RA, Saavedra AP. Fitzpatrick's color atlas and synopsis of clinical dermatology. 7th ed. New York: McGraw-Hill Medical; 2013.

20. Mease PJ. Measures of psoriatic arthritis: Tender and Swollen Joint Assessment, Psoriasis Area and Severity Index (PASI), Nail Psoriasis Severity Index (NAPSI), Modified Nail Psoriasis Severity Index (mNAPSI), Mander/Newcastle Enthesitis Index (MEI), Leeds Enthesitis Index (LEI), Spondyloarthritis Research Consortium of Canada (SPARCC), Maastricht Ankylosing Spondylitis Enthesis Score (MASES), Leeds Dactylitis Index (LDI), Patient Global for Psoriatic Arthritis, Dermatology Life Quality Index (DLQI), Psoriatic Arthritis Quality of Life (PsAQOL), Functional Assessment of Chronic Illness Therapy-Fatigue (FACIT-F), Psoriatic Arthritis Response Criteria (PsARC), Psoriatic Arthritis Joint Activity Index (PsAJAI), Disease Activity in Psoriatic Arthritis (DAPSA), and Composite Psoriatic Disease Activity Index (CPDAI). Arthritis Care Res. 2011;63 Suppl 11:S64–85. doi:10.1002/acr.20577.

21. Rich P, Scher RK. Nail Psoriasis Severity Index: a useful tool for evaluation of nail psoriasis. J Am Acad Dermatol. 2003;49(2):206–12.

22. Aktan S, Ilknur T, Akin C, Ozkan S. Interobserver reliability of the Nail Psoriasis Severity Index. Clin Exp Dermatol. 2007;32(2):141–4. doi:10.1111/j.1365-2230.2006.02305.x.

23. Parrish CA, Sobera JO, Elewski BE. Modification of the Nail Psoriasis Severity Index. J Am Acad Dermatol. 2005;53(4):745–6. doi:10.1016/j.jaad.2004.11.044; author reply 6–7.

24. Cassell SE, Bieber JD, Rich P, Tutuncu ZN, Lee SJ, Kalunian KC, et al. The modified Nail Psoriasis Severity Index: validation of an instrument to assess psoriatic nail involvement in patients with psoriatic arthritis. J Rheumatol. 2007;34(1):123–9.

25. de Jong EM, Menke HE, van Praag MC, van De Kerkhof PC. Dystrophic psoriatic fingernails treated with 1 % 5-fluorouracil in a nail penetration-enhancing vehicle: a double-blind study. Dermatology. 1999;199(4):313–8.

26. Klaassen KM, van de Kerkhof PC, Bastiaens MT, Plusje LG, Baran RL, Pasch MC. Scoring nail psoriasis. J Am Acad Dermatol. 2014;70(6):1061–6. doi:10.1016/j.jaad.2014.02.010.

Psoriatic Arthritis

17

Michaela Koehm and Frank Behrens

Abstract

Psoriatic Arthritis is an inflammatory musculoskeletal disease. Its pathogenesis is still unclear. There is evidence that it results from multiple genetic and environmental factors. Approximately 30 % of the patients with psoriasis will develop the musculoskeletal manifestation in their lifetime. The real estimated number of cases is still unknown. Risk factors for the development of Psoriatic Arthritis in Psoriasis patients contain nail psoriasis. Different subtypes of Psoriatic Arthritis are differentiated. Those subtypes were used for classification of Psoriatic Arthritis in former days. In the meanwhile, it is well known that transitions of subtypes occur frequently. Psoriatic Arthritis can be discriminated from other types of arthritis using clinical characteristic, missing of Rheumatoid Factor and ACPA and imaging findings such as osteoproliferations and osteolysis. For classification of Psoriatic Arthritis the CASPAR-criteria are used nowadays. Due to the distinct patterns of Psoriatic Arthritis, including arthritis, enthesitis, dactylitis, and spondyloarthritis different possibilities for measurement of disease activity are available. The Synovio-Entheseal-complex, detected in animal model, is one of the theories for determination of PsA-origin, especially of the occurrence of the characteristic DIP-Arthritis. Due to the risk-population of Psoriasis patients, tools for early detection of Psoriatic Arthritis are important for clinical routine care for early treatment possibilities. Questionnaires as well as Imaging Biomarkers are developed for early diagnosis and still under examination to determine their use in clinical practice.

M. Koehm, MD (✉) • F. Behrens, MD
Department of Rheumatology, Fraunhofer IME,
Project Group Translational Medicine and
Pharmacology TMP, University Hospital of Frankfurt,
Theodor-Stern-Kai 7,
Frankfurt 60580, Germany
e-mail: Michaela.Koehm@kgu.de

© Springer International Publishing Switzerland 2016
A. Adebajo et al. (eds.), *Psoriatic Arthritis and Psoriasis: Pathology and Clinical Aspects*,
DOI 10.1007/978-3-319-19530-8_17

Keywords

Psoriatic Arthritis • PsA-Subtypes • Synovio-Enthesial-complex • Early detection tools for PsA • PASE-Questionnaire • PEST-Questionnaire • TOPAS-Questionnaire

Clinical Aspects

Psoriatic Arthritis (PsA) is an inflammatory musculoskeletal disease usually proceeding chronically. Although its exact pathogenesis is still unclear, there is evidence that it results from multiple genetic and environmental factors [1]. PsA can be distinguished from rheumatoid arthritis by its distinct clinical manifestations, characteristic radiographic changes and usually the absence of rheumatoid factor and anti-citrullinated protein antibodies (ACPA) [2]. Patients often present with inflammation at multiple sites and musculoskeletal structures, including involvement of skin, joints and the tendon insertion sites or entheses. Due to the fact of its occurrence of axial involvement, it is categorised in the group of the spondyloarthopathies. Clinical appearance, severity of manifestation and disease course of PsA are distinct. First symptoms of PsA are often oligoarticular and mild, wherefore the diagnosis of PsA at early stages is could be difficult. Variations of PsA disease course can include a single manifestation on tendons and their insertions up to arthritis mutilans (<5 %) with severe deformations and osteolysis, keeping in mind, that up to half of PsA-patients show erosive bone changes even after 2-years of manifestation.

Epidemiology

Psoriasis is one of the most common skin diseases worldwide. In Europe, up to 1–3 % of the population is affected. Incidence rates vary due to ethnical background. PsA occurs in about 20–30 % of the psoriasis patients [3]. The real estimated number of cases is unknown. In a multidisciplinary study, 1511 psoriasis patients were included and interviewed in focus on musculoskeletal symptoms. Those, who had musculoskeletal complains were examined by rheumatologist. In 46 of the 1511 patients a PsA had been already diagnosed before. After examination of the rheumatologist, the number of those suffering from musculoskeletal involvement increased up to 312 patients (30 %) [3]. Those results were verified in a recent study, in which 949 patients having affirmed psoriasis were promptly examined by rheumatologist and 30 % of the patients were diagnosed as PsA [4]. Those numbers differ marked from the formally assumed rates, listed with 5–10 % [5] due to the fact that a large percentage of psoriasis patients are treated by GP without access to dermatologic or rheumatologic specialists. To reveal those incidence rates, registries such as PsoBest, the German Psoriasis Registry, or PSOLAR (Psoriasis Longitudinal Assessment and Registry) are important. Moreover, incidence rates are influenced by regional and geographic differences, which are probably caused by different genetic backgrounds [6].

Classification of PsA

In the new ASAS classification criteria [7] SpA with peripheral arthritis is defined as arthritis, enthesitis or dactylitis with additional one or more of the following co-manifestations: psoriasis, inflammatory bowel disease, preceding infection, HLA-B27, uveitis or sacroiliitis on imaging (radiograph or MRI) or two or more of the following co-manifestations: arthritis, enthesitis, dactylitis, inflammatory back pain in the past or positive family history for SpA (Table 17.1).

PsA has been classified among the spondyloarthopathies due to its high frequency of associated spondyloarthritis, the presence of extra-articular features common to other spondyloarthropathies and its association to HLA-B27 [8].

Table 17.1 ASAS classification criteria for SpA with peripheral arthritis

Arthritis or enthesitis or dactylitis	Plus ≥1 of:
	Psoriasis
	Inflammatory bowel disease
	Preceding infection
	HLA-B27
	Uveitis
	Sacroiliitis on imaging (radiograph or MRI)
	or
	Plus ≥2 of the remaining:
	Arthritis
	Enthesitis
	Dactylitis
	Inflammatory back pain in the past
	Positive family history for SpA

Based on data from Ref. [7]

Table 17.2 Moll and wright definition of PsA in the presence of psoriasis

Type	Description
Distal Pattern	Involvement of the distal interphalangeal joints (DIP)
Oligoarticular Pattern	Four or less affected joints
Polyarticular Pattern	More than four joints affected
Spondyloarthritis	Involvement of sacroiliacal joints and the apophyseal joints in the back
Arthritis Mutilans	Including severe deformations

Based on data from Ref. [8]

Moll and Wright described five clinical patterns in PsA [8] (Table 17.2):

1. A distal patterns with involvement of the distal interphalangeal joints (DIP)
2. An oligoarticular pattern where four or less joints are affected
3. A polyarticular pattern which might be indistinguishable from RA
4. A spondyloarthritis, affecting the sacroiliacal joints and the apophyseal joints in the back
5. Arthritis mutilans with severely deformations

In their initial reporting of the pattern, the oligoarticular pattern was the most often described one, occurring in up to 70 % of the PsA patients. The distal pattern and arthritis mutilans, though clinically considered more specific for PsA, occurred only in less than 5 %. In recent studies, the DIP involvement and the polyarticular type are seen more often [9]. This might be due to the fact those disease patterns might change over time. So, for early symptoms it is proposed that an oligoarticular manifestation changes over time to a polyarticular disease, seen in approximately 50 % of the patients [10]. Arthritis mutilans may come up quickly in patients with PsA without evidence of prior inflammation.

Moll and Wright did not mean those patterns to serve either as diagnostic criteria or classification. Even so, many clinicians and investigators still use these patterns to diagnose PsA or to define PsA-patients for clinical trials.

For defining more consistent classification criteria for PsA, several attempts of different working groups were provided. The most common known group, the CASPAR group (Classification of Psoriatic Arthritis), has been collecting disease courses of PsA patients and controls to establish and develop widely accepted classification criteria. The "Classification criteria for the diagnosis of Psoriatic Arthritis" (CASPAR-criteria) are used since 2006 with a sensitivity to diagnose PsA of 95 % and a specificity of 98 % [11]. The CASPAR-criteria extend the criteria of Moll and Wright that were mainly defined to distinguish PsA from RA and Osteoarthritis (OA). In opposite to Moll and Wright, CASPAR indicates active peripheral and axial joint disease, the tendons and entheses and carry on additional factors for disease classification. Additionally, radiographic changes such as characteristic osteoproliferations are displayed in the criteria for the first time (Table 17.3).

Clinical Features

Arthritis

Asymmetric Oligoarthritis

Oligoarthritis is defined as swelling and tenderness as signs for arthritis of less than five small or large joints. In PsA, large joints such as knees or elbows are more frequent affected asymmetrically

Table 17.3 CASPAR-classification criteria for PsA

Criterion	Description
1. Evidence of psoriasis (one of a, b, c)	
(a) Current psoriasis[a]	Psoriatic skin or scalp disease currently present, as judged by rheumatologist or dermatologist
(b) Personal history of psoriasis	A history of psoriasis obtained from patient or family physician, dermatologist, rheumatologist, or other qualified health car professional
(c) Family history of psoriasis	A history of psoriasis in a first or second degree relative by patient report
2. Psoriatic nail dystropy	Typical psoriatic nail dystrophy, including onycholysis, pitting and hyperkeratosis, observed on current physical examination
3. Negative result for rheumatoid factor (RF)	By any method except latex but preferably by ELISA or nephelometry, according to the local reference range
4. Dactylitis (one of a, b)	
(a) Current	Swelling of an entire digit
(b) History	A history of dactylitis recorded by a rheumatologist
5. Radiological evidence of juxta-articular new bone formation	Defined ossification near joint margins (excluding osteophyte formation) on plain x-ray films of hand or foot

To be classified as having PsA, a patient must have inflammatory articular disease (joint, spine, entheseal) with ≥3 of the following 5
[a]Current psoriasis scores 2; all other items 1
Based on data from Ref. [11]

in its onset. Moll and Wright described asymmetric oligoarthritis as the most common clinical presentation of PsA [12], including involvement of a single joint [13]. Moll and Wright also included the occurrence of dactylitis in this group. Clinical occurrence of heel pain (due to enthesitis), dactylitis and oligoarthritis is described as almost characteristic for PsA [14]. In recent studies it was shown that oligoarthrits only occurred in 28 % of the cases, whereas polyarthritis was the most dominant type of arthritis [15].

Polyarthritis

The involvement of the distal interphalangeal joints (DIP), defined as swelling and tenderness in the end joint of the fingers and toes is a clinical characteristic of PsA. It is frequently seen in association with nail involvement of psoriasis. In the absence of psoriasis, clinical involvement of the DIP is mostly associated with inflammatory OA as important differential diagnosis to PsA. However, in PsA inflammation may also present with characteristic involvement in the joints of the thumb and great toes and the DIP joints of the feet, which is clinical untypical for

the presence of OA. Nevertheless, the observer might miss isolated DIP inflammation for PsA diagnosis [16]. If there is clinically doubt of the diagnosis, radiographic examination or MRI should help to separate inflammatory osteoarthritis from psoriatic arthritis. Typical radiographic pattern of PsA are changes in the terminal phalanx, including erosions and osteolysis [17]. In arthrosonography, osteophytes and erosions can be displayed using power doppler signal to demonstrate inflammatory hyper-vascularisation.

Symmetric polyarthritis is defined as affection of five or more joints on both sites of the body. This form of PsA can be misdiagnosed as RA as important differential diagnosis. Arthritis mutilans is the extreme form of PsA occurring with deformations and destructions of the joints. It is often accompanied by a shortening of the affected finger or toe (Fig. 17.1).

Dactylitis

Dactylitis is another characteristic clinical feature of PsA (Fig. 17.2). It causes an entire finger or toe to swell. Dactylitis occurs in approximately 16–48 % of the reported cases [18, 19].

Fig. 17.1 Arthritis mutilans with telescopic fingers (Courtesy of Rheumatology Department, Frankfurt/Main)

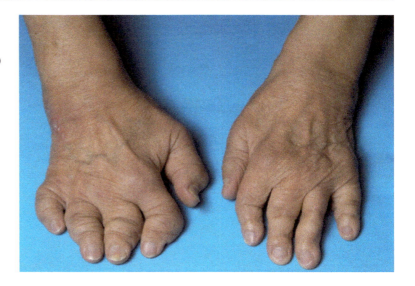

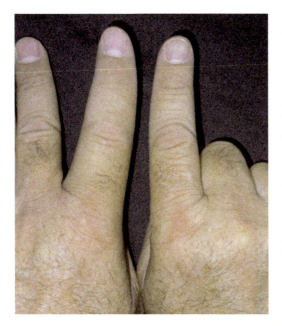

Fig. 17.2 Dactylitis (Courtesy of Rieke Alten, Berlin)

According to some authors, dactylitis is predominantly due to swelling and inflammation in the flexor tendon sheats [20]. Other groups describe it as isolated joint synovitis including tenosynovitis [21]. Enthesitis may also contribute to its clinical feature. Typically for the clinical manifestation of PsA non-tender diffuse swelling may occur as sign of less inflammation.

Enthesitis

Enthesitis (Fig. 17.3) is an inflammation of the entheses, the sites where tendons or ligaments insert into the bone. The entheses are any point of attachment of skeletal muscles to the bone. McGonagle et al. describe enthesitis as the major pathological change underlying PsA [22]. The most common sites in PsA are the bilateral calcaneum (both at the attachement of the Achilles tendon and at the attachement of the plantar fascia), the muscular and tendon attachements around the pelvis, the inferior aspect at the patella, and the elbow. In this contends spondylitis may be regarded as example of enthesial inflammation at multiple sites with formation of syndesmophytes representing bony 'spurs'. Specificity of enthesitis in PsA is still unclear, as it was demonstrated in one study using ultrasound to examine calcaneal enthesitis that bone erosions were more often detected in RA than in PsA [23].

Spondylitis

Classical ankylosing spondylitis is seen in association with Psoriasis. This form of spondylitis shows differences to the PsA typical form of spondylitis. Differences of PsA-associated spondylitis can be described as follows:

Fig. 17.3 Enthesitis
(Courtesy of Rieke Alten,
Berlin)

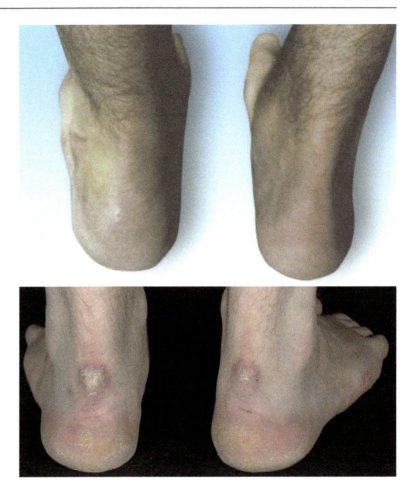

- Asymmetric sacoiliitis
- More frequent pseudosyndesmophytes
- Less frequent marginal syndesmophytes
- Less frequent lumbar spine involvement

In most of the cases spondylitis in PsA is less extensive. The prevalence of spondylitis in PsA depends on the method used to identify spinal involvement. Clinical examination to test sacroiliac joint involvement is usually less sensitive. Williamson et al. [24] demonstrated poor sensitivity (38 %) and specificity (67 %) of the regular clinical tests. Nevertheless, Gladman [25] and Williamson [24] demonstrated a high prevalence of asymptomatic spinal involvement in psoriatic arthritis. Furthermore, Gladman showed that changes typical for inflammatory spondylitis can occur in PsA in the absence of radiological sacroiliitis. This is an important

observation, because the presence of radiographic sacroiliitis is defined as criteria for the diagnosis of ankylosing spondylitis (AS) [26]. Additionally to radiographic examination, MRI is a sensitive method to detect early inflammation in the iliosacral joints.

Other Clinical Features

Due to its belonging to the group of spondyloarthropathies and its association to HLA-B27, ocular involvement is one of the most frequent extra-articular features in PsA after psoriasis. Both conjunctivitis (found in approximately 20 % of the cases) and uveitis (in approximately 7 % of the cases) have been described [27].

In a recent study it was shown that the risk for development of inflammatory bowel disease

(IBD) such as Crohn's disease (CD) and ulcerative colitis (UC) is increased in patients with psoriasis and concomitant psoriatic arthritis [28]. This might be explained due to the fact that genome-wide association studies have found common susceptibility genes.

In numerous case reports secondary amyloidosis affecting renal and gastrointestinal tissues in PsA were described, although it is not clear whether skin or joint disease is responsible for it [29, 30].

The SAPHO syndrome (its acronym stands for synovitis, acne (usually acne conglobata or fulminans), (palmoplantar) pustulosis, (sternoclavicular) hyperostosis and (sterile multifocal) osteomyelitis) is occasionally seen in association with PsA. It may even be a subgroup of this disease. Severity and prevalence of SAPHO differ regional. More severe forms of SAPHO have been described in Japan and the Mediterranean littoral. In the United Kingdom, Helliwell et al. found a high prevalence of sternoclavicular abnormalities in PsA-patients associated with Psoriasis vulgaris, describing it as osteoarticular manifestation of PsA [31].

Hypothesis of the 'Synovio-Entheseal Complex'

Experimental models of inflammatory arthritis with features of Psoriatic Arthritis demonstrate that the disease process starts at the enthesis [32–34]. These models confirm imaging findings in PsA and SpA patients [22, 35]. However, it is difficult to prove this hypothesis because of the limitations in conserving tissue samples easily.

Enthesiopathy can be measured by ultrasound. It is very common in patients with psoriasis without clinical manifestations of arthritis suggesting that it might be a primary abnormality [36]. The presence of clinically silent enthesiopathy in psoriasis appears to be associated with the subsequent development of Psoriatic Arthritis [37]. Synovitis or joint swelling in Psoriatic Arthritis may be linked to dysfunction of the enthesis where it forms tissue structures called 'synovio-entheseal complexes' (SECs) [38]. Osteitis or bone inflammation appears frequently in PsA patients. The enthesis and the underlying bone are functionally integrated with the enthesis being anchored to the underlying bone. Nail disease in psoriasis patients is a risk factor for development of PsA. It has been demonstrated that the nail is anchored directly to the skeleton by ligament and tendon entheses [39]. This may offer a new explanation for a possible link between nail disease and arthritis. Taken together, Psoriatic Arthritis might start at the insertions before spreading to other sites.

Differential Diagnosis

Osteoarthritis

Osteoarthritis is a common type of arthritis due to gradual loss of cartilage from the joints. It is typically located at the distal interphalangeal joints (DIP) and can therefore be mistaken as PsA. Symptoms of osteoarthritis include pain, stiffness, some loss of joint motion and changes in the shape of affected joints. Symptoms improve when less motion is performed. Two forms of osteoarthritis are differentiated: idiopathic osteoarthritis without identifiable cause and secondary osteoarthritis due to for example joint injury, accumulation of calcium inside the joint and bone and joint conditions. Risk factors include age, gender (women are between two and three times more likely than men), obesity, occupation and sports. Osteoarthritis is diagnosed using x-ray and exclusion of other inflammatory diseases. Osteoarthritis generally worsens slowly over time.

Rheumatoid Arthritis

One of the differential diagnoses to PsA is rheumatoid arthritis (RA). The differentiation of both forms of arthritis is sometimes difficult, especially in the rarely courses of both diseases, since patients with rheumatoid arthritis (RA) may suffer from concomitant psoriasis. There are clinical

Table 17.4 Differentiation of psoriatic arthritis from rheumatoid arthritis

Features	Psoriatic arthritis	Rheumatoid arthritis
Gender distribution M:F	1:1	1:3
Age at onset	36–40 year	30–50 year
Joint distribution	Asymmetric	Symmetric
Distal joins involvement	Common	Uncommon
Pattern of involvement	All joints of one digit, "ray"	All joints of the same level
Spinal involvement	Common	Rare
Rheumatoid nodules	Never	Common
Nail lesions	Common	Uncommon
Psoriasis	Almost always	Uncommon
HLA association	HLA-B27, −B17, C0602	HLA-DRB$_1$04

and radiological differences between PsA and RA (Table 17.4). RA affects women more commonly than men, whereas PsA affects both genders equally. Clinically, joint distribution is different, particularly in early disease. RA tends to be a symmetrical arthritis, affecting small, medium and large joints bilaterally. Distal interphalangeal joints are affected in RA rarely. PsA tends to be asymmetric, and to affect all the joints in one digit, in a ray distribution, rather than the same group of joints on both sides. Patients with PsA have less tenderness than patients with RA in their most affected joint [40].

Other Spondyloarthropathies

About 40–50 % of patients with PsA have a spondyloarthritis in addition to their peripheral joint involvement. Other spondyloarthropathies should be excluded as differential diagnosis as well. PsA can be differentiated from other spondyloarthopathies by the presence of marked inflammatory arthritis of peripheral joints, the presence of psoriasis and nail lesions. In PsA there are more often an asymmetric sacroiliitis and the formation of pseudo-syndesmophytes associated [41].

Reactive Arthritis

Reactive arthritis is defined as an arthritis that develops following an infection. Causative are usually gastrointestinal and urogenital pathogens such as Chlamydia trachomatis, Yersinia, Salmonella, Shigella, Campylobacter, Escherichia coli, Clostridium diffiicile and Chlamydia pneumoniae [42–44]. Clinical features of reactive arthritis include a typically mono- or oligoarticular pattern of arthritis, often involving the lower extremities and an interval ranging from several days to weeks between infection and arthritis. It typically occurs in young adults, affecting both men and women equally. In most of the patients, all symptoms resolve in less than 6 months to 1 year. Other musculoskeletal involvements such as enthesitis and dactylitis make a differentiation to PsA worse. Extraarticular manifestations occur more often in reactive arthritis compared to PsA. Those manifestations include conjunctivitis, genitourinary tract symptoms, oral lesion and nail changes. HLA-B27 is frequently detected.

Clinical Assessments

Tools for Early Diagnosis of PsA

For the early diagnosis of disease, for PsA it is an advantage that its risk population is predefined: Screening of patients with psoriasis is of great importance. In 60 % of the cases, PsA occurs after an average of 10-years of disease course of Psoriasis [4]. Because not all of the patients suffering from Psoriasis can be monitored and repeatedly examined by rheumatologists for development of musculoskeletal complains, tools for improvement of early diagnosis of PsA were generated. Questionnaires were created to detect even first symptoms of PsA. These questionnaires can easily be used when the patient visits regularly at the dermatology or GP department. Different questionnaires are validated. Of these four, only the "Toronto PsA Screening Questionnaire" (ToPAS) is suitable for usage in the total population and not limited to Psoriasis patients. The "Psoriatic Arthritis Screening and Evaluation-Questionnaire" (PASE) and the "Psoriasis Epidemiology Screening Tool" (PEST) address patients with psoriasis (Table 17.5). The "German Psoriasis Arthritis Diagnostic Questionnaire" (GEPARD) is a German tool that is still in evaluation.

PASE includes aspects of symptoms and loss of functionality of the patients. In a validation study comparing the three questionnaires, for PASE a sensitivity of 82 % for detection of PsA and a specificity of 73 % was seen. The score correlates with the disease severity [46]. ToPAS was developed for PsA-screening in the total population, so that it can be used at the GP department. It has a sensitivity to detect PsA of 94 % and a specificity of 92 % in the validation cohort [45]. It includes 12 questions and was developed in an integrated approach between dermatologists and rheumatologists. ToPAS involves clinical pictures of skin and nail lesions to simplify the assessment for the patient [47]. With a sensitivity

to detect PsA of 97 % and a specificity of 79 %, the PEST questionnaire is one of the newest tools in early detection of PsA. It includes 18 questions and a description of the involved joints to simplify the identification of PsA in Psoriasis patients [48]. The GEPARD questionnaire is a German approach to detect PsA patients in the psoriasis population. It is still in development and consists of 14 questions [49].

The validation of those four questionnaires in the different target populations to define its value is performed in clinical trials conducted and supervised by GRAPPA (Group for Research and Assessment of Psoriasis and Psoriatic Arthritis).

Measurement of Severity and Disease Activity

After detection and classification of PsA, severity and disease activity should be determined to specify the individual treatment strategy. GRAPPA distinguishes three different grades of severity: mild, moderate and severe (Table 17.6).

Different measurements for determination of disease activity of PsA as well as for psoriasis are available. In contrast to RA, involvement of joints of the feet and the toes can be detected in the majority of cases, so that approximately 2/3 of the disease defining joints are not represented in the disease activity score 28 joints (DAS28) [51].

Table 17.5 Differences of the three Questionnaires for early diagnosis of PsA

Criterion	ToPAS	PASE	PEST
Number of questions	12	15	18
Target population	All	Psoriasis	Psoriasis
Sensitivity (%)	94	82	97
Specificity (%)	92	73	79

Based on data from Ref. [45]

Table 17.6 Grades of severity (GRAPPA)

	Mild	Moderate	Severe
Peripheral arthritis	<5 joints No damage on x-ray No loss of function QoL minimal impact Pt. evaluation mild	≥5 joints (S or T) Damage on x-ray IR to mild Rx Mod. LOF Mod. impact on QoL	≥5 joints (S or T) Severe damage on x-ray IR to mild-moderate Rx Severe LOF Severe impact on QoL
Skin disease	BSA <5, PASI <5, asymptomatic	Pt. evaluation moderate Non-response to topicals, DLQI, PASI <10	Pt. evaluation severe BSA >10, DLQI >10 PASI >10
Spinal disease	Mild pain	Loss of function or BASDAI >4	Failure of response
Enthesitits	No loss of function 1–2 sites	>2 sites or loss of function	Loss of function or >2 sites and failure of response

Based on data from Ref. [50]

Therefore, for determination of disease activity of PsA all of the 64 tender joints (TJC) and 66 swollen joints (SJC) should be examined. Beside the joint count, BASDAI (Bath Ankylosing Spondylitis Disease Activity Index) should be performed when axial involvement is assumed. Serological parameters, such as CRP and ESR are less important for classification of disease activity in the position of Severity but essential for the further prognosis of disease course [52].

Scores for detection of disease activity should be performed either at the dermatology or the rheumatology department. They are used for documentation of disease activity and disease course. Reliability of the scores depends on the examiner, his job specialisation and his experience. Dermatologists are comparable experienced in detecting tender joints in comparison to dactylitis. The other way around, rheumatologists have difficulties to survey Body Surface Area (BSA) to discriminate severity of Psoriasis, but evaluation of PASI or NAPSI are comparable to the dermatologists [53]. Nevertheless, evaluation of scores for discrimination of severity of disease should only be performed by trained personal. This is exclusively possible in integrated work between dermatologists and rheumatologists.

The measurement of enthesitis is difficult because of the lack of a useful gold standard other than histopathological examination using biopsy. The Maastrich Ankylosing Spondylitis Enthesitis Score (MASES) a clinical score was developed during a 2-year period. Thirteen sites that were evaluated as most specific and sensitive for enthesitis were identified and included using a dichotomous 0/1 score for tenderness. MASES correlated with other disease measurements [54]. Although, MASES is not validated for PsA, data from weeks 24 and 52 in the Golimumab PsA trials suggest that MASES is discriminative and responsive [55, 56]. Moreover, the modified MASES score includes the plantar fascia. More recently, a new outcome measure for enthesitis in SpA was created from the Spondyloarthritis Research Consortium of Canada (SPARCC) [57]. Information from Ultrasound and MRI studies in PsA-patients, in healthy controls and AS-patients

were used for its formation. The 16 most frequently affected entheseal sites were identified [58]. Correlation was seen between the score and other disease activity measures. Shortened versions of SPARCC using more commonly involved sites showed larger effect sizes and standardised means. This would be useful in clinical practice as it takes less time for evaluation but still illustrates entheseal involvement [57]. The Leeds Enthesitis Index (LEI) is the only measurement tool specifically created for PsA. In its development the six most commonly involved entheseal sites were identified [59]. In an open-label longitudinal study the LEI was compared to other entheseal indices. The LEI showed closest correlation with other disease activity measures of PsA, a large effect size and the smallest floor effect, indicating a superior possibility for identification of the majority of patients with enthesitis.

Dactylitis can be characterized as active/tender form, including erythematous and warm affection of the joints of one digit in a "ray" as signs for its acute inflammation. It can be discriminated to the sub-acute/non-tender form with swelling but without tenderness. Studies using imaging have confirmed that physical examination can identify pathology in tender dactylitis [20]. The simplest measure used is the simple count of the digits affected. The Leeds Dactylitis Instrument was developed in response to the need for a clinical, objective, validated outcome measure. It is based on the evaluation of the median differences in digital circumference between dactylitic digits and control digit. Dactylitis is defined as an increase in circumference of the digit of more than 10 % compared to contralateral non-affected digit [60].

Imaging

Different imaging methods are available to detect inflammation of PsA. Radiographic imaging is a approved method to detect bone shifts such as erosions, osteo-proliferations or typical nail involvement such as changes in coronal nail parts. Its sensitivity to detect early stages of PsA is limited. Radiographic imaging of the hand and feet in two-layer projection is used for classification and diagnosis of PsA and should be used repeatedly in therapy monitoring. X-Ray imaging of the spine and pelvis region should be added, if axial involvement is suspected in early diagnostic and disease activity.

Arthrosonography is more potent in diagnostic of PsA than radiographic procedures. It can be performed quickly, is less expensive compared to other imaging methods and able to illustrate tendons, synovia, cartilage, bone and blood perfusion as marker for inflammation in power doppler mode (PDA). It is superior in the detection of enthesitis.

Magnet resonance imaging (MRI) is the most sensitive method for imaging of changes in tissue such as synovitis, enthesitis, osteitis and useful in illustration of structural damage. In patients with psoriasis it was shown that structural changes defined as one or more signs of arthritis were detected in 68 % of the patients without diagnosis of manifest PsA in MRI-examination in contrast to x-ray [61]. In MRI 28 % of the cases showed erosive changes compared to 20 % in x-ray examination. In 46 % of the patients with Psoriasis oedema of bone mark in localisation of small joints and the wrist were detected. So, MRI should be used for detection of early stages of PsA and in difficult cases to discriminate PsA from different forms of arthritis.

Performance of szintigraphy is another imaging method used for detection of inflammatory processes. Although it is sensitive in detection of changes in bone metabolism, it only has low specificity.

A new approach in the use of imaging as biomarker for detection and treatment monitoring of PsA is fluorescence-optical imaging. Indo-cyanine-green (ICG) is used as colorant to record changes in micro vascularisation of the hands, which is important in early inflammatory stages of disease. Different patterns for differentiation of types of arthritis were detected [62]. Validation of this method in early diagnosis in PsA and treatment monitoring is actually performed.

References

1. Gladman DD, Rahman P. Psoriatic arthritis. In: Ruddy S, Harris ED, Sledge CB, Budd RC, Sergent JS, editors. Kelly's textbook of rheumatology. 6th ed. Philadelphia: WB Saunders; 2001. p. 1071–9.
2. Gladman DD. Current concept in psoriatic arthritis. Curr Opin Rheumatol. 2002;14:361–6.
3. Reich K, Kruger K, et al. Epidemiology and clinical pattern of psoriatic arthritis in Germany: a prospective interdisciplinary epidemiological study of 1511 patients with plaque-type psoriasis. Br J Dermatol. 2009;160:1040–7.
4. Mease PJ, Gladman DD, Papp KA, Khraishi MM, Thaçi D, Behrens F, et al. Prevalence of rheumatologist-diagnosed psoriatic arthritis in patients with psoriasis in European/North American dermatology clinics. J Am Acad Dermatol. 2013;69(5):729–35.
5. Veale DJ, Fitzgerald O. Psoriatic arthritis - pathogenesis and epidemiology. Clin Exp Rheumatol. 2002;20(6 Suppl 28):S27–33.
6. Hellgren L. Association between rheumatoid arthritis and psoriasis in total populations. Acta Rheumatol Scand. 1969;15:316–26.
7. Lipton S, Deodhar A. The new ASAS classification criteria for axial and peripheral spondyloarthritis: promises and pitfalls. Int J Clin Rheumatol. 2012;7(6): 675–82.
8. Wright V, Moll JMH. Psoriatic arthritis. In: Seronegative polyarthritis. Amsterdam: North Holland; 1976. p. 169–223.
9. Gladman DD Psoriatic arthritis. In: Classification and assessment of rheumatic disease, part 1. In: Silman AJ, Symmons DPM editors. Balliére's clinical rheumatology. International practice and research. London: Balliére's Tindall; 1995. p. 319–29.
10. McHugh NJ, Balachrishnan C, Jones SM. Progression of peripheral joint disease in psoriatic arthritis: a 5-yr prospective study. Rheumatology (Oxford). 2003;42: 778–83.
11. Taylor W, et al. Classification criteria for psoriatic arthritis: development of new criteria from a large international study. Arthritis Rheum. 2006;54: 2665–73.
12. Moll JMH, Wright V. Psoriatic arthritis. Semin Arthritis Rheum. 1973;3:51–78.
13. Helliwell PS, Wright V. Psoriatic arthritis: clinical features. In: Klippel JH, Dieppe PA, editors. Rheumatology. London: Mosby; 1998. p. 6.21.1–8.
14. Eulry F, Diamano J, Launay D, Tabache F, Lechervalier D, Magnin J. Sausage like toe and heel pain value for diagnosing and evaluating the severity of spondylarthropathies defined by Amors's criteria. A retrospective study in 161 patients. Joint Bone Spine. 2002;69:574–9.
15. Gladman DD, Shuckett R, Russell ML, Thorne JC, Schachter RK. Psoriatic arthritis (PSA)--an analysis of 220 patients. Q J Med. 1987;62(238):127–41.

16. Gorter S, van der Heijde DMFM, van der Linden S, Houben H, Rethans JJ, Scerpbier AJJA, et al. Psoriatic arthritis performance of rheumatologists in daily practice. Ann Rheum Dis. 2002;61:219–24.

17. Avila R, Pugh DG, Slocumb CH, Winkelmann RK. Psoriatic arthritis: a roentgenological study. Radiology. 1960;75:691.

18. Fournie B, Crognier L, Arnaud C, Zabraniecki L, Lascaux-Lefebvre V, Marc V, et al. Proposed classification criteria of Proriatic arthritis. Rev Rhum Engl Ed. 1999;66:446–56.

19. Rothschild BM, Pingitore C, Eaton M. Dactyitis: implications for clinical practice. Semin Arthritis Rheum. 1998;28:41–7.

20. Olivieri I, Barozzi U, Favaro L, Pierro A, De Matteis M, Borghi C, et al. Dactylitis in patients with seronegative spondyloarthropathy. Assessment by ultrasonography and magnetic resonance imaging. Arthritis Rheum. 1996;39:1524–8.

21. Kane D, Greanery T, Bresnihan B, Gibney R, Fitzgerald O. Ultrasonography in the diagnosis and management of psoriatic dactylitis [comment]. J Rheumatol. 1999;26:1746–51.

22. McGonagle D, Gibbon W, Emery P. Classification of inflammatory arthritis by enthesitis. Lancet. 1998;352: 1137–40.

23. Falsetti P, Frediani B, Fioravanti A, Acciai C, Baldi F, Filippou G, et al. Sonographical study of calcaneal entheses in erosive osteoarthritis, nodal osteoarthritis, rheumatoid arthritis and psoriatic arthritis. Scand J Rheumatol. 2003;32:229–34.

24. Williamson I, Dockerty JL, Dalbeth N, McNally E, Ostlere S, Wordsworth BP. Clinical assessment of sacroiliitis and HLA-B17 are poor predictors of sacroiliitis diagnosed by magnetic resonance imaging in psoriatic arthritis. Rheumatology. 2004;43:85–8.

25. Khan M, Schentag C, Gladman D. Clinical and radiological changes during psoriatic arthritis disease progression. J Rheumatol. 2003;30:1022–6.

26. The HSG, Steven MM, Van der Linden SM, Cats A. Evaluation of diagnostic criteria for ankylosing spondylitis: a comparison of the Rome, New York, and modified New York criteria in patients with a positive clinical history screening test for ankylosing spondylitis. Br J Rheumatol. 1985;24:242–9.

27. Lambert JR, Wright V. Eye inflammation in psoriatic arthritis. Ann Rheum Dis. 1976;35:354–6.

28. Li WQ, Han JL, Chan AT, Qureshi AA. Psoriasis, psoriatic arthritis and increased risk of incident Crohn's disease in US women. Ann Rheum Dis. 2013;72(7):1200–5.

29. Mpofu S, Teh LS, Smith PJ, Moots RJ, Hawkins PN. Cytostatic therapy for AA amyloidosis complicating psoriatic spondyloarthropathy. Rheumatology. 2003; 42:362–6.

30. Ujfalussy I, Bely M, Koo E, Seztak M. Systemic, secondary amyloidosis in a patient with psoriatic arthritis. Clin Exp Rheumatol. 2001;19:225.

31. Helliwell P, Marchesoni A, Peters M, Baker M, Wright V. A re-evaluation of the osteoarticular manifestations of psoriasis. Br J Rheumatol. 1991;30:339–45.

32. Lories RJ, Matthys P, de Vlam K, Derese I, Luyten FP. Ankylosing enthesitis, dactylitis, and onychoperiostitis in male DBA/1 mice: a model of psoriatic arthritis. Ann Rheum Dis. 2004;63(5):595–8.

33. Sherlock JP, Joyce-Shaikh B, Turner SP, et al. IL-23 induces spondyloarthropathy by acting on ROR-γt+CD3+CD4-CD8- entheseal resident T cells. Nat Med. 2012;18(7):1069–76. doi:10.1038/nm.2817.

34. Armaka M, Apostolaki M, Jacques P, et al. Mesenchymal cell targeting by TNF as a common pathogenic principle in chronic inflammatory joint and intestinal diseases. J Exp Med. 2008;205(2): 331–7.

35. McGonagle D, Conaghan PG, Emery P. Psoriatic arthritis: a unified concept twenty years on. Arthritis Rheum. 1999;42(6):1080–6.

36. Naredo E, Möller I, de Miguel E, Batlle-Gualda E, et al. High prevalence of ultrasonographic synovitis and enthesopathy in patients with psoriasis without psoriatic arthritis: a prospective case-control study. Rheumatology (Oxford). 2011;50(10):1838–48.

37. Tinazzi I, McGonagle D, Biasi D, Confente S, Caimmi C, Girolomoni G, Gisondi P. Preliminary evidence that subclinical enthesopathy may predict psoriatic arthritis in patients with psoriasis. J Rheumatol. 2011;38(12):2691–2.

38. McGonagle D, Lories RJ, Tan AL, Benjamin M. The concept of a "synovio-entheseal complex" and its implications for understanding joint inflammation and damage in psoriatic arthritis and beyond. Arthritis Rheum. 2007;56(8):2482–91.

39. McGonagle D, Tan AL, Benjamin M. The nail as a musculoskeletal appendage – implications for an improved understanding of the link between psoriasis and arthritis. Dermatology. 2009;218(2): 97–102.

40. Buskila D, Langevitz P, Gladman DD, Urowitz S, Smythe H. Patients with rheumatoid arthritis are more tender than those with psoriatic arthritis. J Rheumatol. 1992;19:1115–9.

41. Gladman D, Brubacher B, Buskila D, Langevitz P, Farewell VT. Differences in the expression of spondyloarthropathy: a comparison between ankylosing spondylitis and psoriatic arthritis. Genetic and gender effects. Clin Invest Med. 1993;16:1–7.

42. Braun J, Kingsley G, van der Heijde D, Sieper J. On the difficulties of establishing a consensus on the definition of and diagnostic investigations for reactive arthritis. Results and discussion of a questionnaire prepared for the 4th International Workshop on Reactive Arthritis, Berlin, Germany, July 3–6, 1999. J Rheumatol. 2000;27:2185.

43. Townes JM. Reactive arthritis after enteric infections in the United States: the problem of definition. Clin Infect Dis. 2010;50:247.

44. Rohekar S, Pope J. Epidemiologic approaches to infection and immunity: the case of reactive arthritis. Curr Opin Rheumatol. 2009;21:386.

45. Coates LC, Aslam T, Al Balushi F, Burden AD, et al. Comparison of three screening tools to detect psoriatic arthritis in patients with psoriasis (CONTEST study). Br J Dermatol. 2013;168(4):802–7.

46. Dominguez PL, Husni ME, et al. Validity, reliability, and sensitivity-to change properties of the psoriatic arthritis screening and evaluation questionnaire. Arch Dermatol Res. 2009;301(8):573–9.

47. Gladman DD, Schentag CT, et al. Development and initial validation of a screening questionnaire for psoriatic arthritis: the Toronto Psoriatic Arthritis Screen (ToPAS). Ann Rheum Dis. 2009;68(4):497–501.

48. Ibrahim GH, Buch MH, et al. Evaluation of an existing screening tool for psoriatic arthritis in people with psoriasis and the development of a new instrument: the Psoriasis Epidemiology Screening Tool (PEST) questionnaire. Clin Exp Rheumatol. 2009;27(3):469–74.

49. Härle P, Hartung W, Lehmann P, et al. Detection of psoriasis arthritis with the GEPARD patient questionnaire in a dermatologic outpatient setting. Z Rheumatol. 2010;69(2):157–60. 162–3.

50. Märker-Hermann E, Behrens F. Psoriatic arthritis. Treatment outcome parameters. Z Rheumatol. 2009;68:16–22.

51. Erdem CZ, Tekin NS, et al. MR imaging features of foot involvement in patients with psoriasis. Eur J Radiol. 2008;67:521–5.

52. Gladman DD, Mease PJ, et al. Risk factors for radiographic progression in psoriatic arthritis: sub-analysis of the randomized controlled trial ADEPT. Arthritis Res Ther. 2010;12(3):R113.

53. Chandran V, Schentag CT, Gladman DD. Sensitivity of the classification of psoriatic arthritis criteria in early psoriatic arthritis. Arthritis Rheum. 2007;57(8):1560–3

54. Gladman DD, Inman RD, Cook RJ, et al. International spondyloarthritis interobserver reliability exercise. the INSPIRE study: II. Assessment of peripheral joints, enthesitis, and dactylitis. J Rheumatol. 2007;34:1740–5.

55. Kavanaugh A, McInnes I, Mease P, et al. Golimumab, a new human tumor necrosis factor alpha antibody, administered every four weeks as a subcutaneous injection in psoriatic arthritis: twenty-four-week efficacy and safety results of a randomized, placebo-controlled study. Arthritis Rheum. 2009;60:976–86.

56. Kavanaugh A, Mease P. Treatment of psoriatic arthritis with tumor necrosis factor inhibitors: longer-term outcomes including enthesitis and dactylitis with golimumab treatment in the Longterm Extension of a randomized, placebo-controlled study (Go-Reveal). J Rheumatol. 2012;89(Suppl):90–3.

57. Maksymowych WP, Mallon C, Morrow S, et al. Development and validation of the Spondyloarthritis Research Consortium of Canada (SPARCC) enthesitis index. Ann Rheum Dis. 2009;68:948–53.

58. D'Agostino MA, Said-Nahal R, Hacquard-Bouder C, Brasseur JL, et al. Assessment of peripheral enthesitis in the spondyloarthropathies by ultrasonography combined with power Doppler: a cross-sectional study. Arthritis Rheum. 2003;48:523–33.

59. Healy PJ, Helliwell PS. Measuring clinical enthesitis in psoriatic arthritis: assessment of existing measures and development of an instrument specific to psoriatic arthritis. Arthritis Rheum. 2008;59:686–91.

60. Helliwell PS, Firth J, Ibrahim GH, Melsom RD, et al. Development of an assessment tool for dactylitis in patients with psoriatic arthritis. Arthritis Rheum. 1989;32:531–7.

61. Offidani A, Cellini A, et al. Subclinical joint involvements in psoriasis: magnetic resonance imaging and x-ray findings. Acta Derm Venereol. 1998;78(6):463–5.

62. Wiemann O, Werner SG, Röver H, Lind-Albrecht G et al. Sensitivity and specificity of the "green nail" sign in fluorescence optical imaging in Psoriatic Arthritis, ACR 2014, Abstract 2129.

Part V
Imaging

Arthur Kavanaugh

Imaging Tools in Skin and Nail Psoriasis

Marwin Gutierrez and Chiara Bertolazzi

Abstract

Imaging plays a key role in the assessment of psoriasis. However they findings are not still adequately standardized which reduces the confidence from the clinicians on his application.

Ultrasound (US) is a promising tool for the assessment of both quantification of the disease activity and the treatment responsiveness in patients with psoriasis. The continuous technological advances in this field allowed the development of equipments provided with very sensitive power Doppler (PD), which permit a sensitive detection of blood flow even in small vessels of superficial tissues such as nail and skin.

Over the past few years, videocapillaroscopy (VCP) is also generating a great interest in the assessment of microvascular changes in psoriasis representing an emergent tool for both clinical and research approaches.

This chapter provides data about the potential role of imaging, including US and VCP, in depicting both skin and nail changes in patients with psoriasis.

Keywords

Psorisis • Imaging • Ultrasound • Videocapillaroscopy • Skin • Nail

M. Gutierrez, MD (✉)
Department of Rheumatology,
Instituto Nacional de Rehabilitación,
Calzada Mexico-Xochimilco 289 Colonia Arenal de Guadalupe, CP 143898 Mexico City, Mexico
e-mail: dr.gmarwin@gmail.com

C. Bertolazzi, MD
Department of Rheumatology,
Clinica Reumatologica, Università Politecnica delle Marche, Jesi, Ancona, Italy

Introduction

Psoriasis is a chronic inflammatory skin disease affecting 1–3 % of the world's population [1]. A considerable proportion of patients with psoriasis will develop a psoriatic arthritis (PsA). The prevalence of PsA in patients with psoriasis varies from 7.6 to 36 % according to the different populations' studied and approximately 10–55 %

© Springer International Publishing Switzerland 2016
A. Adebajo et al. (eds.), *Psoriatic Arthritis and Psoriasis: Pathology and Clinical Aspects*,
DOI 10.1007/978-3-319-19530-8_18

of patients with psoriasis will have nail involvement [2, 3].

The diagnosis of psoriasis is routinely based on the clinical history and physical examination, and the severity is determined using the Psoriasis Area and Severity Index (PASI), a specific validated method for assessing the extension of psoriatic lesions [4]. Nevertheless, histological examination remains the reference standard for the final diagnosis.

Imaging may play a key role in the assessment of psoriasis; however it is not yet developed an adequate confidence from the clinicians on his application, in part related to the scarce availability of standardized approaches to assess and interpret the findings.

Ultrasound (US) has demonstrated to be a useful tool for the assessment of both quantification of the disease activity and the treatment responsiveness in patients with psoriasis, but until few years, only a grayscale technique was available limiting its application in routine practice [5–11].

The continuous technological advances in the field of US allowed the development of equipments provided with very sensitive power Doppler (PD), which permit both the detailed study of morphostructural changes (with resolution power of 0.1 mm) and the sensitive detection of blood flow even in small vessels of superficial tissues such as nail and skin.

Over the past few years, there has also been increasing interest by rheumatologists in the use of videocapillaroscopy (VCP) to assess the microvascular changes in psoriasis, including nail psoraisis and psoriatic arthritis [12–19]. This imaging tool is already an established method to assess the microcirculation "status" in patients with Raynaud's phenomenon and connective tissue diseases [20–22]. So, considering that changes in the microcirculation are also key features in the pathogenesis of psoriasis it is easy to consider that VCP represents a promising tool for both clinical and research approaches.

The aim of this chapter is to provide information about the potential role of imaging, especially US using sensitive PD technique, and VCP in depicting both skin and nail changes in patients affected by psoriasis.

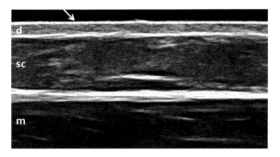

Fig. 18.1 Grayscale image of the normal skin obtained at the forearm. The epidermis appears as a thin homogeneous hyperechoic line (*arrow*). The dermis (*d*) appears as a more echogenic band than the underlying hypoechoic sub-cutaneous tissue (*sc*). *m* muscle

Ultrasound

Healthy Skin

In normal skin, the epidermis appears as a thin hyperechoic and continuous line with homogeneous thickness. The dermis is visualized as a less echoic and homogeneous band, whereas the subcutaneous tissue is characteristically hypoechoic (because of adipose tissue) separated by hyperechoic lines generated by fibrous septa of connective tissue (Fig. 18.1).

Healthy Nail

The components of the nail unit are clearly visible on US. The dorsal and ventral plates appear as two hyperechoic parallel lines with a virtual hypoechoic space in between. The nail bed appears as a hypoechoic band not clearly distinguishable from the underlying subcutaneous tissue. The bony margin of the distal phalanx appears as a continuous hyperechoic line below the nail bed (Fig. 18.2a). A minimal amount of PD may be detectable on PD imaging in some nail beds because of the presence of thin arterial and venous vessels (Fig. 18.2b).

Psoriatic Plaques

The sonographic morphostructural changes in the psoriatic skin are generally easily distinguishable from surrounding healthy skin. In the gray scale examination, the epidermis and dermis appear thicker compared with the normal surrounding skin. Moreover, a hypoechoic band in the upper lesion dermis can be observed very frequently and may represent the inflammatory edema and the

vasodilatation within the papillary dermis (Fig. 18.3a). In active psoriatic plaques, PD imaging allows sensitive detection of an increased blood flow signal that may be seen within the dermis (Fig. 18.3b). The US features of skin and nails in patients with psoriasis are represented in the Table 18.1.

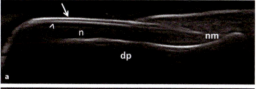
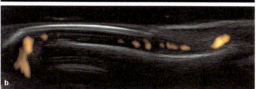

Fig. 18.2 (**a**) Grayscale image of the nail. The dorsal (*arrow*) and ventral (*arrowhead*) nail plates appear as bilaminar structures with a hypoechoic space in between. The nail bed (*n*) appears as a hypoechoic area under the plates. (**b**) Mild quantity of power Doppler in healthy subject. *dp* distal phalanx, *nm* nail matrix

Table 18.1 Ultrasound findings of psoriatic skin and nails in patients with psoriasis

Psoriatic skin	Psoriatic onychopathy
Thickening of epidermis	Focal hyperechoic deposits in the ventral plate (may be subclinical and correlate with subungual keratosis) without involvement of dorsal plate
Thickening of dermis	Loss of definition of both nail plates, adopting a wavy form
Hypoechoic band in upper dermis	Thickening of nail bed
	Increased blood flow detected on PD sonography
	Increased blood flow in nail bed detected on PD sonography

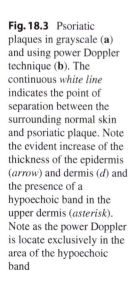

Fig. 18.3 Psoriatic plaques in grayscale (**a**) and using power Doppler technique (**b**). The continuous *white line* indicates the point of separation between the surrounding normal skin and psoriatic plaque. Note the evident increase of the thickness of the epidermis (*arrow*) and dermis (*d*) and the presence of a hypoechoic band in the upper dermis (*asterisk*). Note as the power Doppler is locate exclusively in the area of the hypoechoic band

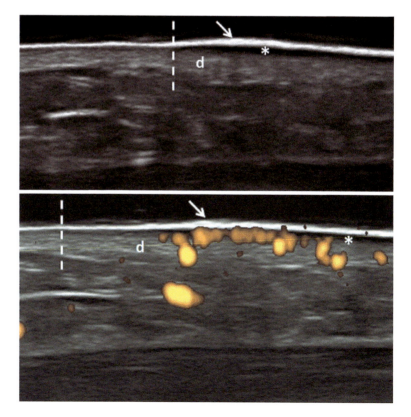

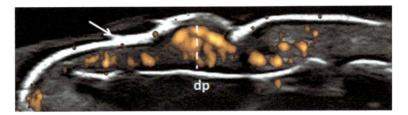

Fig. 18.4 Ultrasound of psoriatic onychopathy showing thickening and irregular undulation of the nail plates, which became a single and wavy hyperechoic layer (*arrow*). The nail bed is clearly thickened (*white vertical line*). The presence of intense power Doppler indicates an evident blood flow increase. *dp* distal phalanx

Psoriatic Onychopathy

In psoriatic onychopathy, the changes are located in both the nail plates and nail bed. The nail plates may show hyperechoic parts or loss of definition, which can involve only the ventral plate or both plates. In later stages, a wavy or thickened appearance of both plates may be visible (Fig. 18.4). The thickening of the nail bed can be measured (i.e., the distance between the ventral plate and the bone margin of the distal phalanx). These changes can be associated with an increase of blood flow observed with the PD technique within the nail bed.

Evidence of US in Psoriatic Skin and Nail

Within the last decade, there has been an increasing interest to assess psoriatic disease by US. Several studies have been conducted, but the majority of these using dated US machines provided with single and fixed frequency probes and only grayscale technique [5–9].

Very high- frequency probes (up to 100 MHz) have also been used in past in the assessment of psoriatic plaques but only in experimental settings unlikely to be feasible in daily practice [7].

El Gammal et al., [8] formulated in the eighties the hypothesis that the hypoechoic band in the upper dermis corresponded to the clinically palpable papule. However, it is not specific for psoriasis because it may be also present in other inflammatory conditions, such as contact dermatitis, atopic eczema, and acanthoma [23].

Thickening of both the epidermis and dermis is the most constant sonographic pathologic finding in psoriatic plaques [24], whereas the hypoechoic band in the upper dermis is particularly detectable in the active stages of the disease [23]. The reduction of both the epidermal and dermal thickness and principally the disappearance of the hypoechoic band at the superficial dermis level were described as the main gray scale sonographic indicators of effective therapy [5, 6, 8, 9]. Some authors have suggested normal US values of thickness in the different layers of the skin [25, 26], but because the normal thickness is widely variable according to the anatomic area, it could be more rational to perform a comparison between the lesion area and normal skin in the same area of the same patient.

The recent availability of new generation top-gamma US machines provided with high and variable frequency probes and a very sensitive PD technique has allowed to re-open the research on its validity in psoriatic skin and nail. Although the way is large towards this goal, interesting preliminary results are strengthening its potential role in the assessment of psoriatic plaque and onychopathy. The results demonstrated the criterion validity and sensitivity to change of PDUS by a positive correlation with the histology findings at psoriatic plaque level in patients receiving TNF-α antagonist therapy [27]. Further investigations regarding both intra- and inter-observer reproducibility and studying larger series are still needed to confirm these preliminary studies.

Therapeutic Monitoring

US offers some advantages with respect to other imaging techniques in therapy monitoring of psoriatic skin and nail since it can reflect

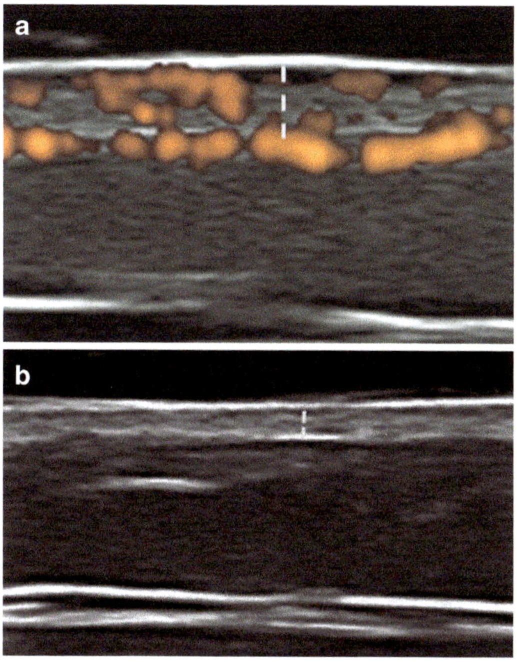

Fig. 18.5 Psoriatic plaque. (**a**) Active psoriatic plaque characterized by epidermis thickening (*white line*), hypoechoic oedema and intense power Doppler. (**b**) Follow-up ultrasound revealed a dramatic reduction of the dermal thickness (*white line*) and marked decrease and disappearance of power Doppler signal at dermal level

contemporaneously morphostructural changes, inflammatory activity and anatomical damage. Moreover US can be easily and safely repeated during the treatment.

Recently our group demonstrated the sensitivity to change of PDUS assessments of psoriatic plaque over an 8 weeks period in a cohort of psoriasis and PsA patients receiving TNF-α antagonist therapy [27] (Fig. 18.5).

To date, the few data available in literature testing the sensitivity to change of PDUS in PsA have depicted its potential assessing only a single domain (i.e. joint, enthesis, tendon or skin). We have recently proposed a preliminary PDUS composite score for the global assessment of blood flow changes after treatment in PsA patients [28]. The PDUS composite score was called "Five Targets Power Doppler for Psoriatic Disease (5TPD)" that includes the assessment of joint, tendon with synovial sheath, enthesis, skin and nail together. PD for each target was graded from 0 to 3 on the basis of the semiquantitative scoring systems previously suggested. The maximum total score of 5TPD is 15 as results of the sum of all the five targets PD scores. The preliminary results showed a significant improvement of global 5TPD scores from baseline to 8 weeks after anti TNF-α treatment.

Nailfold Videocapillaroscopy in Skin Psoriasis

VCP patterns in psoriatic skin lesion consist of tortuous, coiled and bushy capillary formations [29, 30] (Fig. 18.6).

Bushan et al. reported decreased vessel density and a reduction in the size of the capillary loops but found no other morphological abnormalities [31]. On the other hand, Bartosinska et al. evaluated patients with psoriasis vulgaris and psoriatic arthritis and identified four distinct patterns: (a) normal, (b) with coiled capillary loops, (c) a pattern similar to that found in plaque psoriasis; and (d) the presence of thin and fragile capillaries in a pale background [32]. The latter pattern was detected only in patients with psoriatic arthritis.

Brushan et al., [13] conducted an interesting study testing the hypothesis that any abnormalities in nailfold capillaries in psoriasis patients of either a quantitative or qualitative nature might be observed more readily in subjects with pathology adjacent to the nailfold, i.e. distal interphalangeal (DIP) joint changes and/or nail dystrophy, when using this technique. They studied 44 patients with psoriasis with different skin, nail and DIP involvement compared with an age- and sex-matched health control group. There was a decrease in capillary loop density in patients with either psoriasis plus nail disease or nail and DIP joint disease when compared with controls in patients with psoriatic arthritis affecting the DIP joints with or without nail changes, there was a decrease in arterial and venous capillary limb diameters,. However, there was no difference in capillary dimensions between patients with only psoriasis and/or nail changes when compared with normal controls.

De angelis et al., [20] investigate the distribution, morphology and density of capillaries in lesional and perilesional skin of the psoriatic

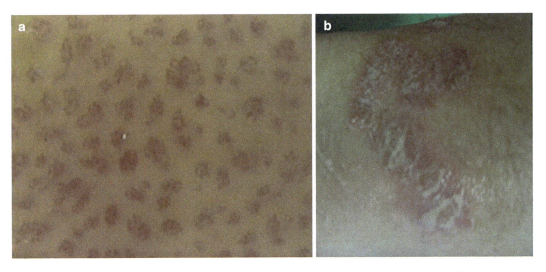

Fig. 18.6 (**a**) Videocapillaroscopy of the psoriatic plaque showing tortuous, coiled and bushy capillary formations. (**b**) Photo of the corresponding psoriatic plaque

plaque in well-delimited psoriatic plaques of the trunk, arms or legs in 15 consecutive untreated patients with chronic psoriasis plaque. The authors described in the lesional skin, capillaries tortuous and dilated, homogeneously appearing as 'bushy' whereas in the perilesional skin, capillary loops seemed to be on a parallel course with respect to the skin surface, with their apex directed towards the marginal zone. The number of capillary loops per area unit was statistically increased in perilesional compared to lesional skin. The authors suggested two different angiogenetic patterns in lesional and perilesional skin.

Ribeiro et al., performed a study to investigate changes at nailfold capillaroscopy in 46 psoriatic patients compared with controls [17]. Patients with psoriasis had lower capillary density increased avascular areas and an increased number of morphologically abnormal capillaries compared to controls. No association was found between capillary density and the duration of the disease or the extent of skin involvement, as measured by the PASI. The presence of avascular areas was more common in psoriatic individuals whose nails were affected by the condition. The study suggested that there is a decreased capillary density and a greater presence of mor-

phologically abnormal capillaries at nailfold level in psoriasis patients when compared to controls.

Differential Diagnosis

This area is still underexplored and there is not sufficient evidence to formulate clear conclusions. However it seems to be a promising topic to address the future researches.

Rosina et al., designed a study in order to evaluate to capability of VCP to differentiate the psoriasis from the dermatitis of the scalp [12]. VCP was performed on histology-confirmed scalp lesions of 30 patients with chronic plaque psoriasis, 30 age- and sex-matched patients with seborrheic dermatitis and 30 healthy subjects. The morphology, mean density per mm [2] and mean diameter of capillary loops was measured. Scalp psoriasis exhibited homogeneously tortuous and dilated capillaries (bushy pattern). In contrast, scalp seborrheic dermatitis presented a multiform pattern, with mildly tortuous capillary loops and isolated dilated capillaries, but a substantial preservation of local microvessel architecture. Mean diameter of capillary loop was significantly lower and similar to that of the scalp of healthy subjects. Capillary loop density was similar in patients with psoriasis seborrheic dermatitis and healthy scalp skin.

Treatment Monitoring

There is a growing interest to explore the potential of VCP in the treatment monitoring. Different treatments were used to describe the morphological changes in the microvascularity of psoriasis [16, 33–36]

Stinco et al., evaluated the modifications of the superficial capillary bed in a psoriatic plaque and healthy perilesional skin during treatment with a topical steroid in 24 patients with psoriasis vulgaris [34]. At the end of the study, the diameters of dilated and convoluted capillaries in the psoriatic plaque were significantly reduced in all subjects. A marked clinical improvement was noted. The perilesional skin showed improvement in VCP alterations, even if the drug had not been applied to those areas. Remarkable half of patients clinically healed at the end of the treatment period, although the capillaroscopic picture returned to normal in only 2 of them.

Rosina et al., conducted a similar study comparing the clinical and capillaroscopic modifications of a psoriatic target lesion during topical therapy [35]. Thirty patients with chronic plaque psoriasis were studied. Clinical and capillaroscopic modifications in comparable lesions of the elbows were analyzed during different topical therapies (calcipotriol, betamethasone dipropionate and calcipotriol plus betamethasone dipropionate) at baseline, and after 15 and 30 days of therapy. The modified PASI, the megapillary density per square mm and the mean diameter of capillary loops were measured. Microvascular restoration to a normal pattern, as detected by VCP, was faster than clinical improvement suggesting that VCP is an easily executable and non-invasive technique that detects early microcirculatory changes in psoriasis during topical therapy.

Stinco et al., assessed the modifications in the superficial capillary bed in psoriatic plaques during treatment with etanercept in 22 patients with plaque psoriasis resistant to conventional therapy [36]. At the beginning of the study, and at weeks 6, 12, 18 and 24, VCP of a selected plaque was performed. The PASI was determined as clinical outcome. Etanercept produced a significant reduction in PASI, plaque severity score and diameter of the basket-weave area at every time point. Four patients had complete remission, although none of the patients regained a normal capillaroscopic pattern.

Imaging techniques have only recently been utilized in combination with clinical observation to objectively quantify psoriasis severity and evaluate therapeutic response (Fig. 18.7). In this way Masumeci et al., evaluated the sensitivity of VCP and US to assess the therapeutic effect of cyclosporine in 22 patients with moderate-to-severe psoriasis [33]. VCP and US were performed at baseline, 2, 4 and 8 weeks. At the end of the study, Both VCP and US strongly correlated with one another. Skin thickness was the first parameter that improved. In contrast, improvement in VCP was delayed. Normalization rate of vascular pattern (assessed by VCP) was relative low in patients, despite virtually complete normalization by clinical and US assessment.

Our group in a case series showed contrasted results from Masumeci et al. since after 8 week of biological treatment a homogeneous clinical, US, histological and VCP response was detected in psoriatic plaque. However the cohort was too short to elaborate concrete conclusions.

Discussion

Currently, US, PDUS and VCP permit a fast and accurate assessment of vascular morphofunctional changes of psoriasis.

The skin (lesional and perilesional), the nail and the nailfold could be suitable anatomic sites to assess by US and VCP imaging for detecting minimal blood flow and capillary changes.

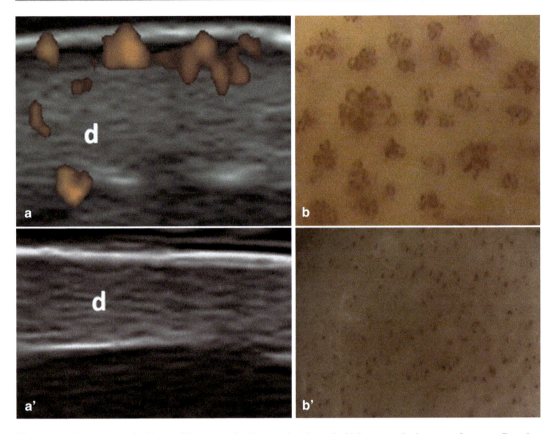

Fig. 18.7 Ultrasound and videocapillaroscopy findings during treatment. (**a**) Ultrasound shows an active psoriatic plaque with an increased epidermis and dermis, and intense power Doppler signal within the dermis. (**a'**). Examination after the treatment revealed a reduction of the dermal thickness and absence of power Doppler. (**b**) Videocapillaroscopy showing the typical tortuous and dilated (bushy) capillaries of the psoriatic plaque. (**b'**) The follow up showed that the bushy loops had disappeared and fewer dilated capillaries remain. *d* dermis

High-resolution grayscale US with PD and VCP are real-time and noninvasive imaging techniques that can be used as an adjunct to the clinical evaluation in assessing the extensión, activity and responsiveness of psoriasis lesions. Nevertheless, further investigations studying larger series of patients in correlation with histologic data may be useful to support these observations.

References

1. Nestle FO. Psoriasis. Curr Dir Autoimmun. 2008;10: 65–75.
2. Salaffi F, De Angelis R, Grassi W, MArche Pain Prevalence, INvestigation Group (MAPPING) Study. Prevalence of musculoskeletal conditions in an Italian population sample: results of a regional community-based study, I: the MAPPING study. Clin Exp Rheumatol. 2005;23:819–28.
3. Salomon J, Szepietowski JC, Proniewicz A. Psoriatic nails: a prospective clinical study. J Cutan Med Surg. 2003;7:317–21.
4. Feldman SR, Krueger GG. Psoriasis assessment tools in clinical trials. Ann Rheum Dis. 2005;64:1165–8.
5. Gupta AK, Turnbull DH, Harasiewicz KA, et al. The use of high-frequency ultrasound as a method of assessing the severity of a plaque of psoriasis. Arch Dermatol. 1996;132:658–62.
6. Vaillant L, Berson M, Machet L, Callens A, Pourcelot L, Lorette G. Ultrasound imaging of psoriatic skin: a noninvasive technique to evaluate treatment of psoriasis. Int J Dermatol. 1994;33:786–90.
7. El Gammal S, El Gammal C, Kaspar K, et al. Sonography of the skin at 100 MHz enables in vivo visualization of stratum corneum and viable epidermis in palmar skin and psoriatic plaques. J Invest Dermatol. 1999;113:821–9.
8. El Gammal S, Auer T, Popp C, et al. Psoriasis vulgaris in 50 MHz B-scan ultrasound: characteristic

features of stratum corneum, epidermis and dermis. Acta Derm Venereol Suppl (Stockh). 1994;186: 173–6.

9. Serup J. Non-invasive quantification of psoriatic plaque: measurement of skin thickness with 15 MHz pulsed ultrasound. Clin Exp Dermatol. 1984;9: 502–8.

10. Olsen LO, Serup J. High-frequency ultrasound scan for noninvasive cross-sectional imaging of psoriasis. Acta Derm Venereol. 1993;73:185–7.

11. Creamer D, Allen MH, Sousa A, Poston R, Barker JN. Localization of endothelial proliferation and micro-vascular expansion in active plaque psoriasis. Br J Dermatol. 1997;136:859–65.

12. Rosina P, Zamperetti MR, Giovannini A, Girolomoni G. Videocapillaroscopy in the differential diagnosis between psoriasis and seborrheic dermatitis of the scalp. Dermatology. 2007;214:21–4.

13. Bhushan M, Moore T, Herrick AL, Griffiths CE. Nailfold video capillaroscopy in psoriasis. Br J Dermatol. 2000;142:1171–6.

14. Sallì L, Raimondi F, Pappalardo A. Periungual capil-laroscopy in psoriatic arthritis. Clin Ter. 1999;150: 409–12.

15. Bull RH, Bates DO, Mortimer PS. Intravital video-capillaroscopy for the study of the microcirculation in psoriasis. Br J Dermatol. 1992;126:436–45.

16. Trevisan G, Magaton Rizzi G, Dal Canton M. Psoriatic microangiopathy modifications induced by PUVA and etretinate therapy. A nail-fold capillary microscopic study. Acta Derm Venereol Suppl (Stockh). 1989; 146:53–6.

17. Ribeiro CF, Siqueira EB, Holler AP, Fabrício L, Skare TL. Periungual capillaroscopy in psoriasis. An Bras Dermatol. 2012;87:550–3.

18. Lambova SN, Müller-Ladner U. Capillaroscopic pattern in inflammatory arthritis. Microvasc Res. 2012;83:318–22.

19. Hegyi J, Hegyi V, Messer G, Arenberger P, Ruzicka T, Berking C. Confocal laser-scanning capillaroscopy: a novel approach to the analysis of skin capillaries in vivo. Skin Res Technol. 2009;15:476–81.

20. De Angelis R, Grassi W, Cutolo M. A growing need for capillaroscopy in rheumatology. Arthritis Rheum. 2009;61:405–10.

21. Cutolo M, Sulli A, Pizzorni C, Smith V. Capillaroscopy as an outcome measure for clinical trials on the peripheral vasculopathy in SSc: is it useful? Int J Rheumatol 2010;2010:pii: 784947.

22. Herrick AL, Cutolo M. Clinical implications from capillaroscopic analysis in patients with Raynaud's phenomenon and systemic sclerosis. Arthritis Rheum. 2010;62(2):595–604.

23. Di Nardo A, Seidenari S, Giannetti A. B-scanning evaluation with image analysis of psoriatic skin. Exp Dermatol. 1992;1:121–5.

24. Seidenari S. High-frequency sonography combined with image analysis: a noninvasive objective method for skin evaluation and description. Clin Dermatol. 1995;13:349–59.

25. Fornage BD, McGavran MH, Duvic M, Waldron CA. Imaging of the skin with 20-MHz US. Radiology. 1993;189:69–76.

26. Guastalla P, Guerci VI, Fabretto A, et al. Detection of epidermal thickening in GJB2 carriers with epidermal US. Radiology. 2009;251:280–6.

27. Gutierrez M, De Angelis R, Bernardini ML, et al. Clinical, power Doppler sonography and histological assessment of the psoriatic plaque: short-term monitoring in patients treated with etanercept. Br J Dermatol. 2011;164:33–7.

28. Gutierrez M, Di Geso L, Salaffi F, et al. Development of a preliminary US power Doppler composite score for monitoring treatment in PsA. Rheumatology. 2012;51:1261–8.

29. Hern S, Mortimer OS. In vivo quantification of microvessels in clinically univoled psoriatic skin and in normal skin. Br J Dermatol. 2007;156:1224–9.

30. Espinoza LR, Vasey FB, Espinoza GG, Bocanegra TS, Germain BF. Vascular changes in psoriatic synovium. A light and electron microscopy study. Arthritis Rheum. 1982;25:677–84.

31. Bhusman M, Moore T, Herrick A, Griffiths CEM. Naildfold video capillaroscopy in psoriasis. Br J Dermatol. 2000;142:1171–6.

32. Bartosinska J, Chodorowska G. Original proposal of capillaroscopic images classification in psoriasis vulgaris and psoriatic arthritis. Adv Dermatol Allergol. 2009;26:17.

33. Musumeci ML, Lacarrubba F, Fusto CM, Micali G. Combined clinical, capillaroscopic and ultrasound evaluation during treatment of plaque psoriasis with oral cyclosporine. Int J Immunopathol Pharmacol. 2013;26:1027–33.

34. Stinco G, Buligan C, Maione V, Valent F, Patrone P. Videocapillaroscopic findings in the microcirculation of the psoriatic plaque during etanercept therapy. Clin Exp Dermatol. 2013;38:633–7.

35. Rosina P, Giovannini A, Gisondi P, Girolomoni G. Microcirculatory modifications of psoriatic lesions during topical therapy. Skin Res Technol. 2009;15: 135–8.

36. Stinco G, Lautieri S, Piccirillo F, Valent F, Patrone P. Response of cutaneous microcirculation to treatment with mometasone furoate in patients with psoriasis. Clin Exp Dermatol. 2009;34:915–9.

Radiographic Assessment of Psoriatic Arthritis (PsA)

Javier Rosa, Percival D. Sampaio-Barros, and Enrique Roberto Soriano

Abstract

Radiographs are accessible, inexpensive and safe, and therefore remain the generally accepted means for imaging assessment of joint disease in PsA. Radiographs can help in making a diagnosis of PsA, are useful in differentiating PsA from other diseases, and have been used as an outcome measure in the clinical trials and observational studies in PsA. Although there are not specific radiographic features in PsA, there are some typical characteristics that are very useful, and should prompt the physician to think about PsA. These are discussed and described in this chapter, and include: predilection for the distal interphalangeal (DIP) joints of the hands and interphalangeal joint of the great toe, the absence of juxta-articular osteopenia, the presence of large erosions with bony proliferation (pencil-in-cup image), the presence of osteolysis and ankylosis (sometimes in the same hand or finger), periostitis, and the presence of enthesal erosions and calcifications. We also discuss the importance of baseline radiographs in disease prognosis, and the different radiographs scoring methods that have been validated for use in PsA clinical trials and observational studies.

Keywords

Radiographic assessment • Psoriatic arthritis • X-Rays

J. Rosa, MD • E.R. Soriano, MD, MSC (✉)
Department of Rheumatology,
Instituto Universitario Hospital Italiano
de Buenos Aires, Peron 4190 (1181). CABA,
Buenos Aires, Argentina
e-mail: enrique.soriano@hospitalitaliano.org.ar

P.D. Sampaio-Barros, MD, PHD
Division of Rheumatology,
Faculdade de Medicina da Universidade
de São Paulo, São Paulo, Brazil

Introduction

Psoriatic arthritis once thought as a benign rheumatic disease, is nowadays considered a progressive disease where a substantial number of patients can develop severe erosive and deforming disease with major structural damage [1–4]. Patients with polyarticular onset

© Springer International Publishing Switzerland 2016
A. Adebajo et al. (eds.), *Psoriatic Arthritis and Psoriasis: Pathology and Clinical Aspects*,
DOI 10.1007/978-3-319-19530-8_19

Table 19.1 Musculoskeletal structures seen with various imaging modalities

	X-ray	Ultrasound	MRI
Bone			
Joint erosion	✓	✓	✓
New bone formation	✓	✓	✓
Osteitis			✓
Synovium			
Synovitis		✓	✓
Cartilage			
Loss	(Indirect)	✓	✓
Tendons			
Tendonitis		✓	✓
Enthesitis		✓	✓
Dactylitis		✓	✓
Effusion		✓	✓
Spondylitis			
Spinal disease	✓		✓
Sacroilitis	✓		✓

Adapted from Anandarajah [7]. With permission from Springer Science

are at increased risk for progression of joint deformities, as are the patients who had been given high doses of medications [5, 6].

Radiographs are accessible, inexpensive and safe, and therefore remain the generally accepted imaging method used for structural assessment of joint disease in PsA [7]. They help in making a diagnosis of PsA and have been used as an outcome measure in the assessment of conventional and biologic therapies for the treatment of PsA. The inability to view the soft tissue structures, the two dimensional views, and the exposure to radiation are limitations that have led to the development of newer imaging technologies, such as ultrasound (US) and magnetic resonance imaging (MRI) [7]. Power Doppler US is especially useful for the assessment of musculoskeletal (joints, tendons, enthesis) and cutaneous (skin, nails) involvement, as well as for monitoring therapy and guiding steroid injections in PsA [8, 9]. MRI has been increasingly used due to its capacity of allowing an early diagnosis through the visualization of inflammation in peripheral and axial joints and enthesis, contributing to the design of the pattern of inflammation in the spondyloarthritis (SpA) [10, 11].

Table 19.1 shows information on the use of conventional radiography, ultrasound (US), and magnetic resonance image (MRI) in the assessment and diagnosis of PsA, according to different structures involved.

Radiographic Features in PsA

There are many axial and peripheral radiographic features in PsA. In 2003, Taylor et al. reported the results of a systematic review of the literature in order to conceptualize and standardize operational definitions for these radiological features (Table 19.2) [12].

Here we describe radiographic characteristics at different levels and joints:

Hands

- *Normal mineralization:* One typical feature of PsA is the lack of periarticular osteopenia. In the early phases of the disease there might be transient juxta-articular osteopenia, however restoration of normal mineralization occurs in the majority of cases.
- *Uniform reduction of joint space:* This is the radiographic expression of cartilage loss, and could be seen at any involved joint, more typically at the distal interphalangeal (DIP) and proximal interphalangeal (PIP) joints, and more infrequently at the metacarpophalangeal (MCP) joints.
- *Erosions:* in early stages erosions occur in the joint margins, resembling "mouse ears" and are different from the central erosion ("gull wings") (Fig. 19.2) of erosive osteoarthritis (EO). Erosions progress over time and may affect the central area. If they are extensive, the subchondral bone can be destroyed, leading to joint space widening. The ends of the bones can become pointed, resulting in the image of "pencil in cup" (Fig. 19.3). This appearance is not specific for PsA or any of the other spondyloarthritis, but it is most commonly seen in these conditions. There

Table 19.2 Operational definitions of the principal plain radiograph features of PsA

Feature	Definition
Axial features	
Marginal syndesmophyte	Classic, thin syndesmophyte arising vertically from annular attachment to vertebral body
Non-marginal syndesmophyte	Vertically oriented or curvilinear syndesmophyte, often thick and chunky, arising from beyond the annular attachment to vertebral body (Fig. 19.1)
Paravertebral ossification	Ossification close to vertebral body, but with a clearly defined gap between the margins of the ossification and the vertebral body
Destructive discovertebral lesión	Irregularity of superior and inferior endplates with erosive changes and adjacent vertebral sclerosis, with or without fracture and angulation (Andersson lesion)
Romanus lesión	Clearly defined erosion of the anterior margin of the discovertebral junction at the superior or inferior portions of the vertebral body
Sacroiliitis.	New York grade ≥ 2 bilaterally, or ≥3 unilaterally
Peripherical features	
Extraarticular entheseal erosion	Erosion at entheseal insertion of calcaneus, ischial tuberosities, iliac crest, femoral trochanters, humeral tuberosity, or patella
Extraarticular entheseal ossification	Irregular bony proliferation at entheseal insertion of calcaneus, ischial tuberosities, iliac crest, femoral trochanters, humeral tuberosity, patella
DIP erosive disease, excluding erosive OA	Clearly defined marginal erosion of DIP joint AND either: evidence of joint destruction (widened joint space or osteolysis) or juxtaarticular periostitis OR absence of osteophytes (Figs. 19.2, 19.3 and 19.4)
Joint osteolysis.	Osteolysis producing a wide, sharply demarcated joint space, including phalangeal whittling (Fig. 19.5)
Loss of tuft cortical definition.	Loss of cortical definition of terminal tuft, often with a "fluffy" appearance
Juxtaarticular bony proliferation	Ill-defined ossification near joint margins, but excluding osteophyte formation (Fig. 19.3)
Periosteal new bone formation	Linear, ill-defined metaphyseal or diaphyseal bony apposition
Bony ankylosis	Bony ankylosis indicated by trabeculae crossing the joint space (Figs. 19.3, 19.5 and 19.6)

Adapted from Taylor et al. [12]. With permission from The Journal of Rheumatology

may be resorption of distal phalangeal tufts (acroosteolysis), almost always accompanied by severe nail lesions. Pronounced osteolysis can also occur and may present as loss of the whole phalanx. The presence of erosions and ankylosis in the same hand and sometimes in the same finger is a unique and intriguing finding in PsA (Fig. 19.3) [7]. The DIP involvement and the asymmetric distribution also can help differentiate PsA from rheumatoid arthritis (RA).

- *Bone proliferation:* irregular overgrowth adjacent to erosions with a fluffy or speculated appearance might be seen. Along the

shaft we can see periostitis, cottony cushion initially that may form solid new bone simulating enlargement of the phalangeal diaphysis.

Feet

- The findings are similar, although with certain peculiarities. The involvement of the interphalangeal joint (IF) of the first finger presents with widespread destruction.
- One characteristic feature of PsA in the foot is the "ivory phalanx," which classically involves the distal phalanges (especially in the first digit) with sclerosis, enthesitis, periostitis, and

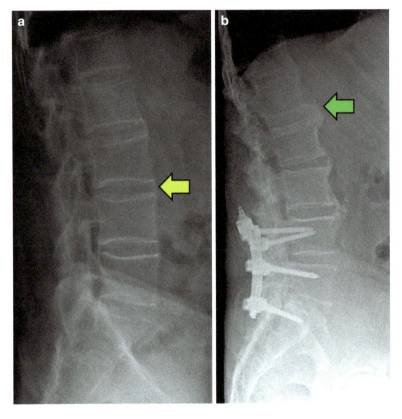

Fig. 19.1 Lateral lumbar spine. (**a**) syndesmophytes in patient with Ankylosing Spondylitis (*yellow arrow*); (**b**) chunky syndesmophytes in a patient with psoriatic arthritis (*green arrow*)

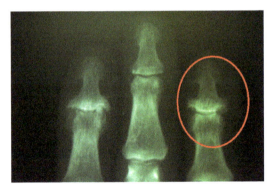

Fig. 19.2 Plain radiograph of the hand with marginal erosions at the 4th distal interphalangeal joint resembling "mouse ears" (*red circle*)

insertion of the plantar aponeurosis; creating irregular spurs.

Other Peripheral Joints

- Involvement of the shoulder, elbow, knee and ankle tends to be asymmetrical, with erosive changes and proliferation of adjacent bone; cartilage loss is uniform. Bone proliferation in the insertion of the rotator cuff, coraco-clavicular ligament, patellar tendon, ischial tuberosities and femoral trochanter could also be seen.
- Hip involvement is uncommon.

soft-tissue swelling [7]. Joint subluxation and luxation may also be present.

- Involvement of the metatarsophalangeal joints (MTF) is more common than MCF joints.
- Calcaneal erosion and bone proliferation occur in the posterior-superior insertion of the Achilles tendon and the lower side by the

Arthritis Mutilans

Recent studies found an arthritis mutilans (AM) prevalence ranging from 1.5 to 4.9 % (Fig. 19.5). Research of AM has been impeded by the rarity of the subphenotype, and the lack of an agreed clinical or radiographic definition. AM

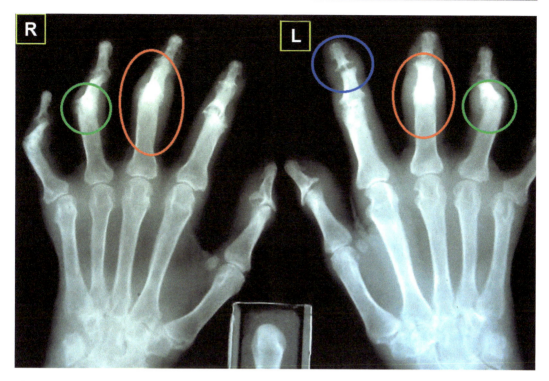

Fig. 19.3 Plain radiograph of both hands showing: extensive erosion, giving the typical "pencil in cup" image at the left 2nd distal interphalangeal joint (*blue circle*); bony ankylosis at bilateral 4th proximal interphalangeal joints (*green circle*); and soft-tissue swelling at bilateral 3rd proximal interphalangeal joints (*red circle*)

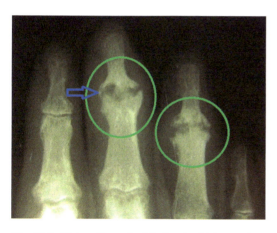

Fig. 19.4 Plain radiograph of the hand, with juxtaarticular bony proliferation at the 3rd distal interphalangeal joint (*blue arrow*), and extensive marginal erosions at the 3rd and 4th distal interphalangeal joints (*green circles*)

represents an aggressive form of arthritis characterized by marked erosion of small joints of hands and feet, progressing to irreversible joint disruption. AM has been defined as osteolysis affecting ≥50 % of the articular surface on both sides of the joint [13]. The resulting finger and toe mutilations severely impair patients' functional capacity. Development of AM has been associated with longer arthritis duration, involvement of distal phalanges, and impaired functional capacity, suggesting these patients should undergo tight disease control and therapy. AM is an infrequent but highly disabling form of PsA. Therapy with DMARD seems unable to prevent its development. A potential role for biologic therapy is expected, and prospective studies are urged [14].

Axial Disease

Psoriatic arthritis may also involve the axial skeleton, a finding that occurs in 20–40 % of patients with peripheral articular disease [15, 16].

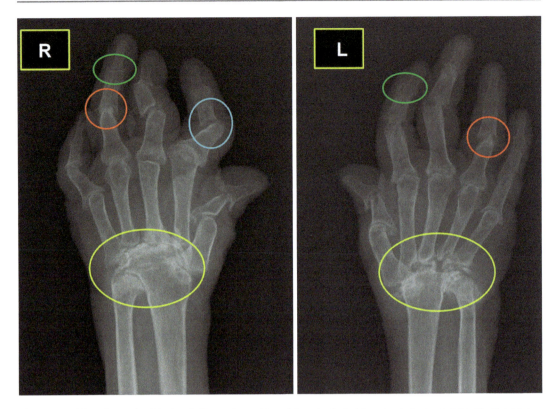

Fig. 19.5 Plain radiograph of the hands in a patient with arthritis mutilans shows bilateral osteolysis on carpal joints (*yellow circles*) and of distal 2nd right phalange, pencil-in-cup lesions in both 4th proximal interphalangeal joints (*red circle*) and ankylosis at right 4th distal interphalangeal joint and left 2nd distal interphalangeal joint (*green circles*) and luxation at the 2nd right proximal interphalangeal joint (blue circle)

Some radiographic features of axial PsA, such as asymmetrical sacroiliitis, nonmarginal and asymmetrical syndesmophytes, paravertebral ossification, and frequent involvement of cervical spine, seem to be so characteristic as to be potentially helpful in diagnosing PsA [15]. The sacroiliac joints will show signs of inflammation, with sclerosis in the subchondral bone plate, osseous erosions, joint space irregularity and mild widening, and eventual joint space narrowing and intraarticular bone ankylosis. Sacroiliac joint involvement in PsA might be unilateral or bilateral, either symmetric or asymmetric in the grade of involvement. Initially it affects the iliac side of the synovial joint. When erosions increase and affect the sacrum side, bone proliferation may be more extensive than in AS. Ossification of ligaments between the sacrum and the ilium is possible, even without synovial joint ankylosis.

Other tendon attachments can become ossified, such as the iliac crest, femoral trochanter and the ischial tuberosity. Radiographic sacroiliitis has been defined using the New York grading system: grade 2–4 bilaterally or grade 3–4 unilaterally [17].

The thoracolumbar spine may show large comma-shaped paravertebral ossifications; however, spondylitis is uncommon in the absence of sacroiliitis. The facet joints are relatively spared, and there is absence of vertebral body "squaring". Cervical spine involvement was found in 45 % of those examined and 36 % of patients X-rayed in one study [18]. The pattern of disease was ankylosing in 85 % of patients, characterized by ankylosis, syndesmophytes and ligamentous ossification [18].

At axial sites, bony proliferation may be manifest as paravertebral ossification,

Fig. 19.6 Plain radiograph of both feet showing: erosions and ankylosis in both 1st left interphalangeal joints (*red circle*); luxation and subluxation of 2nd and 3rd metatarsophalangeal joints in the left foot (*blue circle*), and metatarsophalangeal joints in right foot (*green circle*)

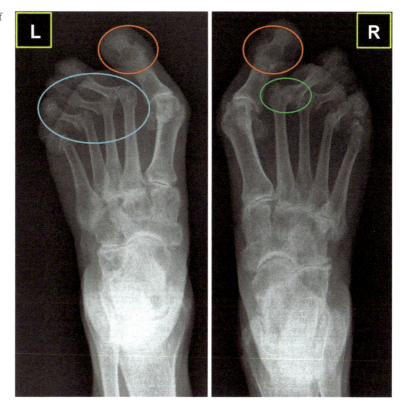

syndesmophytes, or sacroiliac ankylosis. Syndesmophytes may be of three morphologies: marginal, nonmarginal (which includes "chunky" and "comma"), and paravertebral ossification (which may simply be an early stage of non-marginal). Discovertebral lesions such as osteitis, Romanus lesion, vertebral squaring and others are less common in psoriatic SpA than in AS. There are other lesions of the cervical spine reported, including apophyseal joint and disc space narrowing, posterior ligamentous calcification, atlantoaxial subluxation, odontoid erosion, and subaxial erosions. The radiographic features of enthesitis are erosion and/or ossification at entheseal insertions, which might include the following sites: posterior and plantar aspect of the calcaneus, femoral trochanters, ischial tuberosities, ankle malleoli, distal portion of femoral condyles, olecranon of the ulna, iliac crest, inferior margin of clavicle, anterior portion of patella, and spinous processes of verterbrae [15, 16].

Nevertheless, literature concerning radiology in PsA can be somewhat confusing in its terminology [12]. For example, there are several ways in which osteolytic changes have been described, including "resorptive arthritis", "mutilation", "mushrooming", "cup in stem", "pencil in cup deformity", "whittling of terminal phalanges", "pseudowidening of the interosseous joint space", "phalangeal tuft resorption", or "osteolysis producing a widely, sharply demarcated joint space" [12]. Similarly, there is some potential confusion regarding the correct meaning of "non-marginal syndesmophytes" with seeming equivalence between "paramarginal", "parasyndesmophyte", "non-marginal", "comma shaped", and "chunky" [12].

Conventional radiography has some difficulties in defining the cause of the thickening of periarticular soft tissues, for example, in the cases of synovial hypertrophy, tendinitis, tenosynovitis, enthesitis or bursitis. The evaluation of joint space allows assessing articular cartilage indirectly. A severe joint space narrowing can lead to bony ankylosis in late stages of the disease.

X-Rays in the Diagnosis of PsA

Radiographic examination should include AP and lateral views of hands and feet in patients with peripheral joint involvement, and cervical, lower thoracic, lumbar spine and sacroiliac joints when axial symptoms are present.

The distinctive radiographic features of PsA are the result of a combination of erosive and proliferative bone changes. Characteristic findings include "opera-glass" deformity, which consists of telescoping erosive joint destruction; fluffy periostitis caused by periosteal ossification; "pencil in cup" deformity in which simultaneous destruction of the head of the middle phalanx and expansion of the base of the distal phalanx produces the characteristic finding; and acroosteolysis, consisting of resorption of the tuft of the distal phalanx [16].

Findings may be bilateral or unilateral and symmetric or asymmetric. Involvement of several musculoskeletal structures in a single digit, with soft-tissue swelling, produces what appears clinically as a "sausage digit" [19]. The bone proliferation produces an irregular appearance to the marginal bone on the involved joint, characterized as a "fuzzy" appearance or "whiskering". Periostitis may take several forms: it may appear as a thin periosteal layer of new bone adjacent to the cortex, a thick irregular layer, or irregular thickening of the cortex itself [19]. It is important to note that periostitis may occur in an area without bone erosions; one such site is the radial aspect of the wrist extending into the first metacarpal bone.

Marginal erosions at peripheral joints may occur in PsA, and may be distinguished from RA by preservation of juxtaarticular bone density. The juxta-articular osteopenia is uncommon in PsA, although when present is a sign of poor prognosis [20]. However, the assessment of juxtaarticular osteopenia is known to be highly dependent upon radiographic technique.

Bony proliferation is a fairly characteristic feature of PsA. It also occurrs in other SpA, but is rarely seen in RA. Other proliferative features include bony ankylosis, particularly of interphalangeal joints. Asymetric involvement is usually referred as one of the characteristics of PsA. The usual definition of symmetry requires that at least 50 % of involved joints are symmetric pairs. Given this definition, and given that there are a finite number of possible joints that can be involved, it has been argued that the presence of symmetry is strongly influenced by the total number of joints involved [21].

Several proposed PsA classification criteria include radiographic features [7]. The presence of erosions in small joints with a relative lack of osteoporosis was included as one of the criteria by Bennett [22]. McGonagle proposed the presence of radiographic evidence for enthesitis as one the features in his classification criteria for PsA [23]. The radiological evidence of entesitis has been suggested as a discriminatory feature from RA; however, it remains an infrequent radiographic feature. The new developed CASPAR criteria include the presence of bone neoformation phenomenon detected on radiographs [24].

X-Ray in the Differential Diagnosis of PsA

An additional utility of conventional radiography in PsA is that it might be useful in the differential diagnosis with other pathologies.

- *Reactive arthritis (ReA):* The radiographic features of ReA are similar to those of PsA and include joint inflammation, bone proliferation, periostitis, and enthesitis, with a distribution that is unilateral or bilateral and symmetric or asymmetric;
- *Ankylosing spondylitis (AS):* AS affects predominantly the axial skeleton, although large peripheral joints of lower limbs may also be affected. The radiographic presentation of syndesmophytes in AS uses to be symmetrical, regular and from margin to margin, while it is predominantly asymmetrical and irregular in PsA. The distribution along the spine might also be different. Progression of syndesmophytes from lumbar toward cervical is the rule in

AS, while a more random distribution is the most frequent finding in axial PsA [15]. There might also be some differences in syndesmophytes type. In PsA syndesmophytes had a so-called "chunky" shape, meaning a substantial structural difference from those "coarse" marginal and symmetrical ones observed in typical AS (Fig. 19.1).

- **Rheumatoid arthritis (RA):** Compared with RA, PsA has differences in the radiographic features, and sites of involvement. The typical radiographic features of RA include periarticular osteopenia, uniform joint space loss, bone erosions, and soft-tissue swelling. Periostitis, osteolysis, juxtaarticular bony proliferation and ankylosis are not common in RA, and should raise the suspicion of PsA. The proximal distribution of joint involvement in the hands and feet suggests RA. Bone erosions in PsA are often less sharply demarcated, probably due to being obscured by concomitant bone apposition, a feature usually lacking in RA. Furthermore, in PsA the erosions not only occur in the PIP, MCP, and wrist joints, but in DIP joints as well. If joint inflammation is limited to a single joint, infection must first be carefully excluded.
- **Septic arthritis:** The radiographic features of a septic joint encompass those of any inflammatory arthritis namely periarticular osteopenia, uniform joint space narrowing, soft-tissue swelling, and bone erosions [19].
- **Erosive osteoarthritis (EOA):** EOA is characterized by severe IP destruction with relative sparing of the MCP joints and frequent involvement of the trapeziometacarpal joint. Combined MCP and IP arthritis is much more prevalent in PsA than EOA. Furthermore, MCP arthritis is rare in EOA, and it is usually not associated with bone erosions in EOA, whereas such erosions are common in PA [25]. Radiocarpal, radioulnar, and diffuse carpal joint involvement are common in PA (Fig. 19.5), but rare in EOA [25]. Diagnostically significant features of EOA include the configuration of the eroded subchondral cortex of the IP joints and linear periosteal bone apposition. Joint involvement in both PsA and EOA is typically associated with uniform narrow-

ing of the cartilage space. However, in EOA some of the joints, particularly those not severely affected, exhibited non-uniform loss of cartilage [25]. The erosions on the distal surface of the DIP joints in PsA have a characteristic appearance which suggests "mouse ears" (Fig. 19.2). By contrast, the erosions of the IP joints in EOA are largely a consequence of destruction of the articular cartilage. The resultant deformity of the distal subchondral cortex suggests "gull wings" because the most marked bone erosion is peripheral, whereas on the proximal side of the joint, the erosion is usually most marked near the center of the bone.. Periosteal bone apposition is well known in PsA, but is not a widely recognized feature of EOA. It is often irregular and exuberant in PsA, whereas in EOA it is always linear and usually minimal to moderate in degree. In EOA it occurs typically near affected joints. After the inflammatory phase of PsA subsides, fluffy periosteal bone apposition becomes more compact and linear. Hence, smooth cortical thickening may result in both conditions;. Linear bone apposition is extremely common in EOA in the first metacarpal, associated with arthritis of the trapeziometacarpal joint. Another significant diagnostic feature from a radiologic viewpoint is the selective involvement of the joints of a particular ray severely affected with sparing of other joints ("ray-pattern") This ray pattern may be relatively specific for PsA, inasmuch as they have not been described in other rheumatic diseases [25]. The presence of arthritis of one hand with sparing of the contralateral side in EOA is uncommon, but can be seen in PsA [25]. Malalignment of finger joints may be observed in both PsA and EOA. In EOA these are usually restricted to mild flexion deformity and medial or lateral deviation, but in PsA such malalignments may be severe and subluxation also occurs. IP arthritis of the small toes with irregular subchondral bone erosion has not been described in EOA. Well marginated calcaneal spurs, localized to the posterior attachment of the plantar aponeurosis, are commonly the result of mechanical stress. This finding is not necessarily a feature of EOA. Interphalangeal fusion of the fingers is commonly considered to be diagnostic of PsA; however, this may be more common in EOA. Such fusion also occurrs in the feet in PsA, but not typically in EOA [25, 26].

X-Ray in the Prognosis of PsA

Conventional radiographies have also been used in PsA to establish the severity, extent and prognosis of joint damage [27]. Radiographic damage is frequent in PsA, with around 47 % of patients showing joint damage by 1 or 2 years of follow up [28].

Baseline radiological damage in PsA observational studies has proven to be a strong predictor of structural damage and mortality [29]. Given that the clinical examination may underestimate joint damage in PsA, radiography is currently considered a standard measure of assessment for the identification and measurement of the extent of the articular process.

Several studies have shown that biological agents, particularly TNF inhibitors, are able to significantly decrease the progression of joint damage in PsA [30]. More recently, other agetns, including the IL-12/23 inhibitor ustekinumab and the IL-17 inhibitor secukinumab have also beenshown capable of inhibiting structural damage. The evidence of the hault of radiographic progresion with biologics agents has been sumarized in Table 19.3. Therefore, it is imperative to assess the structural damage radiologically at the initiation of therapy, and regularly thereafter in order to evaluate disease progression.

Radiographic Scoring Methods in PsA

Conventional X-ray is a core outcome measure in both randomized control trials for novel therapies, as well as in longitudinal observational studies. Several scoring methods validated for use in RA and subsequently modified for use in PsA have been proposed, including the modified Sharp score (MSS), the Sharp/van der Heijde modified method (SHS), the modified Steinbrocker method, and the PsA Ratingen score [27]. These are summarized in Table 19.4. During the 2012 Group for Research and Assessment of Psoriasis and Psoriatic Arthritis (GRAPPA) annual meeting in Stockholm the choice of radiographic outcome measure to use in PsA randomized controlled trials and longitudinal observational studies was discussed [27, 38]. There was consensus that the SHS was the optimal tool to use in randomized controlled trials (where sensitivity to change is often the most important attribute of the outcome measure), but the most appropriate tool for use in longitudinal observational studies is yet to be determined [27, 38]. Tillet et al. assessed the feasibility, reliability, and sensitivity to change of 4 radiographic scores in PsA [27]. They have shown that none of the existing radiographic measures are both sufficiently feasible and sensitive to change to be easily applied in large longitudinal observational studies. The different radiographic methods in PsA are summarized in Table 19.3 [27].

The time required to apply each method differs considerably from 6.2 to 14.6 min. As may be expected, the global score (the Steinbrocker method) is the most feasible. The SHS is consistently the more sensitive to change than the MSS. Finally, the Ratingen scoring method is more sensitive than the Steinbrocker method as it is a composite rather than a global score, allowing grading of erosion and proliferation [27]. The soft tissue swelling element of the Steinbrocker method is an additional source of variability; particularly at the metatarsophalangeal joints as there is a less clear view of the soft tissues. The scoring of joint space narrowing is not specific to PsA and can occur in concurrent osteoarthritis and thus overestimate progression. The Ratingen score includes a measure of proliferation, which was the only radiographic change sufficiently specific to PsA to justify inclusion in the CASPAR criteria. The smallest detectable change (SDC) of the Ratingen score is close to that of the MSS and SHS, but it is quicker to perform and may be more specific to PsA through inclusion of proliferation [27].

Table 19.3 Effect on radiographic progression of biologics in randomized control trials

Author/year	Biologic agent/Dose	PsA duration years, mean (SD) Biologics/no biologics	Number of patients Biologics/no biologics	mTSS[a] change at week 24 meanm (SD) Biologics/no biologics	Patients without disease progression[b] at week 24, N Biologics/no biologics (%)
Mease at al. 2006 [31]	Etanercept/25 mg twice/weekly	9.0 (ND) 9.2 (ND)	101/104		64/71 (90.1)/48/70 (68.6)
Gladman et al. 2007 (ADEPT) [32]	Adalimumab/40 mg/EOW	9.7 (8.2)/9.1(8.6)	151/162	−0.1 (ND)/0.9 (ND)	131/145 (91.0)/108/153 (71.1)
Mease et al. 2009 (ADEPT) [33]	Adalimumab/40 mg/EOW	9.8 (8.3)/9.2 (8.7)	151/162	−0.1 (1.20)/0.8 (2.42)	
van der Heijde et al. 2007 (IMPACT 2) [34]	Infliximab/5 mg/kg/every 8 weeks	8.4 (7.2)/7.5 (7.8)	100/100	−0.7 (2.53)/0.82 (2.62)	90/100 (90.0)/78/100 (78.0)
Kavanaugh et al. 2012 (GOREVEAL) [35]	Golimumab/50 mg/ Every 4 weeks 100 mg/every 4 weeks	7.2 (6.8)/7.6 (7.9) 7.7 (7.8)/7.6 (7.9)	146/113 146/113	−0.16 (1.31)/0.27 (1.26) −0.02 (1.32)/0.27 (1.26)	104/132 (78.8)/64/102 (62.8) 105/137 (76.6)/64/102 (62.8)
van der Heijde et al. 2013 (RAPID PsA) [36]	Certolizumab/200 mg/EOW OR CZM 400 mg/Every 4 weeks	9.6 (8.5)/7.9 (7.7) 8.1 (8.3)/7.9(7.7)	138/136 135/136	0.01 (0.08)/0.29 (0.08)[c] 0.12 (0.08)/0.29 (0.08)[c]	83.3/34.6[d] 93.5/80.1[e] 76.3/34.6[d] 90.4/80.1[e]
Kavanaugh et al. 2014 (PSUMMIT 1 y PSUMMIT 2) [37]	Ustekinumab/45 mg at week 0, 4 and every 12 weeks thereafter (PSUMMIT 1) 90 mg at week 0, 4 and every 12 weeks thereafter (PSUMMIT 1) Ustekinumab/45 mg at week 0, 4 and every 12 weeks (PSUMMIT 2) 90 mg at week 0, 4 and every 12 weeks thereafter (PSUMMIT 2)	3.4 (1.2–9.2)/3.6 (1.0–9.7) 4.9 (1.7–8.3)/3.6 (1.0–9.7) 5.3 (2.3–12.2)/5.5 (2.3–12.2) 4.5 (1.7–10.3)/5.5 (2.3–12.2)	615 205/206 615 204/206 312 103/104 312 105/104	0.4 (2.1)/1.0 (3.9) (45 mg) 0.4 (2.4)/1.0 (3.)9 (90 mg) 0.4 (2.3)/1.0 (3.9) (combined)[f]	91.7 % (combined) vs 83.8 % (placebo) p=0.005[g]

[a]mTSS, modified total Sharp score. EOW: every other week

[b]It was defined like nonprogressors to patients with increase in mTSS ≤0.5 between baseline and 24 weeks; a 0.5 mTSS change included most of the change attributable to reader error

[c]No imputation

[d]Percentage of patients using the prespecified mTSS non-progressor rate definition (≤0 cut-off, non-responder imputation (NRI), p<0.05 versus placebo)

[e]Proportion of mTSS non-progressors (≤0.5 points cut-off, linear extrapolation)

[f]Integrated data analysis of change from baseline to wk 24 in total vdH-S score in the PSUMMIT-1 and PSUMMIT-2 studies, Mean±SD

[g]Defined by change in total PsA-modified vdH-S score from baseline ≤SDC (=2.01)

Table 19.4 Summary of scoring methods

Scoring methods/scales	Total erosion score	Total joint space narrowing (JSN)	Total score
Steinbrocker method **42 joints of hands and feet: scale 0–4**	NA (not applicable)	NA (not applicable)	168
0 = normal.			
1 = Juxta-articular osteopenia or soft tissue swelling.			
2 = Presence of any erosion.			
3 = Presence of erosion and joint space narrowing.			
4 = Total joint destruction (lysis or ankylosis).			
Modified Sharp method **54 joints (42 hands, 12 feet) for erosion: scale 0–5**	270	216	486
0 = no erosion			
1 = 1 discrete erosion or involvement of 21 % of the joint is by erosion.			
2 = 2 discrete erosions or joint involvement of 21–40 %.			
3 = 3 discrete erosions or joint involvement of 41–60 %.			
4 = 4 discrete erosions or joint involvement of 61–80 %.			
5 = extensive destruction involving > 80 % of the joint.			
54 joints (44 hands, 10 feet) for JSN: scale 0–4			
0 = Normal joint.			
1 = Asymmetrical or minimal narrowing.			
2 = Definite narrowing with loss ≤50 % of the normal space.			
3 = Definite narrowing with loss of 51–99 % of the normal space.			
4 = Absence of a joint space, presumptive evidence of ankylosis.			
5 = Widening.			
Sharp/van der Heijde method **52 joints (42 hands, 10 feet) for erosion: scale 0–5 (hands), 0–10 (feet)**	320	208	528
0 = No erosions.			
1 = Discrete erosion.			
2 = Large erosion not passing midline.			
3 = Large erosion passing midline.			
4 = Combination of above.			
5 = Combination of above.			

52 joints (42 hands, 10 feet) for JSN: scale 0–4

0 = Normal.

1 = Asymmetrical minimal narrowing with loss of maximum 25 %.

2 = Definite narrowing with loss of 50 % of normal space.

3 = Definite narrowing with 50–99 % loss of normal space/subluxation.

4 = Absence of a joint space, presumptive evidence of ankylosis, or complete subluxation.

Ratingen method
40 joints (30 hands, 10 feet) for destruction: scale 0–5   200   160 (Proliferation)   360

0 = Normal.

1 = 1 definite erosion with an interruption of cortical plate of 1 mm, but destruction of 10 % of total joint surface.

2 = Destruction of 11–25 %.

3 = Destruction of 26–50 %.

4 = Destruction of 51–75 %.

5 = Destruction of >75 % of joint surface.

40 joints (30 hands, 10 feet) for proliferation: scale 0–4

0 = Normal.

1 = Bony proliferation measured from the original bone surface of 1–2 mm, or clearly identifiable bone growth not exceeding 25 % of the original diameter of the bone.

2 = Bony proliferation 2–3 mm or bone growth between 25 and 50 %.

3 = Bony proliferation >3 mm or bone growth >50 %.

4 = Bony ankylosis.

Adapted from Tillett et al. [27]. With permission from John Wiley & Sons

Conclusion

Radiographs are worldwide accessible, inexpensive and safe, can also help in making a diagnosis of PsA, are useful in differentiating PsA from other diseases and are accepted outcome measures in clinical trials and observational studies. Radiographs in PsA might show some typical characteristics that should prompt the physician to think about PsA. In spite of the development of new, more sensitivity and specific imaging modalities, x-Rays have still a major role in the diagnosis and management of PsA.

References

1. Torre Alonso JC, Rodriguez Perez A, Arribas Castrillo JM, Ballina Garcia J, Riestra Noriega JL, Lopez Larrea C. Psoriatic arthritis (PA): a clinical, immunological and radiological study of 180 patients. Br J Rheumatol. 1991;30(4):245–50.

2. Gladman DD, Shuckett R, Russell ML, Thorne JC, Schachter RK. Psoriatic arthritis (PSA) – an analysis of 220 patients. Q J Med. 1987;62(238):127–41.

3. Ory PA, Gladman DD, Mease PJ. Psoriatic arthritis and imaging. Ann Rheum Dis. 2005;64 Suppl 2: ii55–7. doi:10.1136/ard.2004.033928.

4. Siannis F, Farewell VT, Cook RJ, Schentag CT, Gladman DD. Clinical and radiological damage in psoriatic arthritis. Ann Rheum Dis. 2006;65(4): 478–81. doi:10.1136/ard.2005.039826.

5. Gladman DD, Farewell VT, Nadeau C. Clinical indicators of progression in psoriatic arthritis: multivariate relative risk model. J Rheumatol. 1995;22(4): 675–9.

6. Queiro-Silva R, Torre-Alonso JC, Tinture-Eguren T, Lopez-Lagunas I. A polyarticular onset predicts erosive and deforming disease in psoriatic arthritis. Ann Rheum Dis. 2003;62(1):68–70.

7. Anandarajah A. Imaging in psoriatic arthritis. Clin Rev Allergy Immunol. 2013;44(2):157–65. doi:10.1007/s12016-012-8304-4.

8. Naredo E, Moller I, de Miguel E, Batlle-Gualda E, Acebes C, Brito E, Mayordomo L, Moragues C, Uson J, de Agustin JJ, Martinez A, Rejon E, Rodriguez A, Dauden E, Ultrasound School of the Spanish Society of R, Spanish ECOAG. High prevalence of ultrasonographic synovitis and enthesopathy in patients with psoriasis without psoriatic arthritis: a prospective case-control study. Rheumatology (Oxford). 2011;50(10):1838–48. doi:10.1093/rheumatology/ker078.

9. Freeston JE, Coates LC, Nam JL, Moverley AR, Hensor EM, Wakefield RJ, Emery P, Helliwell PS, Conaghan PG. Is there subclinical synovitis in early psoriatic arthritis? A clinical comparison with grayscale and power Doppler ultrasound. Arthritis Care Res. 2014;66(3):432–9. doi:10.1002/acr.22158.

10. Ostergaard M, Poggenborg RP. Magnetic resonance imaging in psoriatic arthritis – update on current status and future perspectives: a report from the GRAPPA 2010 annual meeting. J Rheumatol. 2012;39(2):408–12. doi:10.3899/jrheum.111235.

11. Coates LC, Hodgson R, Conaghan PG, Freeston JE. MRI and ultrasonography for diagnosis and monitoring of psoriatic arthritis. Best Pract Res Clin Rheumatol. 2012;26(6):805–22. doi:10.1016/j.berh.2012.09.004.

12. Taylor WJ, Porter GG, Helliwell PS. Operational definitions and observer reliability of the plain radiographic features of psoriatic arthritis. J Rheumatol. 2003;30(12):2645–58.

13. Haddad A, Chandran V. Arthritis mutilans. Curr Rheumatol Rep. 2013;15(4):321. doi:10.1007/s11926-013-0321-7.

14. Bruzzese V, Marrese C, Ridola L, Zullo A. Psoriatic arthritis mutilans: case series and literature review. J Rheumatol. 2013;40(7):1233–6. doi:10.3899/jrheum.130093.

15. Lubrano E, Marchesoni A, Olivieri I, D'Angelo S, Palazzi C, Scarpa R, Ferrara N, Parsons WJ, Brunese L, Helliwell PS, Spadaro A. The radiological assessment of axial involvement in psoriatic arthritis. J Rheumatol Suppl. 2012;89:54–6. doi:10.3899/jrheum.120244.

16. Day MS, Nam D, Goodman S, Su EP, Figgie M. Psoriatic arthritis. J Am Acad Orthop Surg. 2012;20(1):28–37. doi:10.5435/JAAOS-20-01-028.

17. Gofton JP. Report from the subcommittee on diagnostic criteria for ankylosing spondylitis. In: Population studies of the rheumatic diseases. New York: Excerpta Medica; 1966.

18. Jenkinson T, Armas J, Evison G, Cohen M, Lovell C, McHugh NJ. The cervical spine in psoriatic arthritis: a clinical and radiological study. Br J Rheumatol. 1994;33(3):255–9.

19. Jacobson JA, Girish G, Jiang Y, Resnick D. Radiographic evaluation of arthritis: inflammatory conditions. Radiology. 2008;248(2):378–89. doi:10.1148/radiol.2482062110.

20. Sankowski AJ, Lebkowska UM, Cwikla J, Walecka I, Walecki J. Psoriatic arthritis. Pol J Radiol. 2013;78(1):7–17. doi:10.12659/PJR.883763.

21. Helliwell P, Marchesoni A, Peters M, Barker M, Wright V. A re-evaluation of the osteoarticular manifestations of psoriasis. Br J Rheumatol. 1991;30(5): 339–45.

22. Bennett RM. Psoriatic arthritis. In: Arthritis and allied conditions. 9th ed. Philadelphia: Lea & Febiger; 1979.

23. McGonagle D, Conaghan PG, Emery P. Psoriatic arthritis: a unified concept twenty years on. Arthritis Rheum. 1999;42(6):1080–6. doi:10.1002/1529-0131(199906)42:6<1080::AID-ANR2>3.0.CO;2-7.

24. Taylor W, Gladman D, Helliwell P, Marchesoni A, Mease P, Mielants H, Group CS. Classification criteria for psoriatic arthritis: development of new criteria from a large international study. Arthritis Rheum. 2006;54(8):2665–73. doi:10.1002/art.21972.

25. Martel W, Stuck KJ, Dworin AM, Hylland RG. Erosive osteoarthritis and psoriatic arthritis: a radiologic comparison in the hand, wrist, and foot. AJR Am J Roentgenol. 1980;134(1):125–35. doi:10.2214/ajr.134.1.125.

26. Punzi L, Frigato M, Frallonardo P, Ramonda R. Inflammatory osteoarthritis of the hand. Best Pract Res Clin Rheumatol. 2010;24(3):301–12. doi:10.1016/j.berh.2009.12.007.

27. Tillett W, Jadon D, Shaddick G, Robinson G, Sengupta R, Korendowych E, de Vries CS, McHugh NJ. Feasibility, reliability, and sensitivity to change of four radiographic scoring methods in patients with psoriatic arthritis. Arthritis Care Res. 2014;66(2):311–7. doi:10.1002/acr.22104.

28. Kane D, Stafford L, Bresnihan B, FitzGerald O. A prospective, clinical and radiological study of early psoriatic arthritis: an early synovitis clinic experience. Rheumatology (Oxford). 2003;42(12):1460–8. doi:10.1093/rheumatology/keg384.

29. van der Heijde D, Sharp J, Wassenberg S, Gladman DD. Psoriatic arthritis imaging: a review of scoring methods. Ann Rheum Dis. 2005;64 Suppl 2:ii61–4. doi:10.1136/ard.2004.030809.

30. Mease PJ, Antoni CE. Psoriatic arthritis treatment: biological response modifiers. Ann Rheum Dis. 2005;64 Suppl 2:ii78–82. doi:10.1136/ard.2004.034157.

31. Mease PJ, Kivitz AJ, Burch FX, Siegel EL, Cohen SB, Ory P, Salonen D, Rubenstein J, Sharp JT, Dunn M, Tsuji W. Continued inhibition of radiographic progression in patients with psoriatic arthritis following 2 years of treatment with etanercept. J Rheumatol. 2006;33(4):712–21.

32. Gladman DD, Mease PJ, Ritchlin CT, Choy EH, Sharp JT, Ory PA, Perdok RJ, Sasso EH. Adalimumab for long-term treatment of psoriatic arthritis: forty-eight week data from the adalimumab effectiveness in psoriatic arthritis trial. Arthritis Rheum. 2007;56(2):476–88. doi:10.1002/art.22379.

33. Mease PJ, Ory P, Sharp JT, Ritchlin CT, Van den Bosch F, Wellborne F, Birbara C, Thomson GT, Perdok RJ, Medich J, Wong RL, Gladman DD. Adalimumab for long-term treatment of psoriatic arthritis: 2-year data from the Adalimumab Effectiveness in Psoriatic Arthritis Trial (ADEPT). Ann Rheum Dis. 2009;68(5):702–9. doi:10.1136/ard.2008.092767.

34. van der Heijde D, Kavanaugh A, Gladman DD, Antoni C, Krueger GG, Guzzo C, Zhou B, Dooley LT, de Vlam K, Geusens P, Birbara C, Halter D, Beutler A. Infliximab inhibits progression of radiographic damage in patients with active psoriatic arthritis through one year of treatment: results from the induction and maintenance psoriatic arthritis clinical trial 2. Arthritis Rheum. 2007;56(8):2698–707. doi:10.1002/art.22805.

35. Kavanaugh A, van der Heijde D, McInnes IB, Mease P, Krueger GG, Gladman DD, Gomez-Reino J, Papp K, Baratelle A, Xu W, Mudivarthy S, Mack M, Rahman MU, Xu Z, Zrubek J, Beutler A. Golimumab in psoriatic arthritis: one-year clinical efficacy, radiographic, and safety results from a phase III, randomized, placebo-controlled trial. Arthritis Rheum. 2012;64(8):2504–17. doi:10.1002/art.34436.

36. van der Heijde D, Fleischmann R, Wollenhaupt J, Deodhar A, Kielar D, Woltering F, Stach C, Hoepken B, Arledge T, Mease PJ. Effect of different imputation approaches on the evaluation of radiographic progression in patients with psoriatic arthritis: results of the RAPID-PsA 24-week phase III double-blind randomised placebo-controlled study of certolizumab pegol. Ann Rheum Dis. 2014;73(1):233–7. doi:10.1136/annrheumdis-2013-203697.

37. Kavanaugh A, Ritchlin C, Rahman P, Puig L, Gottlieb AB, Li S, Wang Y, Noonan L, Brodmerkel C, Song M, Mendelsohn AM, McInnes IB, Psummit, Study G. Ustekinumab, an anti-IL-12/23 p40 monoclonal antibody, inhibits radiographic progression in patients with active psoriatic arthritis: results of an integrated analysis of radiographic data from the phase 3, multicentre, randomised, double-blind, placebo-controlled PSUMMIT-1 and PSUMMIT-2 trials. Ann Rheum Dis. 2014;73(6):1000–6. doi:10.1136/annrheumdis-2013-204741.

38. Proceedings of the annual meeting of the Group for Research and Assessment of Psoriasis and Psoriatic Arthritis (GRAPPA), June 26–27, 2012, Stockholm, Sweden. J Rheumatol. 2013;40(8):1407–58.

Psoriasis and Psoriatic Arthritis: Ultrasound Applications

20

Santiago Ruta and Magaly Alva

Abstract

Psoriatic arthritis (PsA) is an inflammatory disease with potential involvement of both peripheral and axial skeleton which has variable clinical course and several degrees of severity.

Ultrasound (US) is a rapidly evolving technique that helps to actually determine the anatomical structure involved in the inflammatory process and is one of the imaging method recommended to assess synovitis at any joint and has the potential to be used not only to detect joint synovitis, but also to assess surrounding soft tissues in order to determine the presence of tenosynovitis, dactylitis and/or enthesitis.

Doppler modalities are currently considered an integral part of the global US assessment of the rheumatic patient. This is mainly due to their capability to detect pathological flow within musculoskeletal soft tissues, thereby demonstrating the presence of local active inflammation.

US has several advantages over other imaging techniques: it is patient-friendly, safe, noninvasive, less expensive, and permits multiple target assessment in real time without the need for external referral.

Available data demonstrate that US can be regarded as a feasible and effective imaging technique that can allow early recognition of anatomical changes, inflammatory subclinical findings, differential diagnosis, careful guidance for aspiration and/or local treatment, and short-term therapy monitoring at joint, tendon, enthesis, nail, and skin levels.

Further research is required into implications of the disparity between US and clinical findings, to really determine the significance of subclinical findings to predict structural damage, relapse and progression of the disease. There is also a need to validate PsA specific composite multi-target US scoring systems.

This chapter summarize the main potential applications of US in cutaneous psoriasis and PsA patients.

S. Ruta, MD
Rheumatology Unit, Hospital Italiano
de Buenos Aires, La Plata,
Buenos Aires, Argentina

M. Alva, MD (✉)
Department of Rheumatology, H. Edgardo Rebagliati
Martins, Edgardo Rebagliti 490, Lima LIMA11, Peru
e-mail: maggyalva@yahoo.com

© Springer International Publishing Switzerland 2016
A. Adebajo et al. (eds.), *Psoriatic Arthritis and Psoriasis: Pathology and Clinical Aspects*,
DOI 10.1007/978-3-319-19530-8_20

Keywords

Ultrasound • Ultrasonography • Psoriatic arthritis • Synovitis • Enthesitis • Enthesopathy • Dactylitis • Tenosynovitis

Introduction

Imaging techniques such as magnetic ultrasound (US) and resonance imaging (MRI) have been increasingly used in the assessment of psoriatic arthritis (PsA) [1, 2].

PsA shows significant clinical heterogeneity with potential involvement of both the peripheral and the axial skeleton. In addition to arthritis, inflammatory changes are seen in many other tissues resulting in enthesitis and dactylitis which are considered hallmarks of PsA [1].

US is a rapidly evolving technique that helps to actually determine the anatomical structure involved in the inflammatory process, which is important in diagnostic and therapeutic procedures.

US has several advantages over other imaging techniques: it is patient-friendly, safe, noninvasive, less expensive, and permits multiple target assessment in real time without the need for external referral [2].

The data also demonstrate that US can be regarded as a feasible and effective imaging technique that can allow early recognition of anatomical changes, subclinical findings, careful guidance for aspiration and/or local treatment, and short-term therapy monitoring at joint, tendon, enthesis, nail, and skin levels [1–3].

This chapter summarizes US research in PsA, discussing technical aspects, definitions of US pathology and potential US applications.

Ultrasound Examination: Technical Aspects

Appropriate use of imaging is essential for accurate patient diagnosis and management as well as optimizing the use of healthcare resources [4].

Guidelines for musculoskeletal ultrasound were published in order to standardize, mainly, patient positioning and standard scans to be performed in rheumatology setting [5].

Table 20.1 shows the most common US scans used to assess musculoskeletal inflammatory involvement in PsA patients with both corresponding anatomical structure evaluated and possible US detectable pathology.

Musculoskeletal US typically employs B mode/grey scale (GS) assessment as a structural indicator (for example, synovial hypertrophy, effusion and tendinopathy) and power Doppler (PD) as a sensitive measure of vascular flow (indicating inflammation) [1].

B mode/grey scale US parameters should be set in order to obtain maximal contrast between all the anatomical structures under examination.

Doppler modalities are currently considered an integral part of the global US assessment of the rheumatic patient. This is mainly due to their capability to detect pathological flow within musculoskeletal soft tissues, thereby demonstrating the presence of local active inflammation [6].

Concerning PD assessment, some important technical aspects need to be mentioned.

The patient must be positioned comfortably, and the area under investigation must be completely relaxed. Related to the examiner, the scanning arm and hand must rest in a comfortable position.

Even more importantly, during Doppler examinations very little pressure should be applied with the transducer. Pressure can affect haemodynamics and potentially result in decreased flow. When small joints are being assessed, plenty of gel ought to be used, in order to help avoid compression of the tissues under examination, that could disturb an adequate visualization of the vascularization [7, 8].

In rheumatology, where the goal is to detect as much flow as possible, the settings must be used to adjust the machine to its highest sensitivity

Table 20.1 Ultrasound standard scans used to assess inflammatory involvement in patients with psoriatic arthritis

	Standard scans	Anatomical structure	US detectable pathology
Shoulder	Anterior transverse and longitudinal scans	Bicipital groove, bursa	Bicipital tenosynovitis, bursitis
	Posterior transverse scan	Joint recess	Synovial fluid and/or hypertrophy
Elbow	Anterior longitudinal and transverse scans	Joint recess	Synovial fluid and/or hypertrophy
	Lateral and medial longitudinal scans	Lateral and medial humeral epicondylus	Epicondylitis (lateral and/or medial), enthesopathy
	Posterior longitudinal and transverse scans	Olecranon fossa, triceps tendon	Synovial fluid and/or hypertrophy, enthesopathy
Wrist	Dorsal longitudinal and transverse scans	Joint recess, extensor tendons	Synovial fluid and/or hypertrophy, tenosynovitis
	Volar longitudinal and transverse scans	Flexor tendons	Tenosynovitis
Fingers	Longitudinal dorsal scans at MCP, PIP and DIP joints	Joint recess	Synovial fluid and/or hypertrophy
	Longitudinal ventral scans at MCP, PIP and DIP joints	Joint recess, flexor tendons	Synovial fluid and/or hypertrophy, tenosynovitis, dactylitis
Hip	Anterior longitudinal and transverse scans	Joint recess	Synovial fluid and/or hypertrophy
Knee	Suprapatellar longitudinal and transverse scans	Joint recess, quadriceps tendon, bursa	Synovial fluid and/or hypertrophy, enthesopathy, bursitis
	Infrapetellar longitudinal and transverse scans	Patelar tendon, bursa	Enthesopathy, bursitis
Ankle and heel	Anterior longitudinal and transverse scans	Joint recess, tibial anterior tendon, extensor tendons	Synovial fluid and/or hypertrophy, tenosynovitis
	Perimalleolar medial longitudinal and transverse scans	Posterior tibial tendon, flexor tendons	Tenosynovitis
	Perimalleolar lateral longitudinal and transverse scans	Peroneus brevis and longus tendons	Tenosynovitis
	Posterior longitudinal and transverse scans	Achilles tendon, bursa	Enthesopathy, bursitis
Foot	Dorsal longitudinal scans at MTP, PIP and DIP joints	Joint recess	Synovial fluid and/or hypertrophy
	Plantar longitudinal scans at MCP, PIP and DIP joints	Joint recess, flexor tendons	Synovial fluid and/or hypertrophy, tenosynovitis, dactylitis
	Plantar posterior longitudinal and transverse scans	Plantar fascia	Enthesopathy

without noise artifacts. The following are the recommendations for PD settings in rheumatology: pulse repetition frequency: the lowest possible (500–750 Hz), persistence: the lowest possible (3–4), wall filter: the lowest possible (2–3) and Doppler frequency between: appropriately low or high depending on the machine [7, 9]. Colour gain has to be set just below the level at which colour noise appeared underlying bone (no flow should be visualized at the bony surface). To confirm that the PD signal represented real blood flow and not an artefact, the spectral Doppler should be used [8, 10].

Regarding entheses, knee and heel entheses should be examined in some grades of flexion or dorsal flexion, respectively, in B mode/grey scale

US examination. However, a neutral position should be used when abnormal vascularization at entheseal level needs to be assessed using PD [10, 11].

Ultrasound Definitions for the Most Common Pathological Findings

The OMERACT (Outcomes Measures in Rheumatology) Group proposed for the first time a consensus on US definitions for common pathological lesions seen in patients with inflammatory arthritis [12].

Synovial fluid: abnormal hypoechoic or anechoic (relative to subdermal fat, but may be isoechoic or hyperechoic) intraarticular material that is displaceable and compressible, but does not exhibit Doppler signal (Fig. 20.1a).

Synovial hypertrophy: abnormal hypoechoic (relative to subdermal fat, but may be isoechoic or hyperechoic) intraarticular tissue that is nondisplaceable and poorly compressible and may exhibit Doppler signal (Fig. 20.1a).

Tenosynovitis: hypoechoic or anechoic thickened tissue with or without fluid within the tendon sheath, which is seen in two perpendicular planes and that may exhibit Doppler signal (Fig. 20.1b, c).

Bone erosion: an intraarticular discontinuity of the bone surface that is visible in two perpendicular planes (Fig. 20.2).

Enthesopathy: abnormally hypoechoic (loss of normal fibrillar architecture) and/or thickened tendon or ligament at its bony attachment (may occasionally contain hyperechoic foci consistent with calcification), seen in 2 perpendicular planes that may exhibit Doppler signal and/or bony changes including enthesophytes, erosions, or irregularity (Fig. 20.3).

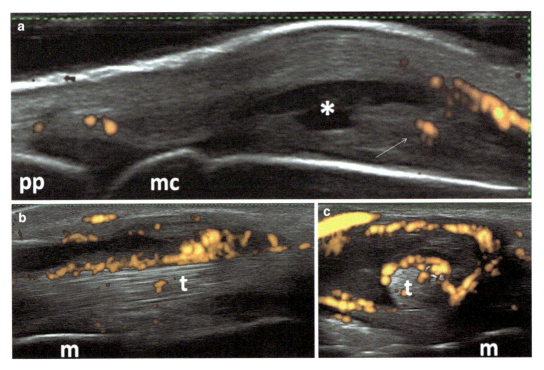

Fig. 20.1 (a) Longitudinal dorsal scan at metacarpophalangeal joint. Joint cavity widening with both anechogenic area representing synovial fluid (*asterisk*) and echogenic area with power Doppler signal representing synovial hypertrophy (*arrow*). *mc* metacarpal head, *pp* proximal phalanx. (b, c) Perimalleolar medial longitudinal and transverse scans, respectively. Tendon sheath distension with power Doppler signal representing tenosynovitis of the posterior tibial tendon (*t*). *m* medial malleolus

US Usefulness

The following are the main potential indications for the use of US in cutaneous psoriasis and PsA patients.

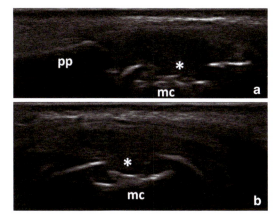

Fig. 20.2 (**a, b**) Longitudinal and transverse lateral scans at metacarpophalangeal joint, respectively. An intraarticular discontinuity (*asterisk*) of the bone surface at metacarpal head (*mc*) that is visible in 2 perpendicular planes representing bone erosion. *pp* proximal phalanx

Assessment of Joint, Tendon and/or Entheseal Involvement

The European Society of Musculoskeletal Radiology evaluated the evidence currently available on the clinical value and indications for musculoskeletal US [4]. US is the imaging method recommended to assess synovitis at wrist/finger, elbow, shoulder, hip, knee and ankle/foot. US has the potential to be used not only to detect joint synovitis, but also to assess surrounding soft tissues in order to determine the presence of tenosynovitis, dactylitis and/or enthesitis.

Peripheral arthritis. Although any peripheral joint can be affected by the inflammatory process in PsA patients, the large joints of the lower limbs and small joints of the hands, including the distal interphalangeal joints, are the preferred ones to be assessed by US.

US has demonstrated the ability to detect inflammatory subclinical findings in patients with inflammatory arthropathies and some authors suggest that this subclinical findings

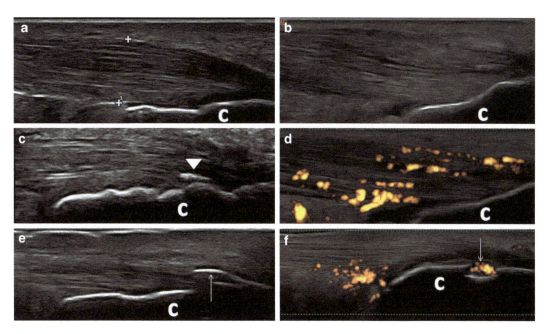

Fig. 20.3   Insertion of the Achilles tendon in the upper pole of the calcaneus (*c*). (**a**) Calipers denoting the presence of thickened Achilles tendon at its bony attachment. (**b**) Marked thickness of Achilles tendon at insertion level with abnormal hypoechoic areas (loss of normal fibrillar architecture). (**c**) Intratendinous hyperechoic linear image (*arrowhead*), in this case without posterior acoustic shadow, indicating the presence of calcification. (**d**) Power Doppler signal over the Achilles tendon denoting increased abnormal vascularization at entheseal level. (**e**) A step up bony prominence at the end of the normal bone contour (*upward arrow*) indicating an enthesophyte. (**f**) A cortical breakage with a step down bone contour defect (*downward arrow*) indicating bone erosion, in this case with increased abnormal vascularization

might predict flares and structural progression, mainly in rheumatoid arthritis patients. Disparity between US and clinical findings was found in a study including US evaluation of joints, tendons, entheses and also dactylitis. The authors concluded that current clinical PsA composite scores (and its joint components) correlate with US-verified synovitis, whereas enthesitis, tenosynovitis and perisynovitis were not adequately represented by these indices [13]. Moreover, another study demonstrated that subclinical synovitis, as identified by US, is very common in early PsA and led to the majority of oligoarthritis patients being reclassified as having polyarthritis [14]. A single study showed that the presence of US determined synovial thickness, enthesitis, and/or onychopathy associated with positive PD signal at baseline and the persistent PD signal over time have relevant prognostic value for the development of articular damage in PsA patients [15]. Further research is required into implications of the disparity between US and clinical findings. For example, what relationship does this subclinical synovitis have with subseqent disease relapses, the progression of structural damage, and change in functional status over time among PsA patients.

Axial disease. Sacroiliac joints may be affected in around 40 % of PsA patients. Although magnetic resonance imaging (MRI) is the gold standard method to assess inflammatory involvement at that level, US has showed good diagnostic test properties for the detection of sacroiliitis [16, 17].

Enthesopathy. Inflammatory involvement of entheses is considered a typical feature in spondyloarthritis. Enthesitis refers to the presence of inflammation of tendons, ligaments and capsules insertions into the bone. These present with abnormal vascularization that can be detected by PD [3, 18]. Knee (mainly proximal and distal insertions of patellar tendon), and heel (distal insertion of Achilles tendon and plantar fascia) are the most frequent involved sites of entheses commonly assessed by US. In the upper limbs, elbow entheses, such as medial and lateral humeral epycondilitis are commonly involved.

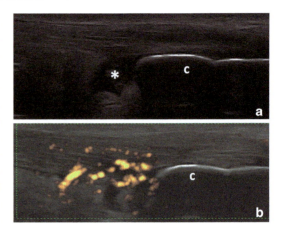

Fig. 20.4 Insertion of the Achilles tendon in the upper pole of the calcaneus (*c*). (**a**) Localized anechoic or hypoechoic area (*asterisk*) compatible with circumscribed increase in diameter of the retrocalcaneal bursa, indicating bursitis. (**b**) Increased abnormal vascularization at entheseal and bursa level

Although bursitis is not included as one of the characteristic lesions used to define enthesopathy according to OMERACT [12], some authors suggest that bursitis is a part of the inflammatory involvement at entheseal level. Burstitis has been included in some entheses score in spondyloarthritis patients [19–21] (Fig. 20.4).

Dactylitis. The literature is scarce, and there is conflicting data describing which tissues contribute to dactylitic inflammation. A systematic review by OMERACT US Task Force provides guidance in defining elementary lesions that may discriminate dactylitic digits from normal digits. The most commonly described features of dactylitis were flexor tendon tenosynovitis and joint synovitis [22]. Inflammatory involvement of surrounded soft tissue and entheses also could be observed in PsA dactylitis [23] (Fig. 20.5).

Assessment of Skin and Nail Involvement

In recent years, US equipment with high frequency transducers (e.g. >15 MHz) have permitted an excellent visualization of all components of skin and nail on B mode/grey scale US assessment. The recent availability of

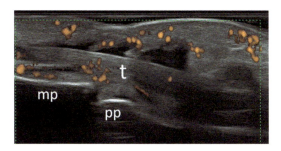

Fig. 20.5 Longitudinal ventral scan at proximal interphalangeal joint. Tenosynovitis of the finger flexor tendon (*t*), synovitis at proximal interphalangeal joint, diffuse soft tissue thickness and increased vascularization by the presence of power Doppler signal, all findings suggesting ultrasound dactylitis. *pp* proximal phalanx, *mp* medial phalanx

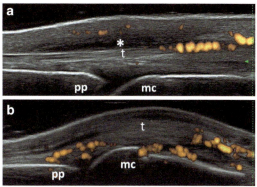

Fig. 20.6 Longitudinal dorsal scan at metacarpophalangeal joint. Differential diagnosis of inflammatory pattern between psoriatic arthritis (**a**) and rheumatoid arthritis (**b**). (**a**) Peritendinous extensor tendon inflammation, "PTI pattern", characterized by a hypoechoic swelling (*asterisk*) and power Doppler signal surrounding the extensor digitorum tendon (*t*). (**b**) Intra-articular inflammatory involvement characterized by synovial hypertrophy within the joint cavity widening with power Doppler signal near to the bone cortex. *mc* metacarpal head, *pp* proximal phalanx, *t* extensor digitorum tendon (Courtesy of Marwin Gutierrez, MD)

US equipment with PD frequency higher than 10 MHz, for its use in clinical practice, also enables a very sensitive visualization of blood flow at dermal level [2, 24].

Further than the ability of US to assess skin and nail involvement in patients with cutaneous psoriasis, the presence of subclinical inflammation at entheseal level has been shown in psoriatic patients without previous history of arthropathy or PsA [25, 26]. Moreover, more subclinical enthesitis was found in psoriasis patients with nail involvement compared to psoriasis patients without nail disease [27]. Another study demonstrate not only the presence of subclinical enthesitis in psoriasis patients but also subclinical inflammatory involvement at joint level [28]. These subclinical inflammatory findings could suggest that this group of patients with cutaneous psoriasis should be carefully followed-up for the development of signs and symptoms that may be consistent with early PsA [29].

Differential diagnosis. There is a little evidence supporting the role of US in the differential diagnosis with other arthropaties. A single study [8] demonstrated a potential role of US in the differential diagnosis between rheumatoid arthritis and PsA at metacarpophalangeal (MCP) joint level. This study showed some differences in the inflammatory pattern, with a peritendinous extensor tendon inflammation (PTI pattern) being more common in PsA patients and intra-articular involvement more frequent in RA patients

(Fig. 20.6). It is interesting to note that the PTI pattern was more frequently observed in patients with shorter disease duration.

It is important to note that other US finding, such as bony proliferations at small joints of the hands (mainly at distal interphalangeal joints), can help to distinguish the inflammatory process between PsA and rheumatoid arthritis patients [30], mainly at early stages of the disease. However, is not always easy to differentiate between RA with secondary osteoarthritis or patients with inflammatory primary osteoarthritis and PsA, since all of these can be associated with bony proliferations.

Finally, it is worth considering that patients with psoriasis may have not only hyperuricemia, but also a higher incidence of gout than the general population, and that sometimes it is not easy to differentiate only with clinical, radiological and biochemical data. US shows good ability to detect monosodium urate crystals, and to do so with high specificity [31, 32], which can be used for differential diagnosis between gout attacks in patients with psoriasis and inflammatory involvement due to psoriatic arthritis.

Therapeutic Monitoring

To date, the role of US in therapeutic monitoring of PsA has not been adequately defined. However, some studies demonstrate that US can be a feasible and effective imaging technique for the short-term monitoring of joints, tendons and entheses in PsA patients. Concerning entheses, US was able to detect both morphological changes on B mode/grey scale assessment (reduction of thickness, hypoechogenicity and bursitis) and a reduction of the abnormal vascularization by PDUS [10, 33]. A global US assessment was proposed in spondyloarthritis patients with peripheral involvement (with a majority of PsA patients) including the examination of joints, tendons and entheses, demonstrating that US features had a good responsiveness to therapy changes [34]. Another study, aimed at developing a composite score for the assessment of inflammatory and structural lesions in PsA patients, showed US to have sufficient convergent construct validity, sensitivity to change, reliability and feasibility [35].

Regarding skin, US with PD technique allows a detailed morphostructural and perfusional assessment of psoriatic plaque, showing remarkable changes in patients undertaking biological therapy [24, 36–38]. Treatment with anti-TNF-α improves the symptoms of patients with PsA at joint and psoriatic skin levels from a clinical and US perspective [37].

A preliminary PDUS composite score for global assessment of PsA patients was developed, including joints, tendons, entheses, skin and nail examination and showed that US could be a feasible, reliable and comprehensive approach to multi-target monitoring of PsA [39].

US Guided Procedures

Aspiration of joint and bursal effusion and intraarticular and soft tissue injection are performed routinely as diagnostic and therapeutic procedures in clinical rheumatology [40]. Some studies showed that conventional (palpation-guided models) approach for aspiration of synovial fluid and/or injections provides a low rate of accurate needle placement [41, 42]. Inaccurate placement can be associated with poor clinical outcomes. US guided injections provide a higher rate of success in comparison with conventional approach for joints and surrounding soft tissue [43]. US-guided needle placement within the target area is an accurate and safe approach for patients with PsA who require aspiration of synovial fluid or injection therapy. Under US guidance it is possible to visualize the progression of the needle in the soft tissues toward the target area [2].

Conclusions

US is a reliable imaging technique that may be considered a powerful tool for assessment of patient with PsA. It complements and improves the evaluation of joints, tendons, enthesie, skin and nails, reflecting both morphostructural changes and inflammatory activity .

Moreover, US could potentially be useful in shortening the time required for early diagnosis and may also have a role in therapeutic monitoring. Finally, US has the capability to guide properly diagnostic and therapeutic procedures.

Research Agenda

- More studies of US in PsA are needed to: determine the significance of subclinical findings to predict structural damage, relapse and progression of the disease.
- Define its the role in early diagnosis and therapy monitoring
- Validate PsA specific composite multi-target US scoring systems

References

1. Coates LC, Hodgson R, Conaghan PG, Freeston JE. MRI and ultrasonography for diagnosis and monitoring of psoriatic arthritis. Best Pract Res Clin Rheumatol. 2012;26(6):805–22.
2. Grassi W, Gutierrez M. Psoriatic arthritis: need for ultrasound in everyday clinical practice. J Rheumatol Suppl. 2012;89:39–43.

3. Riente L, Carli L, Delle Sedie A. Ultrasound imaging in psoriatic arthritis and ankylosing spondylitis. Clin Exp Rheumatol. 2014;32(1 Suppl 80):S26–33.

4. Klauser AS, Tagliafico A, Allen GM, et al. Clinical indications for musculoskeletal ultrasound: a Delphi-based consensus paper of the European Society of Musculoskeletal Radiology. Eur Radiol. 2012;22(5): 1140–8.

5. Backhaus M, Burmester GR, Gerber T, et al. Guidelines for musculoskeletal ultrasound in rheumatology. Ann Rheum Dis. 2001;60(7):641–9.

6. Porta F, Radunovic G, Vlad V, et al. The role of Doppler ultrasound in rheumatic diseases. Rheumatology (Oxford). 2012;51(6):976–82.

7. Torp-Pedersen ST, Terslev L. Settings and artefacts relevant in colour/power Doppler ultrasound in rheumatology. Ann Rheum Dis. 2008;67(2):143–9.

8. Gutierrez M, Filippucci E, Salaffi F, Di Geso L, Grassi W. Differential diagnosis between rheumatoid arthritis and psoriatic arthritis: the value of ultrasound findings at metacarpophalangeal joints level. Ann Rheum Dis. 2011;70(6):1111–4.

9. Naredo E, Monteagudo I. Doppler techniques. Clin Exp Rheumatol. 2014;32(1 Suppl 80):S12–9.

10. Naredo E, Batlle-Gualda E, Garcia-Vivar ML, et al. Power Doppler ultrasonography assessment of entheses in spondyloarthropathies: response to therapy of entheseal abnormalities. J Rheumatol. 2010;37(10): 2110–7.

11. Gutierrez M, Filippucci E, Grassi W, Rosemffet M. Intratendinous power Doppler changes related to patient position in seronegative spondyloarthritis. J Rheumatol. 2010;37(5):1057–9.

12. Wakefield RJ, Balint PV, Szkudlarek M, et al. Musculoskeletal ultrasound including definitions for ultrasonographic pathology. J Rheumatol. 2005; 32(12):2485–7.

13. Husic R, Gretler J, Felber A, et al. Disparity between ultrasound and clinical findings in psoriatic arthritis. Ann Rheum Dis. 2014;73(8):1529–36.

14. Freeston JE, Coates LC, Nam JL, et al. Is there subclinical synovitis in early psoriatic arthritis? A clinical comparison with gray-scale and power Doppler ultrasound. Arthritis Care Res (Hoboken). 2014;66(3): 432–9.

15. El Miedany Y, El Gaafary M, Youssef S, Ahmed I, Nasr A. Tailored approach to early psoriatic arthritis patients: clinical and ultrasonographic predictors for structural joint damage. Clin Rheumatol. 2015;34(2): 307–13.

16. Ghosh A, Mondal S, Sinha D, Nag A, Chakraborty S. Ultrasonography as a useful modality for documenting sacroiliitis in radiographically negative inflammatory back pain: a comparative evaluation with MRI. Rheumatology (Oxford). 2014;53(11): 2030–4.

17. Klauser A, Halpern EJ, Frauscher F, et al. Inflammatory low back pain: high negative predictive value of contrast-enhanced color Doppler ultrasound in the detection of inflamed sacroiliac joints. Arthritis Rheum. 2005;53(3):440–4.

18. Terslev L, Naredo E, Iagnocco A, et al. Defining enthesitis in spondyloarthritis by ultrasound: results of a Delphi process and of a reliability reading exercise. Arthritis Care Res (Hoboken). 2014;66(5): 741–8.

19. Falcao S, de Miguel E, Castillo-Gallego C, Peiteado D, Branco J, Martin Mola E. Achilles enthesis ultrasound: the importance of the bursa in spondyloarthritis. Clin Exp Rheumatol. 2013;31(3):422–7.

20. Balint PV, Kane D, Wilson H, McInnes IB, Sturrock RD. Ultrasonography of entheseal insertions in the lower limb in spondyloarthropathy. Ann Rheum Dis. 2002;61(10):905–10.

21. de Miguel E, Cobo T, Munoz-Fernandez S, et al. Validity of enthesis ultrasound assessment in spondyloarthropathy. Ann Rheum Dis. 2009;68(2):169–74.

22. Bakewell CJ, Olivieri I, Aydin SZ, et al. Ultrasound and magnetic resonance imaging in the evaluation of psoriatic dactylitis: status and perspectives. J Rheumatol. 2013;40(12):1951–7.

23. Fournie B, Margarit-Coll N, Champetier de Ribes TL, et al. Extrasynovial ultrasound abnormalities in the psoriatic finger. Prospective comparative power-doppler study versus rheumatoid arthritis. Joint Bone Spine. 2006;73(5):527–31.

24. Gutierrez M, Wortsman X, Filippucci E, De Angelis R, Filosa G, Grassi W. High-frequency sonography in the evaluation of psoriasis: nail and skin involvement. J Ultrasound Med. 2009;28(11):1569–74.

25. Gisondi P, Tinazzi I, El-Dalati G, et al. Lower limb enthesopathy in patients with psoriasis without clinical signs of arthropathy: a hospital-based case–control study. Ann Rheum Dis. 2008;67(1):26–30.

26. Gutierrez M, Filippucci E, De Angelis R, et al. Subclinical entheseal involvement in patients with psoriasis: an ultrasound study. Semin Arthritis Rheum. 2011;40(5):407–12.

27. Ash ZR, Tinazzi I, Gallego CC, et al. Psoriasis patients with nail disease have a greater magnitude of underlying systemic subclinical enthesopathy than those with normal nails. Ann Rheum Dis. 2012; 71(4):553–6.

28. Naredo E, Moller I, de Miguel E, et al. High prevalence of ultrasonographic synovitis and enthesopathy in patients with psoriasis without psoriatic arthritis: a prospective case–control study. Rheumatology (Oxford). 2011;50(10):1838–48.

29. Tinazzi I, McGonagle D, Biasi D, et al. Preliminary evidence that subclinical enthesopathy may predict psoriatic arthritis in patients with psoriasis. J Rheumatol. 2011;38(12):2691–2.

30. Wiell C, Szkudlarek M, Hasselquist M, et al. Ultrasonography, magnetic resonance imaging, radiography, and clinical assessment of inflammatory and destructive changes in fingers and toes of patients with psoriatic arthritis. Arthritis Res Ther. 2007;9(6): R119.

31. Filippucci E, Riveros MG, Georgescu D, Salaffi F, Grassi W. Hyaline cartilage involvement in patients with gout and calcium pyrophosphate deposition disease. An ultrasound study. Osteoarthritis Cartilage. 2009;17(2):178–81.

32. Thiele RG, Schlesinger N. Diagnosis of gout by ultrasound. Rheumatology (Oxford). 2007;46(7):1116–21.

33. Aydin SZ, Karadag O, Filippucci E, et al. Monitoring Achilles enthesitis in ankylosing spondylitis during TNF-alpha antagonist therapy: an ultrasound study. Rheumatology (Oxford). 2010;49(3):578–82.

34. Ruta S, Acosta Felquer ML, Rosa J, Navarta DA, Garcia Monaco R, Soriano ER. Responsiveness to therapy change of a global ultrasound assessment in spondyloarthritis patients. Clin Rheumatol. 2015;34(1):125–32.

35. Ficjan A, Husic R, Gretler J, et al. Ultrasound composite scores for the assessment of inflammatory and structural pathologies in Psoriatic Arthritis (PsASon-Score). Arthritis Res Ther. 2014;16(5):476.

36. Gutierrez M, Filippucci E, Bertolazzi C, Grassi W. Sonographic monitoring of psoriatic plaque. J Rheumatol. 2009;36(4):850–1.

37. De Agustin JJ, Moragues C, De Miguel E, et al. A multicentre study on high-frequency ultrasound evaluation of the skin and joints in patients with psoriatic arthritis treated with infliximab. Clin Exp Rheumatol. 2012;30(6):879–85.

38. Gutierrez M, De Angelis R, Bernardini ML, et al. Clinical, power Doppler sonography and histological assessment of the psoriatic plaque: short-term monitoring in patients treated with etanercept. Br J Dermatol. 2011;164(1):33–7.

39. Gutierrez M, Di Geso L, Salaffi F, et al. Development of a preliminary US power Doppler composite score for monitoring treatment in PsA. Rheumatology (Oxford). 2012;51(7):1261–8.

40. Balint PV, Kane D, Sturrock RD. Modern patient management in rheumatology: interventional musculoskeletal ultrasonography. Osteoarthritis Cartilage. 2001;9(6):509–11.

41. Eustace JA, Brophy DP, Gibney RP, Bresnihan B, FitzGerald O. Comparison of the accuracy of steroid placement with clinical outcome in patients with shoulder symptoms. Ann Rheum Dis. 1997;56(1):59–63.

42. Jones A, Regan M, Ledingham J, Pattrick M, Manhire A, Doherty M. Importance of placement of intra-articular steroid injections. BMJ. 1993;307(6915):1329–30.

43. Balint PV, Kane D, Hunter J, McInnes IB, Field M, Sturrock RD. Ultrasound guided versus conventional joint and soft tissue fluid aspiration in rheumatology practice: a pilot study. J Rheumatol. 2002;29(10):2209–13.

Magnetic Resonance Imaging in Psoriatic Arthritis

21

René Panduro Poggenborg, Daniel Glinatsi, and Mikkel Østergaard

Abstract

Psoriatic arthritis (PsA) is an inflammatory joint disease characterised by presence of arthritis and often enthesitis in patients with psoriasis, but presenting a wide range of disease manifestations in various patterns. Imaging is an integral part of management of PsA, and is used for multiple reasons including establishing or confirming a diagnosis of inflammatory joint disease, determining the extent of disease, monitoring activity and damage, assessing therapeutic efficacy, and identifying complications of disease or treatment, in the setting of clinical practice or clinical studies. Magnetic resonance imaging (MRI) allows assessment of all peripheral and axial joints involved in PsA, and can visualise both inflammation and structural changes. In this paper, we will provide an overview of the status, strengths and limitations of MRI in PsA, in routine clinical practice and clinical trials.

Keywords

Psoriatic arthritis • Magnetic resonance imaging

Introduction

Psoriatic arthritis (PsA) is a chronic inflammatory joint disease associated with the skin disease psoriasis [1]. It is characterised by arthritis, enthesitis

R.P. Poggenborg, MD, PhD (✉)
D. Glinatsi, MD • M. Østergaard, MD, PhD, DMSc
Copenhagen Center for Arthritis Research,
Center for Rheumatology and Spine Diseases,
Rigshospitalet Glostrup, 57 Nordre Ringvej,
Copenhagen 2600, Denmark
e-mail: Poggenborg@dadlnet.dk

and/or dactylitis. PsA was first described as a distinct rheumatic disease in the 1950s and subsequently in the 1970s as part of the spondyloarthropathy (SpA) concept [2–4]. Differential diagnoses include rheumatoid arthritis (RA), SpA including ankylosing spondylitis (AS), osteoarthritis (OA), gout and fibromyalgia.

Different imaging procedures, primarily conventional radiography, ultrasonography and magnetic resonance imaging (MRI), all having different strengths and limitations, can be used in suspected or established PsA and provide

© Springer International Publishing Switzerland 2016
A. Adebajo et al. (eds.), *Psoriatic Arthritis and Psoriasis: Pathology and Clinical Aspects*,
DOI 10.1007/978-3-319-19530-8_21

important information on the disease process. Conventional MRI allows high-resolution visualization of all structures involved in arthritis, and is sensitive for peripheral and axial disease manifestations. However, MRI in PsA has received less attention than in RA and most knowledge is derived from studies of broader groups of SpA patients, including limited number of patients with PsA [5]. Research into improved techniques and novel imaging methods such as whole-body MRI and dynamic contrast-enhanced MRI are exciting future options. Below, MRI is reviewed organised into MRI technique and findings, peripheral and axial disease in clinical practice, monitoring PsA in clinical trials, new MRI methods and research agenda.

MRI Technique and Findings

T_1-weighted sequences (signal mainly reflecting fat content and presence of gadolinium-contrast) in one (axial joints) or two (peripheral joints) planes, supplemented by a T_2-weighted fat-suppressed or Short Tau Inversion Recovery (STIR) sequence (signal mainly reflecting water content) in two planes are generally performed for visualizing inflammation and structural damage in PsA [6, 7]. Additional acquisition of T_1-weighted sequences after intravenous injection of gadolinium-containing contrast agent aids identification of inflamed tissue in peripheral joints, and can be done with or without fat suppression (FS), while contrast injection is generally not used in axial disease. General agreement on which joints to examine with MRI to assess PsA activity and damage has not been established.

The main inflammatory and structural lesions visualised on MRI in peripheral PsA are synovitis, enthesitis, tenosynovitis, periarticular inflammation, bone marrow oedema (BMO), bone erosion and bone proliferation [5, 6]. Synovitis on MRI is characterised by increased post-contrast enhancement in a thickened synovial compartment (see Fig. 21.1). Enthesitis, tenosynovitis and periarticular inflammation are characterised by high signal intensity on T_1-weighted sequences and/or T_2-weighted FS or STIR sequences, whereas BMO is seen as high signal intensity on STIR images. Bone erosions are seen on T_1-weighted sequences as loss of the dark signal of the cortical bone and the bright signal of the underlying bone marrow fat tissue signal. Bone proliferations are seen on T_1-weighted sequences as abnormal bone formation in the periarticular region, such as at the entheses (enthesophytes) and across the joint (ankylosis).

The main inflammatory and structural lesions visualised on MRI in axial PsA are BMO/osteitis, enthesitis, fat infiltration, bone erosion, bone proliferation and ankylosis. Axially, BMO/osteitis is seen as high signal intensity on STIR or post-contrast T_1-weighted sequences [8]. Sacroiliitis on MRI is important in SpA, and form part of the Assessment of SpondyloArthritis international Society (ASAS) classification criteria for axial SpA [9], in which it is required that BMO is highly suggestive for SpA, and is defined as BMO located at subchondral or periarticular marrow in the sacroiliac joints (SIJ), and is present in at least two sites in one slice, or at least one site in two consecutive slices [10]. Axial enthesitis on MRI lacks a widely accepted definition, but may be characterised in the same way as peripheral enthesitis, or as a high signal on STIR sequences in the marrow at the entheseal insertion, or in the surrounding soft tissue [11, 12]. Fat infiltration is characterised by focal bright signal on a T_1-weighted sequence. Axially, bone erosions are characterised by full-thickness loss of dark appearance of cortical bone and loss of normal bright appearance of adjacent bone marrow on T_1-weighted sequence. Bone proliferations are characterised by a bright signal on T_1-weighted images extending from the vertebral endplate towards the adjacent vertebra, or into the SIJ space. Ankylosis is characterised by bright signal on T_1-weighted images extending from a vertebra and being continuous with the adjacent vertebra, or across the SIJ space [13].

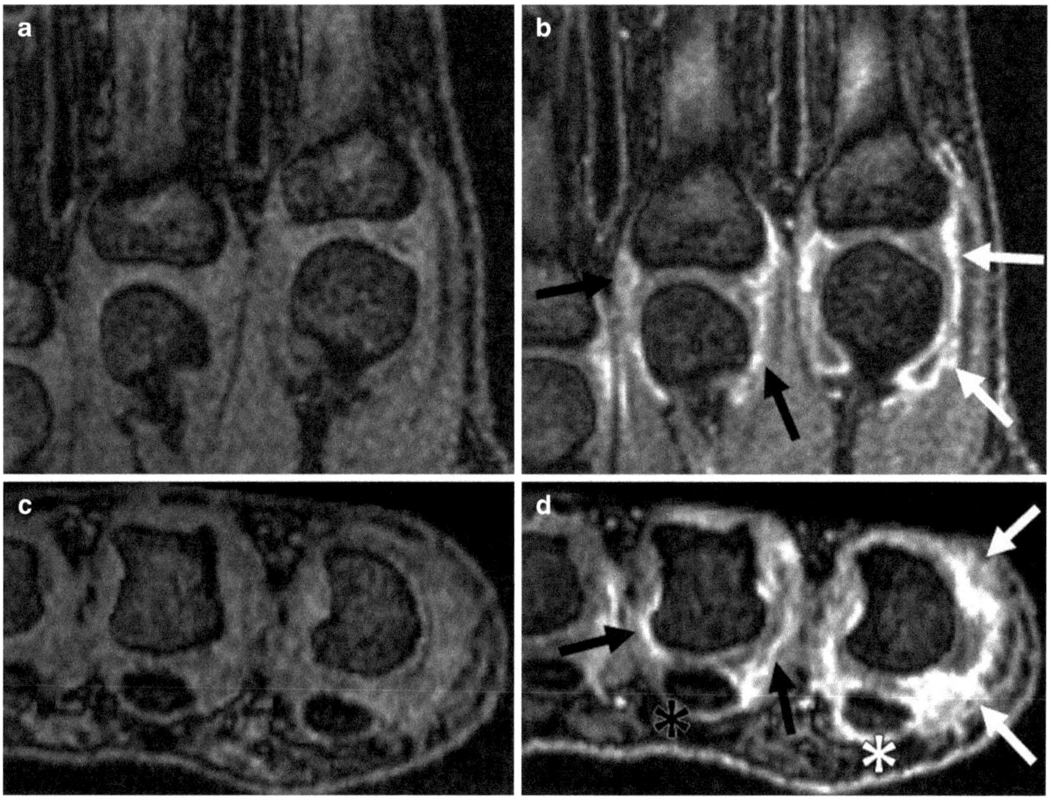

Fig. 21.1 MRI of the second and third metacarpophalangeal (MCP) joints. Images are T_1 weighted in coronal (**a**, **b**) and axial (**c**, **d**) slice orientation, obtained at three tesla before (*left*) and after (*right*) i.v. contrast agent injection (post-gadolinium, Gd). Synovitis is seen at the second (*white arrows*) and third (*black arrows*) MCP joints. Tenosynovitis is seen at the second (*white asterisk*) and third (*black asterisk*) MCP joints. Synovitis is defined as an area in the synovial compartment that shows increased post-Gd enhancement of a thickness greater than the width of the normal synovium. Tenosynovitis is defined as increased water content or abnormal post-Gd enhancement adjacent to a tendon, in an area with a tendon sheath. Enhancement (signal intensity increase) is judged by comparison between T_1-weighted images obtained before and after intravenous Gd contrast

MRI for Diagnosis, Monitoring and Prognostication of PsA in Clinical Practice

MRI for Diagnosing Peripheral PsA

Inflammatory and destructive changes can be seen by MRI in PsA [14–16], and findings such as synovitis, tenosynovitis and/or BMO document the presence of an inflammatory disease, but no changes are specific for PsA. In a literature review, McQueen et al. found that MRI could not distinguish between peripheral PsA and RA, when synovitis and erosions were evaluated [5]. However, in a comparative MRI study of the hand and wrist in PsA and RA patients bone erosions were more frequent in RA, and periostitis more frequent in PsA [17]. In 17 PsA and 20 RA patients with early disease, Narváez et al. found that MRI of the hand detected diaphyseal BMO and/or enthesitis in 71 % of PsA patients, whereas no RA patients had these features [18]. BMO in PsA is often located close to the entheses, in contrast to RA, where BMO often is located close to the capsular attachments, and in OA, where bone marrow lesions are mainly located close to sub-chondral areas [19]. Bone erosions in PsA are more often seen adjacent to collateral ligament insertions, whereas erosions in OA are more often located centrally [20]. Although only lim-ited numbers of psoriasis patients without arthri-tis have been investigated, all studies found higher frequency of arthritic and entheseal changes by MRI in psoriasis patients than in healthy subjects [21–23]. This suggests that MRI may detect PsA before it becomes clinically apparent.

MRI for Prognosticating Peripheral PsA

Only few studies are available on the use of MRI for prognosticating PsA. Based on a cross-sectional MRI study of 11 patients with the aggressive arthritis mutilans form of PsA, and 17 erosive PsA without arthritis mutilans, in which there was close relation between presence of ero-sion and BMO, it has been suggested that BMO is a 'forerunner' of structural joint damage in PsA [24]. In a longitudinal study of 41 PsA patients, BMO detected by MRI was related to subsequent erosive progression as detected by computed tomography [25]. More studies are needed to clarify whether MRI can be used to determine the prognosis in PsA.

MRI for Monitoring Peripheral PsA

MRI can assess joint inflammation and damage and changes therein (see paragraph on monitor-ing in clinical trials, below). In clinical practice, qualitative assessment, i.e. presence or absence, of different pathologies is most often used. Further research is needed to clarify how (e.g. which anatomical areas) and when MRI is best used to optimize clinical follow-up of PsA.

MRI in Axial PsA

Axial PsA can affect the SIJ and/or the spine. In the spine, inflammatory changes, visualized as BMO or soft tissue oedema/enthesitis, are char-acteristic, and can be seen at the anterior and pos-terior corners of the vertebral bodies, at the discovertebral junction, and at the costovertebral, facet and costotransverse joints [26–28]. In the SIJ, inflammation is seen as BMO, but also soft tissue inflammation at entheses occurs frequently [8, 29]. Few studies are available in axial PsA, but findings are overall comparable to AS find-ings, where MRI has proven sensitive for detec-tion of sacroiliitis and spondylitis, although more frequently asymmetric [30–32]. Bollow et al. have reported a correlation between MRI signs of sacroiliac osteitis and cellularity on correspond-ing biopsies [33]. In 2004, a study of PsA patients attending rheumatology out-patient clinics found sacroiliitis on MRI in 38 % [31]. More recently, Castillo-Gallego et al. reported that 70 % of PsA patients with inflammatory back pain had no inflammatory lesion on MRI, but only sacroiliac joints and lumbar spines, not thoracic and cervi-cal spines, were examined [34]. In the latter study, HLA-B27 positivity was significantly related to more severe MRI inflammation. More MRI research is needed on separate PsA popula-tions with axial disease [35].

Combined MRI Assessment of Peripheral and Axial Joints – Whole-Body MRI

Whole-body MRI is a novel imaging method, which allows MRI of the whole body in one scan-ning session, but at the cost of lower image reso-lution than conventional MRI (see Fig. 21.2). Radiologists have applied whole-body MRI for screening for bone marrow malignancies and sys-temic muscle diseases [36]. Weckbach et al. reported the results of whole-body MRI in 30 patients with PsA, and found that the most often detected pathology was enthesitis [37]. Recently, seven clinical enthesitis indices were examined by whole-body MRI in patients with PsA, axial SpA and healthy subjects and compared with entheseal tenderness [38]. A moderate agreement between MRI enthesitis and clinical examination was reported, suggesting a role for whole-body MRI in detecting subclinical inflammation. Furthermore, a new whole-body MRI enthesitis

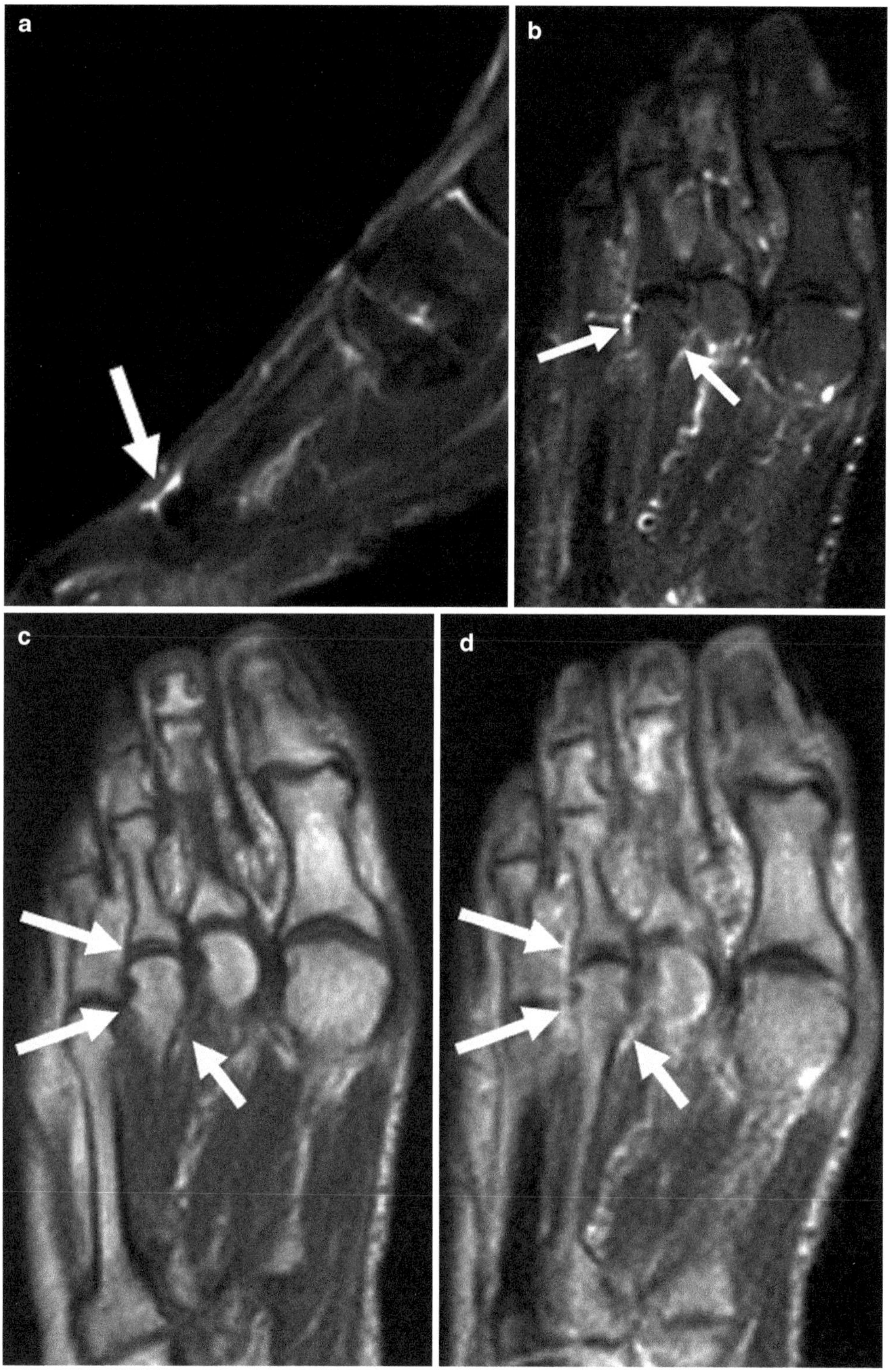

Fig. 21.2 Zoomed view of whole-body MRI of the fore-foot. Images are STIR (**a**, **b**) and T$_1$-weighted (**c**, **d**) images in sagittal (**a**) and coronal (**b–d**) slice orientation, obtained at three tesla before (**a–c**) and after (**d**) i.v. con-trast agent injection. *Arrows* on **a** and **b** shows a bright signal which reflects synovitis and/or joint effusion at the third toe. *Arrows* on **c** and **d** shows synovitis at the third toe

index was proposed, as a potential additional tool for assessing disease activity. An exciting possibility of whole-body MRI is the assessment of the distribution of inflammation and structural damage in the entire body, and the possibility of providing global scores of inflammation and damage in all peripheral and axial joints [39].

MRI for Monitoring PsA in Clinical Trials

Methods for MRI Assessment of Peripheral PsA in Clinical Trials

PsA disease manifestations may be assessed by qualitative, semiquantitative, or quantitative methods. There is no consensus on which joints to assess, neither in practice nor trials, and while it should probably be individualized based on the pattern of involvement, most studies have assessed the wrist and fingers [25, 40–44].

The international MRI in arthritis group of OMERACT [6] has recommended that T_1-weighted MRI before and after intravenous contrast and STIR or T_2-weighted FS images, preferably in two planes, be acquired (see above for details) [6].

Qualitative Methods

Most studies only report *qualitative* MRI assessments, i.e., presence versus absence of the different pathologies of PsA [5] (see Fig. 21.3). The simplicity of this approach may favor implementation in clinical practice, particularly for diagnostic purposes, but the lack of detail, and ensuing lack of sensitivity to change, limits its use in clinical trials when only few joints are examined by conventional MRI. In contrast, if many joints were assessed, as by whole-body MRI counts of inflamed joints, qualitative assessment of each joint may be sufficient. Whole-body MRI has, as described above, been introduced as a potential method for simultaneous assessment of peripheral and axial joints and entheses [37–39]. The method still needs improved image quality and more validation, but seems very promising for use in PsA trials in the future.

Quantitative Methods

Quantitative assessment of contrast enhancement by dynamic contrast-enhanced MRI has been reported [25, 40–43, 45, 46], and allows the assessor to estimate the rate of enhancement on several consecutive fast MRIs obtained at the time of contrast injection, using computer software. However, the PsA data from this method are still limited, and its advantage in clinical trials has not yet been documented.

Semiquantitative Methods, Including the PsAMRIS

Several *semiquantitative* scoring systems for synovitis, BMO, and/or erosions have been introduced [6, 16, 47], but most of these have only been used in a few patients. In a study of 11 PsA patients treated with the anti-tumor necrosis factor (TNF) agent adalimumab for 24 weeks, MRI of a wrist or knee showed significant improvements from baseline at 24 weeks in both clinical measures of disease activity and in MRI BMO and effusion, but not in synovitis [47]. The international MRI in arthritis group of OMERACT has developed the Psoriatic Arthritis Magnetic Resonance Image Score (PsAMRIS) for evaluation of inflammatory and destructive changes in PsA hands [6, 48, 49]. This is the most validated assessment system available and has a documented good intra- and inter-reader reliability for status scores of all parameters. For inflammatory parameters, the intra- and inter-reader reliability was high for change scores and the sensitivity to change was moderate. The damage parameters, bone erosion and bone proliferation, showed very limited change after 1 year of anti-TNF therapy [48].

In a recent 48-week follow-up study of 41 PsA patients initiating adalimumab therapy, MRIs were acquired of the metacarpophalangeal, proximal and distal interphalangeal joints of the hand most clinically involved at baseline, and scored according to the PsAMRIS. In patients fulfilling the modified PsA Response Criteria (PsARC) at follow-up, a statistically significant improvement was seen for all inflammatory parameters except periarticular inflammation. Bone damage showed very little change over time [25].

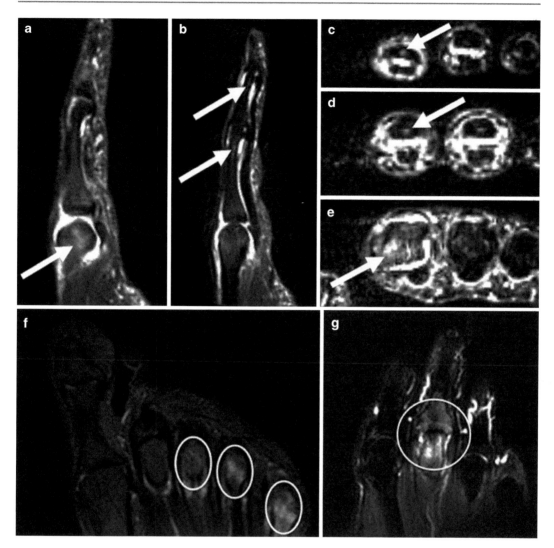

Fig. 21.3 MRI of the hand (**a–e, g**) and forefoot (**f**) showing bone marrow oedema (BMO). Images are STIR sequences in sagittal (**a, b**), axial (**c–e**) and coronal slice orientation (**f, g**). **a** and **e** shows BMO (*arrows*) in the second metacarpophalangeal (MCP) joint. **b, c** and **d** shows BMO (*arrows*) in the proximal (**d**) and distal (**c**) interphalangeal joints. (**f**) Shows BMO (*circles*) in the third, fourth and fifth metatarsophalangeal joints. **g** shows BMO (*circle*) in the second MCP joint

In a placebo-controlled trial, 22 PsA patients were randomized to receive zoledronic acid, or placebo. Bone oedema scored according to PsAMRIS decreased significantly in the zoledronic acid group, but not in the placebo group. No differences in MRI bone proliferation or bone erosion progression could be identified [50].

A subgroup of patients from another randomized controlled PsA trial [51], comparing abatacept and placebo, has recently been assessed by the PsAMRIS method [52]. Three readers from the OMERACT MRI in arthritis group applied the PsAMRIS to MRIs from 40 patients (20 of the foot and 20 of the hand) initiating either abatacept or placebo. In the abatacept group, a statistically significant improvement in synovitis score was seen in the metatarsophalangeal joint of the foot and for the summed synovitis score of the hands and feet at 6 months follow-up. All other inflammatory parameters showed a numerical (but statistically insignificant) improvement in the abatacept group, but not the placebo group. The bone damage parameters did overall not change over 6 months. Intra- and inter-reader intra-class correlation coefficients were generally high for all or some readers, especially for the inflammatory parameters. The responsiveness of the PsAMRIS was excellent for tenosynovitis (hand), synovitis (foot), and periarticular inflammation (hand and foot) [52]. Further application of the PsAMRIS in other MRI data sets from longitudinal randomized controlled trials would be highly relevant.

Methods for Assessment of Axial PsA in Clinical Trials

No PsA-specific MRI scoring systems are available for assessing axial disease. MRIs of the spine can be scored using scoring systems used in AS and axial SpA in general [32]. For SIJ inflammation and damage, the most used methods are The Spondyloarthritis Research Consortium of Canada (SPARCC) scoring system and the Berlin-activity method [32, 53, 54]. SIJ damage has rarely been assessed in clinical trials, but validated systems are available [32, 53, 55, 56]. For assessment of spine inflammation, the Canadian (SPARCC) and the German (Berlin) methods are again the most used [57, 58]. Both these methods assess inflammation in the vertebral bodies of the spine. Another approach, the Canada-Denmark system, assesses not only individual parts of the vertebral bodies, but also separately assesses the posterior elements of the spine, i.e. the facet joints, and the transverse and spinous processes [13, 28], which are often affected, not the least in early disease [27].

Conclusion

In summary, MRI can be used both in clinical practice and in clinical trials, for multiple purposes, including establishing or confirming a diagnosis of inflammatory joint disease, determining the extent of the disease, monitoring change in inflammation and structural damage, assessing therapeutic efficacy and potentially prognostication. Although technical improvements and increasing evidence has been established in the last years, further research is needed to clarify the full potential and the role of MRI in PsA trials and clinical practice.

References

1. Moll JM, Wright V. Psoriatic arthritis. Semin Arthritis Rheum. 1973;3:55–78.
2. Moll JM. Psoriatic arthritis. Br J Rheumatol. 1984;23:241–4.
3. Moll JM, Wright V. Familial occurrence of psoriatic arthritis. Ann Rheum Dis. 1973;32:181–201.
4. Moll JM, Haslock I, Macrae IF, et al. Associations between ankylosing spondylitis, psoriatic arthritis, Reiter's disease, the intestinal arthropathies, and Behcet's syndrome. Medicine (Baltimore). 1974;53: 343–64.
5. McQueen F, Lassere M, Ostergaard M. Magnetic resonance imaging in psoriatic arthritis: a review of the literature. Arthritis Res Ther. 2006;8:207.
6. Østergaard M, McQueen F, Wiell C, et al. The OMERACT psoriatic arthritis magnetic resonance imaging scoring system (PsAMRIS): definitions of key pathologies, suggested MRI sequences, and preliminary scoring system for PsA Hands. J Rheumatol. 2009;36:1816–24.
7. Tan AL, McGonagle D. Imaging of seronegative spondyloarthritis. Best Pract Res Clin Rheumatol. 2008;22:1045–59.
8. Sieper J, Rudwaleit M, Baraliakos X, et al. The Assessment of SpondyloArthritis international Society (ASAS) handbook: a guide to assess spondyloarthritis. Ann Rheum Dis. 2009;68 Suppl 2:ii1–44.
9. Rudwaleit M, van der Heijde D, Landewe R, et al. The development of Assessment of SpondyloArthritis international Society classification criteria for axial spondyloarthritis (part II): validation and final selection. Ann Rheum Dis. 2009;68:777–83.
10. Rudwaleit M, Jurik AG, Hermann KG, et al. Defining active sacroiliitis on magnetic resonance imaging (MRI) for classification of axial spondyloarthritis: a consensual approach by the ASAS/OMERACT MRI group. Ann Rheum Dis. 2009;68:1520–7.
11. Eshed I, Bollow M, McGonagle DG, et al. MRI of enthesitis of the appendicular skeleton in spondyloarthritis. Ann Rheum Dis. 2007;66:1553–9.
12. Althoff CE, Sieper J, Song IH, et al. Active inflammation and structural change in early active axial spondyloarthritis as detected by whole-body MRI. Ann Rheum Dis. 2013;72:967–73.
13. Ostergaard M, Maksymowych W, Pedersen SJ, et al. Structural lesions detected by magnetic resonance imaging in the spine of patients with spondyloarthritis – definitions, assessment system, and reference image set. J Rheumatol. 2009;36 Suppl 84:18–34.

14. Ghanem N, Uhl M, Pache G, et al. MRI in psoriatic arthritis with hand and foot involvement. Rheumatol Int. 2007;27:387–93.

15. Wiell C, Szkudlarek M, Hasselquist M, et al. Ultrasonography, magnetic resonance imaging, radiography, and clinical assessment of inflammatory and destructive changes in fingers and toes of patients with psoriatic arthritis. Arthritis Res Ther. 2007;9: R119.

16. Tehranzadeh J, Ashikyan O, Anavim A, et al. Detailed analysis of contrast-enhanced MRI of hands and wrists in patients with psoriatic arthritis. Skeletal Radiol. 2008;37:433–42.

17. Schoellnast H, Deutschmann HA, Hermann J, et al. Psoriatic arthritis and rheumatoid arthritis: findings in contrast-enhanced MRI. AJR Am J Roentgenol. 2006;187:351–7.

18. Narvaez J, Narvaez JA, de Albert M, et al. Can magnetic resonance imaging of the hand and wrist differentiate between rheumatoid arthritis and psoriatic arthritis in the early stages of the disease? Semin Arthritis Rheum. 2012;42:234–45.

19. Totterman SM. Magnetic resonance imaging of psoriatic arthritis: insight from traditional and three-dimensional analysis. Curr Rheumatol Rep. 2004;6: 317–21.

20. Braum LS, McGonagle D, Bruns A, et al. Characterisation of hand small joints arthropathy using high-resolution MRI – limited discrimination between osteoarthritis and psoriatic arthritis. Eur Radiol. 2013;23:1686–93.

21. Offidani A, Cellini A, Valeri G, et al. Subclinical joint involvement in psoriasis: magnetic resonance imaging and X-ray findings. Acta Derm Venereol. 1998;78:463–5.

22. Erdem CZ, Tekin NS, Sarikaya S, et al. MR imaging features of foot involvement in patients with psoriasis. Eur J Radiol. 2008;67:521–5.

23. Emad Y, Ragab Y, Bassyouni I, et al. Enthesitis and related changes in the knees in seronegative spondyloarthropathies and skin psoriasis: magnetic resonance imaging case–control study. J Rheumatol. 2010;37: 1709–17.

24. Tan YM, Østergaard M, Doyle A, et al. MRI bone oedema scores are higher in the arthritis mutilans form of psoriatic arthritis and correlate with high radiographic scores for joint damage. Arthritis Res Ther. 2009;11:R2.

25. Poggenborg RP, Wiell C, Boyesen P, et al. No overall damage progression despite persistent inflammation in adalimumab-treated psoriatic arthritis patients: results from an investigator-initiated 48-week comparative magnetic resonance imaging, computed tomography and radiography trial. Rheumatology (Oxford). 2014;53:746–56.

26. Queiro R, Tejon P, Alonso S, et al. Erosive discovertebral lesion (Andersson lesion) as the first sign of disease in axial psoriatic arthritis. Scand J Rheumatol. 2013;42:220–5.

27. Bochkova AG, Levshakova AV, Bunchuk NV, et al. Spinal inflammation lesions as detected by magnetic resonance imaging in patients with early ankylosing spondylitis are more often observed in posterior structures of the spine. Rheumatology (Oxford). 2010;49:749–55.

28. Lambert RG, Pedersen SJ, Maksymowych W, et al. Active inflammatory lesions detected by magnetic resonance imaging in the spine of patients with spondyloarthritis – definitions, assessment system and reference image set. J Rheumatol. 2009;36 Suppl 84:3–17.

29. Poggenborg RP, Eshed I, Pedersen SJ, et al. Whole-body MRI for assessment of enthesitis in psoriatic arthritis, axial spondyloarthritis and healthy subjects – a comparison with 7 clinical enthesitis indices [abstract]. Ann Rheum Dis. 2012;71 Suppl 3:110.

30. Helliwell PS, Hickling P, Wright V. Do the radiological changes of classic ankylosing spondylitis differ from the changes found in the spondylitis associated with inflammatory bowel disease, psoriasis, and reactive arthritis? Ann Rheum Dis. 1998;57:135–40.

31. Williamson L, Dockerty JL, Dalbeth N, et al. Clinical assessment of sacroiliitis and HLA-B27 are poor predictors of sacroiliitis diagnosed by magnetic resonance imaging in psoriatic arthritis. Rheumatology (Oxford). 2004;43:85–8.

32. Østergaard M, Poggenborg RP, Axelsen MB, et al. Magnetic resonance imaging in spondyloarthritis--how to quantify findings and measure response. Best Pract Res Clin Rheumatol. 2010;24:637–57.

33. Bollow M, Fischer T, Reisshauer H, et al. Quantitative analyses of sacroiliac biopsies in spondyloarthropathies: T cells and macrophages predominate in early and active sacroiliitis- cellularity correlates with the degree of enhancement detected by magnetic resonance imaging. Ann Rheum Dis. 2000;59:135–40.

34. Castillo-Gallego C, Aydin SZ, Emery P, et al. Magnetic resonance imaging assessment of axial psoriatic arthritis: extent of disease relates to HLA-B27. Arthritis Rheum. 2013;65:2274–8.

35. Gossec L, Smolen JS, Gaujoux-Viala C, et al. European league against rheumatism recommendations for the management of psoriatic arthritis with pharmacological therapies. Ann Rheum Dis. 2012;71:4–12.

36. Weckbach S. Whole-body MRI, for inflammatory arthritis and other multifocal rheumatoid diseases. Semin Musculoskelet Radiol. 2012;16:377–88.

37. Weckbach S, Schewe S, Michaely HJ, et al. Whole-body MR imaging in psoriatic arthritis: additional value for therapeutic decision making. Eur J Radiol. 2011;77:149–55.

38. Poggenborg RP, Eshed I, Ostergaard M, et al. Enthesitis in patients with psoriatic arthritis, axial spondyloarthritis and healthy subjects assessed by 'head-to-toe' whole-body MRI and clinical examination. Ann Rheum Dis. 2014;74(5):823–9. doi:10.1136/annrheumdis-2013-204239.

39. Poggenborg RP, Pedersen SJ, Eshed I, et al. Head-to-toe whole-body MRI in psoriatic arthritis, axial spondyloarthritis and healthy subjects: first steps towards global inflammation and damage scores of peripheral and axial joints. Rheumatology (Oxford). 2014;54(6):1039–49.

40. Cimmino MA, Parodi M, Innocenti S, et al. Dynamic magnetic resonance of the wrist in psoriatic arthritis reveals imaging patterns similar to those of rheumatoid arthritis. Arthritis Res Ther. 2005;7:R725–31.

41. Marzo-Ortega H, Tanner SF, Rhodes LA, et al. Magnetic resonance imaging in the assessment of metacarpophalangeal joint disease in early psoriatic and rheumatoid arthritis. Scand J Rheumatol. 2009;38:79–83.

42. Schraml C, Schwenzer NF, Martirosian P, et al. Assessment of synovitis in erosive osteoarthritis of the hand using DCE-MRI and comparison with that in its major mimic, the psoriatic arthritis. Acad Radiol. 2011;18:804–9.

43. Schwenzer NF, Kotter I, Henes JC, et al. The role of dynamic contrast-enhanced MRI in the differential diagnosis of psoriatic and rheumatoid arthritis. AJR Am J Roentgenol. 2010;194:715–20.

44. Strube H, Becker-Gaab C, Saam T, et al. Feasibility and reproducibility of the PsAMRIS-H score for psoriatic arthritis in low-field-strength dedicated extremity magnetic resonance imaging. Scand J Rheumatol. 2013;42:379–82.

45. Cimmino MA, Barbieri F, Boesen M, et al. Dynamic contrast-enhanced magnetic resonance imaging of articular and extraarticular synovial structures of the hands in patients with psoriatic arthritis. J Rheumatol Suppl. 2012;89:44–8.

46. Antoni C, Dechant C, Hanns-Martin Lorenz PD, et al. Open-label study of infliximab treatment for psoriatic arthritis: clinical and magnetic resonance imaging measurements of reduction of inflammation. Arthritis Rheum. 2002;47:506–12.

47. Anandarajah AP, Ory P, Salonen D, et al. Effect of adalimumab on joint disease: features of patients with psoriatic arthritis detected by magnetic resonance imaging. Ann Rheum Dis. 2010;69:206–9.

48. Boyesen P, McQueen FM, Gandjbakhch F, et al. The OMERACT Psoriatic Arthritis Magnetic Resonance Imaging Score (PsAMRIS) is reliable and sensitive to change: results from an OMERACT workshop. J Rheumatol. 2011;38:2034–8.

49. McQueen F, Lassere M, Bird P, et al. Developing a magnetic resonance imaging scoring system for peripheral psoriatic arthritis. J Rheumatol. 2007;34:859–61.

50. McQueen F, Lloyd R, Doyle A, et al. Zoledronic acid does not reduce MRI erosive progression in PsA but may suppress bone oedema: the Zoledronic Acid in Psoriatic Arthritis (ZAPA) Study. Ann Rheum Dis. 2011;70:1091–4.

51. Mease P, Genovese MC, Gladstein G, et al. Abatacept in the treatment of patients with psoriatic arthritis: results of a six-month, multicenter, randomized, double-blind, placebo-controlled, phase II trial. Arthritis Rheum. 2011;63:939–48.

52. Østergaard M, Glinatsi D, Pedersen SJ, et al. Utility in Clinical Trials of Magnetic Resonance Imaging for Psoriatic Arthritis: A Report from the GRAPPA 2014 Annual Meeting. J Rheumatol June 2015 42(6):1044–1047.

53. Hermann KG, Braun J, Fischer T, et al. Magnetic resonance tomography of sacroiliitis: anatomy, histological pathology, MR-morphology, and grading. Radiologe. 2004;44:217–28.

54. Maksymowych WP, Inman RD, Salonen D, et al. Spondyloarthritis research consortium of Canada magnetic resonance imaging index for assessment of sacroiliac joint inflammation in ankylosing spondylitis. Arthritis Rheum. 2005;53:703–9.

55. Maksymowych WP, Wichuk S, Chiowchanwisawakit P, et al. Fat metaplasia and backfill are key intermediaries in the development of sacroiliac joint ankylosis in patients with ankylosing spondylitis. Arthritis Rheumatol. 2014;66:2958–67.

56. Maksymowych WP, Wichuk S, Chiowchanwisawakit P, et al. Development and preliminary validation of the spondyloarthritis research consortium of Canada magnetic resonance imaging sacroiliac joint structural score. J Rheumatol. 2015;42:79–86.

57. Haibel H, Rudwaleit M, Brandt HC, et al. Adalimumab reduces spinal symptoms in active ankylosing spondylitis: clinical and magnetic resonance imaging results of a fifty-two-week open-label trial. Arthritis Rheum. 2006;54:678–81.

58. Maksymowych WP, Inman RD, Salonen D, et al. Spondyloarthritis research consortium of Canada magnetic resonance imaging index for assessment of spinal inflammation in ankylosing spondylitis. Arthritis Rheum. 2005;53:502–9.

Future Trends in Imaging Modalities for Psoriasis and Psoriatic Arthritis

Marwin Gutierrez and Carlos Pineda

Abstract

Imaging features have a valuable role in psoriatic disease; in spite this they are not firmly established in daily clinical practice. The necessity to integrate clinical and imaging findings in PsA patients, from a rheumatological and dermatological perspective, has been recently underlined by the international Group for Research in Psoriasis and Psoriatic Arthritis.

Ultrasound (US) and Magnetic Resonance Imaging (MRI) have been demonstrated to be sensitive for the assessment of anatomical changes, disease activity, and the efficacy of therapy in patients with PsA, especially in the early detection of aggressive arthritis.

Over the last years there has been a rapid progress in the imaging technologies, including the availability of high-end US devices with greater spatial resolution. In addition there has been progress in sophisticated software modalities (i.e. three-dimensional, elastosonography, automated cardiovascular software, and fusion imaging) that has generated growing interest in their use and/or advantages in evaluating several rheumatic diseases. This chapter is focus on the current potential applications of these new imaging modalities and provides evidence supporting its use in the daily practice.

Keywords

Psoriatic disease • Imaging • Ultrasound • Magnetic resonance imaging

M. Gutierrez,
Research Direction,
Instituto Nacional de Rehabilitación Calzada
Mexico-Xochimilco 289 Colonia Arenal de
Guadalupe, CP 143898, Mexico City, Mexico
e-mail: dr.gmarwin@gmail.com

C. Pineda, M.D., PhD (✉)
Research Director, Instituto Nacional de
Rehabilitación, Mexico City, Mexico

© Springer International Publishing Switzerland 2016
A. Adebajo et al. (eds.), *Psoriatic Arthritis and Psoriasis: Pathology and Clinical Aspects*,
DOI 10.1007/978-3-319-19530-8_22

Science is often distinguished from other domains of human culture by its progressive nature – The Stanford Encyclopedia of Philosophy.

Introduction

Psoriatic arthritis (PsA) is a chronic inflammatory disease with a variable intra- and inter-individual clinical course and outcome that may develop in 5–40 % of individuals with psoriasis [1]. Its heterogeneity is such that the term "psoriatic disease" has been recently suggested to encompass the involvement at different tissue level including joint, tendon, enthesis, skin and nail [2, 3].

A variety of clinical instruments are currently used for measuring the disease activity in patients with PsA such as Disease Activity index for Psoriatic Arthritis (DAPSA), PsA Response Criteria (PsARC), Composite Psoriatic Disease Activity Index (CPDAI) and Disease Activity Score using 28 joint count (DAS 28) that was originally developed for patients with rheumatoid arthritis (RA) [4–8].

Imaging features have a valuable role in PsA; in spite this, they are not firmly established in the assessment of effectiveness of treatment and in monitoring patient's outcomes in daily clinical practice. The necessity to integrate clinical and imaging findings in PsA patients, from a rheumatological and dermatological perspective, has been recently underlined by the international Group for Research in Psoriasis and Psoriatic Arthritis (GRAPPA) [9].

Ultrasound (US) and Magnetic Resonance Imaging (MRI) are the imaging techniques that have generated the most evidence in recent years. Both techniques have been demonstrated to be sensitive for the assessment of anatomical changes, disease activity, and the efficacy of therapy in patients with PsA [9–17]. Compared to other imaging techniques, MRI and US also have the great potential as regards the early detection of aggressive arthritis and surveillance of disease activity.

There has been rapid progress in the imaging technologies, including the availability of high-end US devices with greater spatial resolution that allows for the detection of even minimal blood flow changes at different superficial tissues including nail and skin. In addition there has been progress in sophisticated software modalities (i.e. three-dimensional, elastosonography, automated cardiovascular software, and fusion imaging) that has generated growing interest in their use and/or advantages in evaluating several rheumatic diseases. This chapter is focus on the current potential applications of these new imaging modalities, in particular US, and provides evidence supporting its use in the daily rheumatological practice.

Three-Dimensional US

Three-dimensional (3D) US, since its first application in medical practice, appeared to be a useful tool to carry out diagnosis and follow-up in various medical areas including the musculoskeletal diseases.

3D US image is acquired automatically using a volumetric probe in few seconds, due to the automatic sweeping scan movement of the piezoelectric crystals located inside the volumetric probe [18]. It can be performed in both grayscale and power Doppler (PD) mode (Fig. 22.1). Moreover longitudinal, transverse, and coronal planes (by producing a 3D reconstruction of the anatomic area) can also be accurately obtained.

Various studies comparing the findings between 2D and 3D US have been performed. They have been mainly focused on bone erosions, synovial hypertrophy, peripheral enthesitis and bursitis in patients with RA and spondyloarthritis (SpA) including PsA [19–25].

Bone erosions can be accurately assessed by 3D US since it is able to display multiplanar images (longitudinal, transverse, coronal) particularly useful to confirm their presence (Fig. 22.2). Most studies have been performed in RA; however they could be considered as reference also in PsA due to its similar erosive characteristic. Filippucci et al. demonstrated good-to-excellent agreement rates in the detection of presence/absence of bone erosions and in their semiquantitative assessment between 3D centralized reading and conventional 2D US imaging in

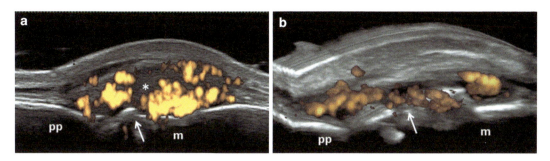

Fig. 22.1 (**a**) Metacarpophalangeal joint. The 2D image shows a proliferative synovitis (*) with intense intra-articular power Doppler. Note also the bone irregularities at metacarpal level (*arrow*). However the image do not permits to confirm clearly the cortical brake. (**b**) 3D image of the same patient confirming the power Doppler and depicting more clearly the bone erosion (*arrow*). *m* metacarpal head, *pp* proximal phalanx

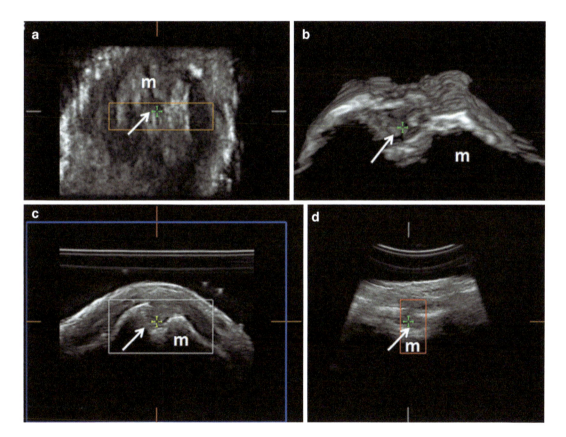

Fig. 22.2 Metacarpophalangeal joint. 3D US image showing contemporaneously coronal (**a**), volumetric reconstruction (**b**) longitudinal (**c**) and transverse (**d**) views of the bone erosion (*arrows*). *mc* metacarpal head

patients with RA [20]. Naredo et al. also reported that 3D US reliability for bone erosions of the wrist joint in patients with RA was almost similar to 2D reliability [26]. Moreover, De Miguel et al. evaluated the accuracy of 3D US compared to 2D US in detecting erosions of the calcaneal bone in patients with SpA. The results showed that 3D US visualized more bone erosions than 2D US and detected more structural changes of bone erosion during the follow up period in SpA [27].

3D PD has been described as a valid method to quantify the synovial perfusion since it allows a spatial visualization of synovial blood vessels in both peri- and intra-articular inflamed regions.

The studies using 3D PD for synovitis in patients with chronic arthritis showed that the quantification of 3D PD images resulted in higher intra- and inter-observer agreement compared with 2D analyses [19, 21, 26]. Moreover, Strunk et al., compared 3D PD US with contrast MRI in their capability to visualize synovial vascularity in inflamed wrists of chronic arthritis. Interestingly, the results showed that 3D PD is a reliable imaging technique for assessing synovial vascularity compared with the clinical symptoms and the gold standard of dynamic MRI [27].

To date, there are still few prospective longitudinal studies using quantitative 3D US to assess the inflammatory process in patients with chronic inflammatory arthritis. Moreover, these studies have included small number of patients and short time follow-up.

Although quantitative 3D US showed a good performance for inflammation assessment, the inter-observer agreement and the responsiveness rates were similar to those obtained with 2D PD US.

Elastosonography

Elastosonography (ES) is an imaging technique that allows a non-invasive evaluation of tissue elasticity in addition to information obtained from conventional B-mode. It is based on the principle that the compression of tissue produces different degree of tissue displacement according to the stiffness of each tissue. The degree of the tissue displacement is calculated in real-time and the elasticity information can be displayed as colour-coded elasticity map, so-called elastograms, superimposed on the B-mode images, in which each colour is representative of a different level of elasticity (Fig. 22.3).

There are no specific studies in PsA; however the recent data may suppose its future application in these patients. Initial results showed that the symptomatic tendons usually present softer ES patterns than healthy tendons [28]. Until recently, application of ES in tendon pathology was poorly considered since high-resolution 2D US seemed to be sufficient to depict accurately the morphostructural changes at tendon level that included: loss of its fibrillar pattern, thickening of the tendon and partial or complete tendon rupture as well as intra-tendinous blood flow changes. However, Klauser et al. reported that 2D US alone may shows false-negative findings in at least 14 % of cases of Achilles tendinopathy. The authors showed an increase in ES diagnostic accuracy by a positive correlation with the histological findings and concluded that it is potentially more sensitively than 2D US in the assessment of Achilles tendinoapthy in the daily clinical setting [29]. Additionally, some studies proposed that ES had greater capability to detect subclinical degenerative tendon abnormalities and to depict accurately the subacromial subdeltoid bursa not detected by 2D US in patients with polymyalgia rheumatica [30, 31].

More recently, studies have also evaluated the utility of ES utility in treatment monitoring of psoriatic plaque [32].

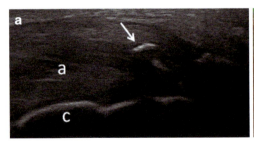
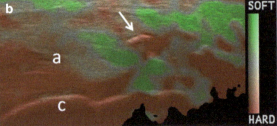

Fig. 22.3 Longitudinal dorsal scan of Achilles tendon in grey-scale showing a calcific tendinopathy (**a**) and the corresponding elastosonography (**b**). Note as the elastosonography depicts clearly the different tissue elasticity within the tendon, in particular shows the hard composition of the calcifications (*arrows*); *a* achilles tendon, *c* calcaneous bone

Automated US Intima-Media Thickness Assessment

The accelerated atherosclerosis leading to premature cardiovascular disease (CVD) is widely recognized as a relevant cause of both morbidity and mortality in patients affected by chronic autoimmune inflammatory disorders such as chronic PsA. Early detection of atherosclerosis is quite important in patients with rheumatic diseases before the development of CVD.

Carotid intima-media thickness (IMT), is a marker of atherosclerosis risk that can improve the individual risk assessment and quantify pathology and to monitor the efficacy of therapy.

Conventionally, the measurement of IMT is performed by manual tracing of the interfaces between tissue layers. Of note this method requires high competency, adequate training and a consolidated level of expertise. Traditionally, primarily cardiologists or radiologists perform IMT examination. In spite the conventional approach to assess carotid IMT there are still some aspects that should be overcome such as the wide inter- and intra-observer variability among experts (because it is dependent of the judgment of them) and time-consuming in IMT measurements.

Recently, US technology based on radio frequency (RF) has been proposed for measuring carotid IMT (QIMT, Quality Intima-Media Thickness). This method seems to be less dependent of the experience in vascular US of the examiner as it provides an automated measure of IM interface [33] (Fig. 22.4). In this way, some rheumatologists have explored its potential application in the cardiovascular risk assessment of the rheumatic patients. Naredo et al., [34] performed a study aimed to assess the reliability of the automated RF-based US QIMT and to evaluate the variability between this method and the conventional B-mode US measurement of carotid IMT in RA patients. The remarkable aspect of the study was the fact that the US examinations were performed by rheumatologists with different degree of experience in vascular US (from none examination to 50 previous examinations). Their findings were compared with those obtained by an expert cardiologist who adopted the conventional method. The results showed good to excellent reliability (ICCs 0.85 and 0.61 for inter- and intra-observer respectively) that indicated that the automated RF-based US QIMT performed by rheumatologist could be a reliable method for assessing cardiovascular risk in patients with chronic arthritis. Di Geso et al., conducted a single-center study in order to compare the performance of conventional and RF-based US QIMT in 32 patients with chronic SpA including PsA. Two sonographers performed the US examinations. A cardiologist employing the conventional manual approach and a rheumatologist, who adopted the automated RF-based US QIMT. They found a high agreement between the two methods. The feasibility in the use of the RF-based US QIMT in evaluating the cardiovascular risk assessment of rheumatic patients was also demonstrated [35]. Gutierrez et al., performed a study to determine the prevalence of increased carotid IMT, as sign of pre-clinical atherosclerosis, in patients with RA and PsA using an automated RF-QIMT in 108 patients (68 with RA and 40 with PsA). In 45 (66 %) out of the 68 patients with RA and 26 (67 %) out of the 39 patients with PsA, US detected an increased carotid IMT. A significant correlation between increased carotid IMT and both disease duration and age of the patients was found. The reliability results were also acceptable [36].

Fusion Imaging – Virtual Navigator

This innovative system allows increasing the diagnostic value of the US, displaying simultaneously in the monitor, the US image and the corresponding CT/MRI image. In practice fusion imaging (FI) combines information obtained by CT or MRI to the great usability and simplicity of US [37].

FI has been largely adopted in several fields such as radiotherapy, interventional radiology, nuclear medicine, and neurosurgery. By incorporating information from previously performed CT or MRI assessments into real-time US, this method has been explored in order to refine the potential clinical applications. It has been tested

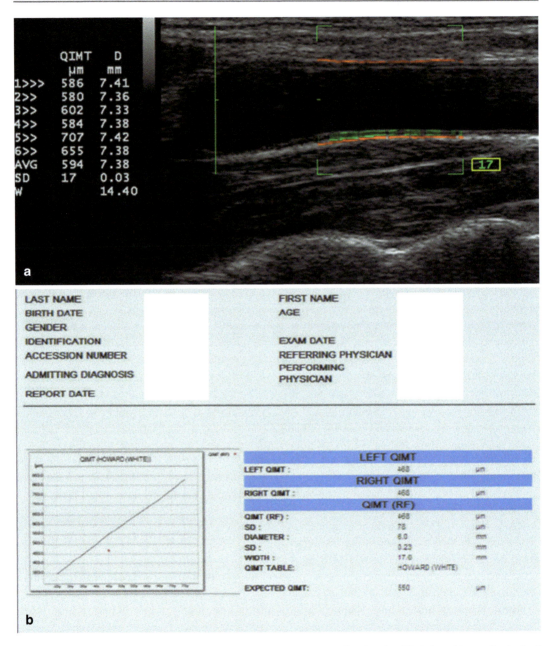

Fig. 22.4 (a) Automatic measurement of carotid Intima Media Thickness. The *green horizontal line* is superimposed on the B-mode image to measure the thickness of intima-media complex. The *orange line* indicates the adventitia. The data are displayed on the *left side* of the screen, which are computed and continuously updated by the system. (b) Vascular Worksheet. Report is obtained automatically after the cIMT assessment. Note as the software reports the intima media thickness by site and an offers an expected value of IMT for each patient. The report in this case is normal

in several conditions including: abdominal pathology, US-guided targeted liver ablation, breast diseases and cerebrovascular abnormalities [38–43].

In the rheumatological field, FI application is still in its investigational stages. There are few reports that tested its advantages in different conditions; no studies have been performed in

PsA. Liu et al. [44], performed a study to evaluate the feasibility of US-MRI virtual navigation in shoulder pathology. They selected 4-points internal marks in the shoulder to combine the US and MRI images. The observed targets included coincidence, stability, and accuracy in the US and MRI by two radiologists. They showed that the 4-points internal marks are considered a valid method and the application of US-MRI virtual navigation is regarded feasible in the shoulder.

Iagnocco et al., [45] investigated the role of US/MRI FI in the hand and wrist joints of osteoarthritis (OA) and RA patients. Image US/MRI superposition was carried out, with real-time contemporary visualization of the US and related MRI images. Randomly selected stored images of different joints were subsequently re-analyzed by a different operator. Concordance between the static and dynamic evaluations was assessed. The real-time MRI/US overlap provided fusion images of both tools. A striking concordance in the visualization of the bony profile was found with evidence of pronounced osteophytes in OA and bone erosions in RA. The analysis of stored selected images demonstrated a high concordance between real-time and static assessment. Additional advantage was that MRI/US fusion imaging provided a composite set of information with accurate anatomical correlations. Other applications of FI could be hypothesized, for instance a precise needle placement in peripheral joints and sacroiliac joints in PsA patients, can be achieved under US/MRI guidance; in cases where avoidance of radiation exposure is imperative, these modalities, can replace fluoroscopy or CT guidance.

High-Resolution Transducers to Assess Psoriatic Skin and Nail Involvement

The recent availability of US equipment with PD frequency higher than 10 MHz, enables a very sensitive visualization of the blood flow also at dermal level.

Preliminary results demonstrating the potential role of PDUS in the assessment of psoriatic plaque and onychopathy in patients with psoriasis and/or PsA have been recently published [14, 46–48]. The PD criterion validity and responsiveness to change has been demonstrated by a positive correlation with the histology findings at psoriatic plaque level in patients receiving TNF-α antagonist therapy [46]. Further investigations regarding both intra- and inter-observer reproducibility and studying larger series are still needed to confirm these preliminary studies.

Conclusion

Advances in imaging technology over the last 5 years have revolutionized almost every aspect of medicine. Nowadays, imaging is considered an important tool for the practicing rheumatologist due to its potential to provide early and more accurate diagnoses, to assess and evaluate response to therapy, and to monitor disease activity for several rheumatic diseases.

As usually occurs, technological change in the US field is under continuous progress, providing exciting instruments that expand the imaginary range of applications of imaging in rheumatology. Although several of these new modalities have been successful and have made a contribution to physician education and patient care, much more effort is still required to explore all the potential advantages and clinical indications of these elusive, but fascinating and challenging advanced imaging techniques.

References

1. Gladman DD, Antoni C, Mease P, et al. Psoriatic arthritis: epidemiology, clinical features, course, and outcome. Ann Rheum Dis. 2005;64 Suppl 2:ii14–7.
2. Ritchlin CT. From skin to bone: translational perspectives on psoriatic disease. J Rheumatol. 2008;35: 1434–7.
3. McGonagle D, Conaghan P, Emery P. Psoriatic arthritis-aunified concept 20 years on. Arthritis Rheum. 1999;42:1080–6.
4. Clegg DO, Reda DJ, Mejias E, et al. Comparison of sulfasalazine and placebo in the treatment of psoriatic arthritis. A Department of Veterans Affairs Cooperative Study. Arthritis Rheum. 1996;39: 2013–20.

5. Fransen J, Antoni C, Mease PJ, et al. Performance of response criteria for assessing peripheral arthritis in patients with psoriatic arthritis: analysis of data from randomised controlled trials of two tumour necrosis factor inhibitors. Ann Rheum Dis. 2006;65:1373–8.

6. Nell-Duxneuner VP, Stamm TA, Machold KP, et al. Evaluation of the appropriateness of composite disease activity measures for assessment of psoriatic arthritis. Ann Rheum Dis. 2009;2010(69):546–9.

7. Schoels M, Aletaha D, Funovits J, et al. Application of the DAREA/DAPSA score for assessment of disease activity in psoriatic arthritis. Ann Rheum Dis. 2010;69:1441–7.

8. Mumtaz A, Gallagher P, Kirby B, et al. Development of a preliminary composite disease activity index in psoriatic arthritis. Ann Rheum Dis. 2011;70:272–7.

9. Coates LC, Anderson RR, Fitzgerald O, et al. Clues to the pathogenesis of psoriasis and psoriatic arthritis from imaging: a literature review. J Rheumatol. 2008;35:1438–42.

10. Weiner SM, Jurenz S, Uhl M, et al. Ultrasonography in the assessment of peripheral joint involvement in psoriatic arthritis: a comparison with radiography, MRI and scintigraphy. Clin Rheumatol. 2008;27:983–9.

11. Wiell C, Szkudlarek M, Hasselquist M, et al. Ultrasonography, magnetic resonance imaging, radiography, and clinical assessment of inflammatory and destructive changes in fingers and toes of patients with psoriatic arthritis. Arthritis Res Ther. 2008;10:402.

12. Delle Sedie A, Riente L, Filippucci E, et al. Ultrasound imaging for the rheumatologist. XXXII. Sonographic assessment of the foot in patients with psoriatic arthritis. Clin Exp Rheumatol. 2011;29:217–22.

13. Gutierrez M, Filippucci E, De Angelis R, Filosa G, Kane D, Grassi W. A sonographic spectrum of psoriatic arthritis: "the five targets". Clin Rheumatol. 2010;29:133–42.

14. Filippucci E, De Angelis R, Salaffi F, Grassi W. Ultrasound, skin, and joints in psoriatic arthritis. J Rheumatol Suppl. 2009;83:35–8.

15. Østergaard M, Bird P, Gandjbakhch F, et al. The OMERACT MRI in arthritis working group – update on status and future research priorities. J Rheumatol. 2015 Feb 15. pii: jrheum.141248. [Epub ahead of print]

16. Tan AL, Fukuba E, Halliday NA, Tanner SF, Emery P, McGonagle D. High-resolution MRI assessment of dactylitis in psoriatic arthritis shows flexor tendon pulley and sheath-related enthesitis. Ann Rheum Dis. 2015;74:185–9.

17. Orbai AM, Weitz J, Siegel EL, et al., GRAPPA Enthesitis Working Group. Systematic review of treatment effectiveness and outcome measures for enthesitis in psoriatic arthritis. J Rheumatol. 2014;41:2290.

18. Meenagh G, Filippucci E, Abbattista T, et al. Three-dimensional power Doppler sonography in short-term therapy monitoring of rheumatoid synovitis. Rheumatology (Oxford). 2007;46:1736.

19. Watanabe T, Takemura M, Sato M, et al. Quantitative analysis of vascularization in the finger joints in patients with rheumatoid arthritis using three-dimensional volumetric ultrasonography with power Doppler. Clin Rheumatol. 2012;31:299–307.

20. Filippucci E, Meenagh G, Delle Sedie A, et al. Ultrasound imaging for the rheumatologist. XX. Sonographic assessment of hand and wrist joint involvement in rheumatoid arthritis: comparison between two- and three-dimensional ultrasonography. Clin Exp Rheumatol. 2009;27:197–200.

21. Strunk J, Strube K, Rumbaur C, et al. Interobserver agreement in two- and three-dimensional power Doppler sonographic assessment of synovial vascularity during anti-inflammatory treatment in patients with rheumatoid arthritis. Ultraschall Med. 2007;28:409–15.

22. Ju JH, Kwok SK, Seo SH, et al. Visualization of extensor digitorum tenosynovitis with three-dimensional ultrasonography. Rheumatology (Oxford). 2007;46:886–7.

23. Mérot O, Guillot P, Maugars Y, et al. Three-dimensional versus two-dimensional ultrasonographic assessment of peripheral enthesitis in spondylarthritis. Clin Rheumatol. 2014;33:131–5.

24. Iagnocco A, Riente L, Delle Sedie A, et al. Ultrasound imaging for the rheumatologist. XXII. Achilles tendon involvement in spondyloarthritis. A multi-centre study using high frequency volumetric probe. Clin Exp Rheumatol. 2009;27:547–51.

25. Falcao S, de Miguel E, Castillo-Gallego C, et al. Achilles enthesis ultrasound: the importance of the bursa in spondyloarthritis. Clin Exp Rheumatol. 2013;31:422–7.

26. Naredo E, Möller I, Acebes C, et al. Three-dimensional volumetric ultrasonography. Does it improve reliabililty of musculoskeletal ultrasound? Clin Exp Rheumatol. 2010;28:79–82.

27. De Miguel E, Falcao S, Castillo C, et al. Enthesis erosion in spondyloarthritis is not a persistent structural lesion. Ann Rheum Dis. 2011;70:2008–10.

28. Ahn KS, Kang CH, Hong SJ, et al. Ultrasound elastography of lateral epicondylosis: clinical feasibility of quantitative elastographic measurements. AJR Am J Roentgenol. 2014;202:1094–9.

29. Klauser AS, Miyamoto H, Tamegger M, et al. Achilles tendon assessed with sonoelastography: histologic agreement. Radiology. 2013;267:837–42.

30. Pedersen M, Fredberg U, Langberg H. Sonoelastography as a diagnostic tool in the assessment of musculoskeletal alterations: a systematic review. Ultraschall Med. 2012;33:441–6.

31. Silvestri E, Garlaschi G, Bartolini B, et al. Sonoelastography can help in the localization of soft tissue damage in polymyalgia rheumatica. Clin Exp Rheumatol. 2007;25:796.

32. Cucoş M, Crişan M, Lenghel M, et al. Conventional ultrasonography and sonoelastography in the assessment of plaque psoriasis under topical corticosteroid treatment – work in progress. Med Ultrason. 2014;16:107–13.

33. Hoeks AP, Willekes C, Boutouyrie P, et al. Automated detection of local artery wall thickness based on M-line signal processing. Ultrasound Med Biol. 1997;23:1017–23.

34. Naredo E, Möller I, Gutiérrez M, et al. Multi-examiner reliability of automated radio frequency-based ultrasound measurements of common carotid intima-media thickness in rheumatoid arthritis. Rheumatology (Oxford). 2011;50:1860–4.

35. Di Geso L, Zardi EM, Afeltra A, et al. Comparison between conventional and automated software-guided ultrasound assessment of bilateral common carotids intima-media thickness in patients with rheumatic diseases. Clin Rheumatol. 2012;31:881–4.

36. Gutierrez M, Naredo E, Di Geso L, et al. Prevalence of sub-clinical carotid atherosclerosis in patients with rheumatoid arthritis and psoriatic arthritis: a new automated radiofrequency-based ultrasound measurement of common intima-media thickness. Ann Rheum Dis. 2014;71 Suppl 3:301–2.

37. Klauser AS, Peetrons P. Developments in musculoskeletal ultrasound and clinical applications. Skeletal Radiol. 2010;39:1061–71.

38. Mauri G, De Beni S, Forzoni L, et al. Virtual navigator automatic registration technology in abdominal application. Conf Proc IEEE Eng Med Biol Soc. 2014;2014:5570–4.

39. Skoloudik D, Kuliha M, Roubec M, et al. Comparison of brain vessel imaging from transtemporal and transcondylar approaches using contrast-enhanced transcranial color-coded duplex sonography and Virtual Navigator. Biomed Pap Med Fac Univ Palacky Olomouc Czech Repub. 2014 dec 5. doi: 10.5507/bp.2014.064

40. Di Mauro E, Solbiati M, De Beni S, et al. Virtual navigator real-time ultrasound fusion imaging with positron emission tomography for liver interventions. Conf Proc IEEE Eng Med Biol Soc. 2013;2013: 1406–9.

41. Forzoni L, De Beni S, D'Onofrio S, et al. Virtual navigator 3D panoramic for breast examination. Conf Proc IEEE Eng Med Biol Soc. 2013;2013:1394–7.

42. Zamboni P, Menegatti E, Viselner G, et al. Fusion imaging technology of the intracranial veins. Phlebology. 2012;27:360–7.

43. Crocetti L, Lencioni R, Debeni S, et al. Targeting liver lesions for radiofrequency ablation: an experimental feasibility study using a CT-US fusion imaging system. Invest Radiol. 2008;43:33–9.

44. Liu J, Zhan W, Zhou M, et al. The feasibility study of US-MRI virtual navigation in the shoulder. Clin Imaging. 2012;36:803–9.

45. Iagnocco A, Perella C, D'Agostino MA, et al. Magnetic resonance and ultrasonography real-time fusion imaging of the hand and wrist in osteoarthritis and rheumatoid arthritis. Rheumatology. 2011;50: 1409–13.

46. Gutierrez M, De Angelis R, Bernardini ML, Filippucci E, Goteri G, Brandozzi G, et al. Clinical, power Doppler sonography and histological assessment of the psoriatic plaque: short-term monitoring in patients treated with etanercept. Br J Dermatol. 2011;164: 33–7.

47. Gutierrez M, Filippucci E, Bertolazzi C, Grassi W. Sonographic monitoring of psoriatic plaque. J Rheumatol. 2009;36:850–2.

48. Gutierrez M, Wortsman X, Filippucci E, De Angelis R, Filosa G, Grassi W. High-frequency sonography in the evaluation of psoriasis: nail and skin involvement. J Ultrasound Med. 2009;28:1569–74.

Part VI

Laboratory Tests

Alice B. Gottlieb

Relevant Laboratory Tests and Therapeutic Monitoring in Psoriasis

Aleksandra Florek and April W. Armstrong

Abstract

Although psoriasis does not require any diagnostic laboratory tests, physicians need to keep in mind the variety of laboratory studies for both screening as well as ongoing monitoring of psoriasis therapies. A multitude of laboratory tests exists to examine the safety of these therapies, including topical therapies, phototherapy, oral medications, and/or biologic agents. Knowledge of the available tests is important to screen vulnerable selected populations prior to initiating psoriasis treatment, such as pregnant women, immunocompromised patients, or patients with certain medical conditions. Screening labs are important in identifying these patients. Most importantly, familiarity with the available laboratory studies will ensure timely management of any anticipated side effects of the various psoriasis therapies.

Keywords

Laboratory tests • Laboratory markers • Therapeutic monitoring • Psoriasis

Psoriasis is a common, chronic, inflammatory, immune-mediated disorder that results from a combination of polygenic susceptibility and environmental influences [1]. It is a systemic disease with predominantly skin and joint manifestations in which approximately 20–30 % of patients have or will eventually develop psoriatic arthritis [2, 3]. Psoriasis may also be associated with several other medical comorbidities, including Crohn's disease, ulcerative colitis, multiple sclerosis, metabolic syndrome, atherosclerotic cardiovascular disease, and lymphomas [4–6]. These comorbidities need to be taken into account when monitoring psoriasis patients in routine clinical and research settings.

A. Florek, MD (✉)
Department of Dermatology,
Northwestern University, 676 N. St Clair Street,
Suite 1600, Chicago, IL 60611, USA
e-mail: aleksandra.florek@northwestern.edu

A.W. Armstrong, MD, MPH
Department of Dermatology,
University of Colorado Denver, Aurora, CO, USA

© Springer International Publishing Switzerland 2016
A. Adebajo et al. (eds.), *Psoriatic Arthritis and Psoriasis: Pathology and Clinical Aspects*,
DOI 10.1007/978-3-319-19530-8_23

Although the differential diagnosis of psoriasis is broad, a diagnosis of psoriasis can be made by history and physical examination in the vast majority of cases. Psoriasis is mainly diagnosed clinically through visual inspection of the skin lesions by dermatologists. Occasionally, a punch biopsy is performed in order to rule out other similar appearing conditions. There are no specific laboratory tests that either confirm or exclude the diagnosis of psoriasis. However, a multitude of laboratory tests exists to examine the safety of psoriasis therapies. Knowledge of the available laboratory diagnostic and therapeutic tests is important for a number of reasons. For example, some therapies are contraindicated in selected populations, such as pregnant women, immunocompromised patients, or patients with certain medical conditions. Screening labs are important in identifying these patients. In addition, laboratory information allows for monitoring of therapies to ensure safety and timely management of any anticipated side effects.

A number of treatments are currently available for the treatment of psoriasis, including topical therapies, phototherapy, oral medications, and/or biologic agents. The majority of patients with mild psoriasis can be managed with topical agents, which include topical corticosteroids, vitamin D analogues, topical calcineurin inhibitors, keratolytics, tar, or a combination of some of these agents [7]. Patients with moderate to severe psoriasis are typically treated with phototherapy, oral agents, or biologic therapy.

Typically, topical therapies do not require any baseline or ongoing laboratory monitoring. However, if a patient had been receiving frequent, high-potency topical steroids to extensive areas of the skin, he or she may experience feelings of fatigue, muscle weakness, depression, or hypotension immediately after withdrawal from the therapy. In contrast, signs or symptoms associated with prolonged exposure to high levels of cortisol, including glucosuria or hyperglycemia, may also occur during treatment due to percutaneous absorption of high potency steroids. In these instances, physicians need to rule out hypothalamic-pituitary-adrenal abnormalities by performing adrenocorticotropic hormone

Table 23.1 Recommended baseline laboratory studies prior to initiating oral agents in psoriasis patients

Oral agents and laboratory tests required prior to their initiation	
Methotrexate	CBC with differential
	Creatinine
	Liver function tests (LFTs)
	Urine pregnancy test
	HIV antibodies
	Hepatitis B and C serology in patients with elevated LFTs
	PPD test
Cyclosporine	Blood urea nitrogen and creatinine on at least 2–3 separate occasions Urinalysis
	CBC count
	Magnesium
	Potassium
	Uric acid
	Lipids
	Liver enzymes
	Bilirubin
	Urine pregnancy test
Acitretin	Lipid tests
	Liver function test
	Urine pregnancy test
	Renal function tests

Based on data from Ref. [9]

(ACTH) stimulation test also known as the cosyntropin stimulation test, checking morning or random plasma cortisol and urinary free cortisol levels.

Treatment with phototherapy does not usually necessitate baseline or ongoing monitoring, with an exception of screening a selected population. Psoralen plus ultraviolet A (PUVA) and UVB are generally contraindicated in patients with lupus erythematous. Therefore, baseline liver enzymes, antinuclear antibodies, and anti-Ro/La antibodies need to be obtained in this population [8].

Among oral agents, methotrexate is probably the most commonly prescribed medication for psoriasis (Table 23.1). The toxicities that are of greatest concern in patients treated with this drug include pulmonary fibrosis, myelosuppression, and hepatotoxicity. According to the 2009 American Academy of Dermatology (AAD) Guidelines, prior to initiation of therapy, baseline laboratory tests which need to be obtained include a complete blood count (CBC) with differential, creatinine, liver function tests (LFTs), purified protein derivative (PPD) test, and HIV tests in selected patients. Pregnancy tests must be performed in women of reproductive potential [9]. Screening for hepatitis B and C is only recommended in those patients with elevated LFTs. According to the 2012 guidelines by the National Psoriasis Foundation, patients without the risk factors for hepatotoxicity from methotrexate (history of diabetes, obesity, abnormal LFT results, excessive ethanol ingestion, chronic liver disease, family history of heritable liver disease) should not undergo a baseline liver biopsy [10]. In these patients, LFT's should be monitored monthly for the first 6 months and then every 1–3 months thereafter. For elevations of LFT's less than two-fold the upper limit of normal, LFTs need to be repeated in 2–4 weeks. For elevations more than twofold but less than threefold the upper limit of normal, clinicians should closely monitor, repeat LFTs in 2–4 weeks, and then decrease the dose as needed. Finally, for persistent elevations in five out of nine AST levels during a 12-month period or if there is a decline in the serum albumin below the normal range with normal nutritional status in a patient with well-controlled disease, a liver biopsy should be performed. Furthermore, liver biopsies should be considered after 3.5–4.0 g total cumulative dosage [9]. Ongoing laboratory monitoring in patients being treated with methotrexate includes obtaining CBC and platelets counts initially every 2–4 weeks for first few months and then every 1–3 months depending on dosage adjustments, symptoms, and previous counts. LFTs should be obtained on a monthly basis, while BUN and creatinine every 2–3 months depending on dosage adjustments, symptoms, and previous levels [9]. Finally it is important to state that the dermatology guidelines for monitoring laboratory markers during methotrexate treatment are stricter compared to the rheumatology ones, as the hepatotoxicity is greater in patients with psoriasis than in patients with rheumatoid arthritis [11].

Cyclosporine is yet another oral medication used in the treatment of psoriasis (Table 23.1). According to the American Academy of Dermatology 2009 Guidelines for treatment of psoriasis, baseline tests prior to initiation of therapy include accurate measurement of renal function (BUN and creatinine measure on two or three separate occasions), urinalysis, CBC count, magnesium, potassium, uric acid, lipids, liver enzymes, bilirubin, and pregnancy test when indicated. After starting therapy, patients should have BUN and creatinine measured every other week, along with monthly levels of CBC count, uric acid, potassium, lipids, liver enzymes, serum bilirubin, and magnesium. After 3 months of every-other-week monitoring of BUN and creatinine, the monitoring frequency can be changed to monthly. Patients who are taking greater than 3 mg/kg/d of CSA over the long term, CSA blood levels should be obtained. Ongoing monitoring should also include periodic pregnancy testing [9].

Acitretin is the third and final most common oral agent used in psoriasis patients (Table 23.1). Pretreatment laboratory studies include pregnancy testing, lipid studies to evaluate for hypertriglyceridemia and hypercholesterolemia, and liver and renal function tests. After starting therapy, patients should be monitored with every other week lipid profiles and liver enzymes. After about 8 weeks of every other week monitoring, the frequency can be changed to every 6–12 weeks [9].

Six biologics are currently FDA-approved for the treatment of psoriasis and/or psoriatic arthritis, including adalimumab, etanercept, infliximab, golimumab, secukinumab, and ustekinumab. Five biologics are currently FDA-approved for psoriasis, including etanercept, adalimumab, infliximab, secukinumab, and ustekinumab. This book chapter will primarily focus on laboratory monitoring in patients treated with psoriasis. A 2008 consensus statement from the Medical Board of the National Psoriasis Foundation addressed the appropriate monitoring of patients with psoriasis who are being treated with biologic agents (Table 23.2) [12].

Prior to starting biologic therapy, it is important to obtain a consistent set of baseline

Table 23.2 Recommended baseline laboratory studies prior to initiating therapy with biologic agents in psoriasis patients

Laboratory tests and their components	
Complete blood count	White blood cell count with a differential (WBC count with differential)
	Red blood cell count (RBC count)
	Hematocrit (Hct)
	Hemoglobin (Hbg)
	Platelet count
	Mean platelet volume (MPV)
	Mean corpuscular volume (MCV)
	Mean corpuscular hemoglobin (MCH)
	Mean corpuscular hemoglobin concentration (MCHC)
	Red cell distribution width (RDW)
Basic metabolic panel	Blood urea nitrogen (BUN)
	Carbon dioxide
	Creatinine
	Glucose
	Sodium
	Chloride
	Potassium
Liver function tests	Alkaline phosphatase
	Aspartate transaminase
	Alanine transaminase
	Albumin
	Total bilirubin
	Direct bilirubin
	Prothrombin time (PT/INR)
Hepatitis panel	Hepatitis C antibody
	Hepatitis B surface antigen
	Hepatitis B surface antibody
	Hepatitis B core antibody, IM and total
Pregnancy test	Urine pregnancy test for women of child-bearing potential
HIV test	Anti-HIV 1 and 2 immunoassay
Tuberculosis tests	PPD test and/or interferon-gamma release assays such as QuantiFERON-TB gold

Based on data from Refs. [6, 12]

laboratory studies to determine the general health of the patient as well as to detect conditions that may present as contraindications to biologic therapy (Table 23.2). TB testing is required prior to initiation and annually thereafter on all patients who will be treated with any biologics, as there are reports of tuberculosis reactivation in patients treated with this class of drug. Baseline LFT's and CBC are also recommended prior to beginning the TNF inhibitors. Thereafter, ongoing monitoring consists of a yearly PPDs, and periodic CBC and LFTs. For example, CBC can be considered every 2–6 months in patients being treated with adalimumab, etanercept, or infliximab. Chemistry screen along with liver function tests should be checked at intervals varying from 3 to 6 months in patients taking these biologic agents. The monitoring should be adjusted per each individual patient, and if a patient develops signs or symptoms of liver disease, then frequency of monitoring should be altered accordingly. As TNF inhibitors have been known to cause reactivation or worsening of hepatitis B, members of the medical board check hepatitis serologies prior to initiating biologic therapy, but usually not thereafter unless laboratory tests or signs or symptoms warrant otherwise. Data concerning the use of biologics in patients with hepatitis C virus infection is lacking, and some findings suggest that they may actually be safe to use. In patients with HCV who are concurrently receiving long-term biologic treatment, it is recommended to check for markers of hepatocellular carcinoma and regular monitoring of serum aminotransferase and HCV RNA levels [10]. Finally, while circulating antinuclear antibodies have been detected in a small proportion of patients on biologics, there are currently no recommendations to screen or monitor patients for antinuclear antibodies [12].

As stated before, psoriasis may be associated with metabolic syndrome, diabetes mellitus, hypertension, or atherosclerotic cardiovascular disease [5, 6]. Routine tests for such comorbidities in psoriasis patients include monitoring blood pressure at each office visit in patients who are 21 years old or older, checking fasting blood glucose every 3 years in patients who are 45 years old or older (earlier and more frequent if diabetes mellitus risk factors are present), and checking fasting lipids every 5 years in patients who are 20 years old or older [13–15].

While the monitoring we have just described focuses on routine clinical setting, there are also several laboratory or diagnostic tests solely used in clinical research setting. For example, a number of genetic tests or cardiometabolic or inflammatory markers can be tested during clinical trials. Previous studies have profiled hundreds of differentially expressed genes related to psoriasis, however, no unique psoriasis profile has been made available yet. Genome-wide association studies have identified multiple susceptibility loci for psoriasis, many of which contain genes involved in regulation of the immune system [16]. The psoriasis-susceptibility (PSORS1) locus within the major histocompatibility complex (MHC) on chromosome 6p21 (location of the HLA genes) is considered the major genetic determinant of psoriasis [17, 18]. Among other MHC genes that have been associated with psoriasis, HLA-Cw6 is the most important allele for susceptibility to early-onset psoriasis [18]. HLA-Cw6 also demonstrates a strong association with guttate psoriasis, while HLA-B17 may be associated with a more severe phenotype.

In a clinical research setting, many additional laboratory tests may be performed which are not typically done during a routine clinical setting. Given that psoriasis is a systemic inflammatory disease, some clinical research studies aim to obtain specific cardiometabolic markers including biomarkers for dyslipidemia (lipoprotein particle, apolipoprotein A1, HDL inflammatory index, serum cholesterol efflux capacity), biomarkers for metabolic dysfunction (adiponectin, leptin, fasting glucose and insulin), or biomarkers for systemic inflammation (high-sensitivity C-reactive protein, tumor necrosis factor- α, IL-6, IL-18, IL-12). As more research is being done in this area, perhaps some of these laboratory tests may be used in a routine clinical setting in the future.

Although psoriasis does not require any diagnostic laboratory tests, physicians need to keep in mind the variety of laboratory studies for both screening as well as ongoing monitoring of psoriasis therapies. Knowledge of the available tests is important to screen vulnerable selected populations prior to initiating psoriasis treatment, such as pregnant women or immunocompromised patients. Most importantly, familiarity with the available laboratory studies will ensure timely management of any anticipated side effects of the various psoriasis therapies.

References

1. Enamandram M, Kimball AB. Psoriasis epidemiology: the interplay of genes and the environment. J Invest Dermatol. 2013;133(2):287–9.
2. Mease PJ, et al. Comparative performance of psoriatic arthritis screening tools in patients with psoriasis in European/North American dermatology clinics. J Am Acad Dermatol. 2014;71:649–55.
3. Gottlieb A, et al. Guidelines of care for the management of psoriasis and psoriatic arthritis: Section 2. Psoriatic arthritis: overview and guidelines of care for treatment with an emphasis on the biologics. J Am Acad Dermatol. 2008;58(5):851–64.
4. Armstrong AW, et al. Infectious, oncologic, and autoimmune comorbidities of psoriasis and psoriatic

arthritis: a report from the GRAPPA 2012 annual meeting. J Rheumatol. 2013;40(8):1438–41.

5. Armstrong AW, et al. Cardiovascular comorbidities of psoriasis and psoriatic arthritis: a report from the GRAPPA 2012 annual meeting. J Rheumatol. 2013;40(8):1434–7.

6. Menter A, et al. Guidelines of care for the management of psoriasis and psoriatic arthritis: section 1. Overview of psoriasis and guidelines of care for the treatment of psoriasis with biologics. J Am Acad Dermatol. 2008;58(5):826–50.

7. Menter A, et al. Guidelines of care for the management of psoriasis and psoriatic arthritis. Section 3. Guidelines of care for the management and treatment of psoriasis with topical therapies. J Am Acad Dermatol. 2009;60(4):643–59.

8. Menter A, et al. Guidelines of care for the management of psoriasis and psoriatic arthritis: section 5. Guidelines of care for the treatment of psoriasis with phototherapy and photochemotherapy. J Am Acad Dermatol. 2010;62(1):114–35.

9. Menter A, et al. Guidelines of care for the management of psoriasis and psoriatic arthritis: section 4. Guidelines of care for the management and treatment of psoriasis with traditional systemic agents. J Am Acad Dermatol. 2009;61(3):451–85.

10. Hsu S, et al. Consensus guidelines for the management of plaque psoriasis. Arch Dermatol. 2012;148(1): 95–102.

11. Helliwell PS, Taylor WJ, Group CS. Treatment of psoriatic arthritis and rheumatoid arthritis with disease modifying drugs – comparison of drugs and adverse reactions. J Rheumatol. 2008;35(3): 472–6.

12. Lebwohl M, et al. From the Medical Board of the National Psoriasis Foundation: monitoring and vaccinations in patients treated with biologics for psoriasis. J Am Acad Dermatol. 2008;58(1): 94–105.

13. Expert Panel on Detection, E. and A. Treatment of High Blood Cholesterol in Adults. Executive summary of the third report of the National Cholesterol Education Program (NCEP) expert panel on detection, evaluation, and treatment of high blood cholesterol in adults (Adult Treatment Panel III). JAMA. 2001;285(19):2486–97.

14. Sheridan S, Pignone M, Donahue K. Screening for high blood pressure: a review of evidence for the U.S. Preventative Services Task Force. Am J Prev Med. 2003;25(2):151–158.

15. Kavanaugh A, van der Heijde D, Beutler A, et al. Patients with psoriatic arthritis who achieve minimal disease activity in response to golimumab therapy demonstrate less radiographic progression: Results through 5 years of the randomized, placebo-controlled, GO-REVEAL study. Arthritis Care Res. 2015. doi: 10.1002/acr.22576. [Epub ahead of print].

16. Stuart PE, et al. Genome-wide association analysis identifies three psoriasis susceptibility loci. Nat Genet. 2010;42(11):1000–4.

17. Trembath RC, et al. Identification of a major susceptibility locus on chromosome 6p and evidence for further disease loci revealed by a two stage genome-wide search in psoriasis. Hum Mol Genet. 1997;6(5):813–20.

18. Nair RP, et al. Sequence and haplotype analysis supports HLA-C as the psoriasis susceptibility 1 gene. Am J Hum Genet. 2006;78(5):827–51.

Laboratory Tests for Psoriatic Arthritis

24

Deepak R. Jadon and Neil John McHugh

Abstract

Laboratory testing is a key component in the management of psoriatic arthritis (PsA) patients. Baseline laboratory tests have a prognostic value, aid the assessment of a patient's general health thereby guiding treatment choices, and in the long-term help monitor disease activity, response to, and tolerability of pharmacological therapies. Laboratory testing complements the clinical suspicion of PsA raised by history, examination and imaging. Whilst there is no pathognomic diagnostic laboratory test specific to PsA, several tests help differentiate PsA from other forms of arthritis.

Keywords

Psoriatic arthritis • Rheumatoid factor • Anti-citrullinated cyclical peptide antibodies • C-reactive protein • Methotrexate • Sulfasalazine • Leflunomide • Biomarkers • Genetic testing • *HLA-B27*

Acute Phase Reactants

Acute-phase reactants, including erythrocyte sedimentation rate (ESR), C-reactive protein (CRP) and plasma viscosity (PV) are elevated in approximately 50 % of PsA cases at diagnosis

D.R. Jadon, MBBCh, MRCP (✉)
Department of Rheumatology, Royal National Hospital for Rheumatic Diseases,
Upper Borough Walls, Bath BA11RL, UK
e-mail: jadondr@yahoo.com

N.J. McHugh, MBChB, MD, FRCP, FRCPath
Pharmacy and Pharmacology, University of Bath,
Bath, UK

and during disease course. A 5-year prospective longitudinal study demonstrated that 50/87 (57 %) of consecutive new PsA clinic attendees had an elevated PV at baseline visit (median 1.74 cP), compared with 45/87 (52 %) at follow-up (median 1.76 cP) [1]. CRP was elevated (>0.01 g/l) at follow-up in 20/87 (23 %) PsA patients [1].

Acute-phase response may be determined by the age at PsA onset, according to a prospective study of 66 consecutive PsA clinic attendees in Italy (disease duration less than 1 year). This study showed that elderly-onset PsA cases (age >60 years at onset; n = 16) have higher levels of

© Springer International Publishing Switzerland 2016
A. Adebajo et al. (eds.), *Psoriatic Arthritis and Psoriasis: Pathology and Clinical Aspects*,
DOI 10.1007/978-3-319-19530-8_24

CRP than young-onset PsA cases (age ≤60 years at onset; n = 50), both at presentation (3.9 *vs.* 1.33 mg/dl, respectively; p < 0.001) and at 2-years follow-up (2.2 *vs.* 0.9 mg/dl, respectively; p < 0.001) [2]. An identical pattern was seen for ESR at presentation (64.2 *vs.* 30.5 mm/h, respectively; p < 0.001) and at 2-years follow-up (38.4 *vs.* 26.3 mm/h, respectively; p < 0.001) [2]. Further research is needed to corroborate these findings, and the classification of PsA cases as elderly- *vs.* young-onset is not routine practice.

Elevated ESR and CRP during disease course appear to be markers of poor prognosis in PsA. This was documented by a prospective 14-year longitudinal study with 6-monthly assessments of 305 PsA cases with a median disease duration at study entry of 6.9 years [3]. Patients with a high ESR (>30 mm/h) were more likely to experience peripheral radiographic progression (relative risk, RR 1.19) compared to those with a low ESR (<15 mm/h; RR 0.67). A decade later, the same group published further results from a now larger cohort of 625 PsA cases followed for up to 27 years [4]. A high ESR (>30 mm/h) at initial presentation was predictive of peripheral clinical and radiographic damage progression [4]. These findings were replicated in an independent cohort, where a significant correlation was shown between initial PV and the rate of progression of joint damage (Spearman, p < 0.01) [1]. Using the even stricter end-point of sustained minimal disease activity, a study of 344 PsA cases from the Toronto cohort (median disease duration of 6.6 years at study entry) showed that an elevated ESR (>15 mm/h for males and >20 mm/h for females) was associated with a lower probability of achieving sustained minimal disease activity (odds ratio, OR 0.55; p = 0.02) [5].

An elevated CRP has been shown to be a predictor of poor cardiovascular outcome in psoriatic disease. A study including PsA and psoriasis cases showed that CRP levels predict all-cause mortality, after adjusting for traditional risk factors [6]. Another study demonstrated that PsA may be associated with the metabolic syndrome (comprising obesity, hypertension, dyslipidaemia and insulin resistance) through shared inflammatory pathways related to high-sensitivity CRP (hsCRP) [7].

PsA patients with a high CRP may have the most to gain from anti-tumour necrosis factor-alpha (anti-TNF) therapy. A post-hoc sub-analysis of a randomised placebo-controlled trial of adalimumab for PsA, investigated risk factors for radiographic progression, defined as a change in modified total Sharp score of >0.5 units from baseline to week 24, in 144 adalimumab-treated and 152 placebo-treated PsA patients [8]. Univariate analyses of 24-week time-averaged CRP showed a strong association between elevated time-averaged CRP and radiographic progression in placebo-treated patients, but not in adalimumab-treated patients (who had negligible radiographic progression) [8]. Multivariate analysis showed that an elevated CRP at baseline is an independent risk factor for radiographic progression (for CRP ≥1.0 mg/dl: OR 3.28; p < 0.001) [8]. PsA cases with the highest CRP at baseline were at greatest risk for joint damage if untreated, and gained most radiographic benefit with adalimumab.

Plasma viscosity (Pv) has an advantage over ESR, as PV is adjusted for age and sex of the individual, as well as concomitant anaemia. Compared to traditional CRP assays, hsCRP assays are able to detect lower concentrations (<5 mg/l) of serum CRP, and hsCRP is therefore a more sensitive marker of inflammation [9]. hsCRP levels have been shown to be elevated in PsA patients compared with healthy controls [7, 10], and hsCRP levels were higher in PsA compared to psoriasis-only cases (3.47 *vs.* 2.11 mg/l, respectively; OR 2.06; p = 0.02) [10].

Haematological Parameters

Leucocytosis is reported in up to 40 % of PsA cases [11]. A normocytic normochromic anaemia of chronic disease may be observed especially during periods of prolonged active disease, and the use of non-steroidal anti-inflammatory drugs (NSAIDs) may induce a microcytic hypochromic anaemia requiring cessation of NSAIDs [11].

Serology

Rheumatoid Factor

The majority of PsA cases are rheumatoid factor (RF) negative. This helps differentiate PsA from rheumatoid arthritis (RA), especially in patients presenting with polyarticular or symmetrical joint involvement. RF appears not to be associated with phenotypes of PsA.

In a 5-year prospective longitudinal study, only 4/87 (5 %) PsA cases were RF positive [1]. A subsequent cross-sectional case–control study from the same group found a similar prevalence of RF of 11/126 (8.7 %) in PsA cases, as compared with 2/40 (5 %) age and sex-matched healthy random blood donors [12]. RF was more common in older PsA patients, which parallels the pattern seen in healthy cohorts. RF serology did not correlate with sex, phenotypes of PsA (polyarthritis, monoarthritis or spondyloarthritis), tender/swollen joint counts, peripheral radiographic erosive disease, DMARD use, or the *HLA-DRB1* shared epitope.

Univariate analyses of a cross-sectional study of 102 PsA patients demonstrated that RF-positive patients were more likely to have used a DMARD than RF-negative patients (15/19 *vs*. 50/83, respectively; p=0.04) [13]. RF was not associated with the five major subsets of PsA, swollen joint count, enthesitis, dactylitis, sex, disease duration, or acute phase response (CRP or ESR). Multivariate analyses did not show an association between RF and either radiographic erosive disease or with polyarticular joint involvement (≥10 involved joints).

Vander Cruyssen et al. demonstrated a prevalence of RF-positivity of 16/192 (8.3 %) in PsA cases [14]. Thirteen of these RF-positive patients also had anti-citrullinated cyclical peptide antibodies.

Anti-citrullinated Cyclical Peptide Antibodies

In RA, anti-citrullinated cyclical peptide antibodies (ACPA) are biomarkers of prognosis. The major antigenic determinants for these antibodies are peptides containing citrulline, a post-translationally modified amino acid, that can be detected in serum using enzyme-linked immunosorbent assay (ELISA). ACPA appears to offer similar prognostic value in PsA, but not to the magnitude seen in RA. The low prevalence of ACPA in PsA compared to RA, gives it some utility in differentiating polyarthritic PsA from RA, especially in the early stages of undifferentiated seronegative arthritis.

A case–control study demonstrated a prevalence of ACPA in PsA cases of 7/126 (5.6 %), compared with 97 % in RF-positive RA patients and 0 % in age and sex-matched random blood donor controls (the difference between PsA and controls was not statistically significant) [12]. Interestingly, ACPA serology was not consistently associated with RF serology; it was rare for both antibodies to be present. The sex and age of ACPA-positive PsA patients were no different from ACPA-negative cases. Compared to ACPA-negative cases, ACPA-positivity was associated with peripheral radiographic erosive disease (RR 1.6; p<0.05), swollen joint count (p<0.02), DMARD use (RR 1.6; p<0.05) and the *HLA-DRB1* shared epitope (p<0.005). Collectively, this implies that ACPA is a marker of poor prognosis in PsA. Compared with the ACPA-negative cases, ACPA-positive PsA cases were just as likely to exhibit features specific to PsA (osteoproliferation, distal interphalangeal joint involvement and/or sacroiliitis).

A cross-sectional study of 192 PsA cases in Belgium (mean disease duration 10 years) found a similar ACPA prevalence of 15/192 (7.8 %) [14]. However, these ACPA-positive cases were more likely to be RF-positive than ACPA-negative cases (4/15 *vs*. 0/177; p<0.001). ACPA-positive cases had a higher number of eroded joints (median 3 *vs*. 0; p=0.03), but no significant differences in swollen joint count at the date of sampling, typical peripheral radiographic features, radiographic sacroiliitis, use of DMARDs, or use of Biologicals.

Another cross-sectional study of 102 PsA patients (median disease duration 36 months; IQR 21–81 months) in Italy, found a higher prevalence of ACPA (16/102; 15.7 %), and all were of high titre (median >100 U/ml) [13]. ACPA-positivity did not associate with any of the five major subsets of PsA (8/68 with symmetric polyarthritis were ACPA positive, as were 1/8 with asymmetric polyarthritis, 2/20 with mono-oligoarthritis, 1/2 with arthritis mutilans, and 0/4 with exclusive axial or distal interphalangeal joint involvement), sex, or the occurrence during disease course of dactylitis or enthesitis. Univariate analyses showed that ACPA positive patients were more likely to have been treated with a DMARD (p=0.01), have higher number of involved joints (p<0.0001), have a higher frequency of erosive arthritis (p=0.01) and be RF-positive (p<0.01). Multivariate analyses demonstrated ACPA to be significantly associated with erosive arthritis (OR 9.8; 95 % CI 1.87–51.8; p=0.007) and polyarticular (≥10) joint involvement (OR 17.99; 95 % CI 3.6–89.2; p=0.0004).

Other Serological Tests

Other autoantibody tests have limited use in the work-up of PsA. A study of 94 biological-naïve PsA patients investigated auto-antibody profiles in cases with established disease (mean disease duration 15.3 years) [15]. Low titre (>1/40) antinuclear antibodies (ANA) were demonstrated in 47 % of PsA cases, with clinically significant titres (≥1/80) evident in 14 % of cases, compared with the reported frequency of ANA (>1/40) in the general population of approximately 30 % [16]. ANA serology status did not correlate with the arthritis pattern at assessment, age at psoriasis onset, age at arthritis onset, active joint count, clinically damaged joint count, radiographic damaged joint count, or psoriasis severity (as measured by the psoriasis area and severity index, PASI). Anti-double-stranded DNA (dsDNA) antibodies were found in 3 % of cases, 2 % had anti-Ro antibodies, and 1 % had anti-RNP antibodies. None had anti-La or anti-Smith antibodies.

ANA, dsDNA and anti-histone antibodies have some utility for detecting and monitoring drug-induced lupus due to either synthetic DMARDs or anti-TNF therapy.

Other Laboratory Tests

Given that PsA patients are more prone to the metabolic syndrome (dyslipidaemia, hypertension, insulin insensitivity, and elevated body mass index) and have an excess burden of cardiovascular disease [17], although unproven, there may be value in performing a blood lipid profile and fasted/un-fasted blood glucose at baseline, and intermittently during disease course as a primary prevention strategy.

Hyperuricemia was evident in 21 % of PsA cases in a prospective 6-year follow-up study [18] and may reflect byproducts of the excess skin cell turnover of psoriasis.

Laboratory Tests Before and During Pharmacological Interventions

Baseline Blood Tests and Monitoring During Synthetic DMARD Therapy

Commonly used disease-modifying antirheumatic drugs (DMARDs) for PsA include methotrexate, sulfasalazine and leflunomide. The British Society of Rheumatology published national guidelines for DMARD monitoring in 2008 [19], and are detailed below for these three agents (Table 24.1).

Methotrexate
Pre-treatment full blood count (FBC), urea and electrolytes (U&Es), creatinine and liver function tests (LFTs) should be performed [19].

Monitoring should include FBC, U&Es, creatinine and LFTs every 2 weeks until the dose of methotrexate and results are stable for 6 weeks [19]. Thereafter monthly testing should be performed until the dose and disease is stable for 1 year. Thereafter the monitoring may be reduced in frequency, based on clinical judgment and due consideration of risk factors for deterioration. Risk factors including age, comorbidity, renal impairment, *etc.* may justify continuation of monthly monitoring.

Whilst liver fibrosis and cirrhosis have been reported in psoriasis-only patients with normal liver enzymes [20], a liver biopsy is not

Table 24.1 Laboratory testing prior to initiation and during pharmacological intervention

Agent	Baseline tests	Monitoring tests	Frequency of monitoring	Comments
Methotrexate	FBC, U&Es, creatinine and LFTs	FBC, U&Es, creatinine, and LFTs	Two-weekly for 6 weeks Then monthly for 1 year Then one/two-monthly thereafter according to risk	Two-weekly testing for 6 weeks after dose increases. Liver biopsy in high-risk cases only. Acute phase reactant testing to monitor response to treatment.
Sulfasalazine	FBC, U&Es, creatinine and LFTs.	FBC and LFTs.	Monthly for 3 months Then three-monthly thereafter	Test 1 month after dose increases. Acute-phase reactant testing to monitor response to treatment
Leflunomide	FBC, U&Es, creatinine and LFTs	FBC and LFTs	Monthly for 6 months, and two-monthly thereafter or monthly if co-prescribed with another hepatotoxic or immunosuppressant agent	Blood pressure and weight should be checked at each monitoring visit Acute-phase reactant testing to monitor response to treatment
Anti-TNF	FBC, U&Es, creatinine, LFTs, CRP, ANA, and dsDNA TB testing HIV, HBV and HCV virology	FBC, U&Es, creatinine, LFTs and CRP	Three-monthly if on monotherapy, or in accordance with synthetic DMARD monitoring if on combination therapy	Acute phase reactant testing to monitor response to treatment

Based on data from Chakravarty et al. [19]

Anti-TNF anti-tumour necrosis factor-alpha, *DMARD* disease-modifying anti-rheumatic drug, *FBC* full blood count, *U&Es* urea and electrolytes, *CRP* C-reactive protein, *LFTs* liver function tests, *TB* tuberculosis, *HIV* human immunodeficiency virus, *HBV* hepatitis B virus, *HCV* hepatitis C virus

recommended in the absence of pre-existing liver disease [19]. The role of serum procollagen III testing in PsA is unclear, and is therefore not routinely recommended [19]. An unexplained fall in albumin in the absence of active PsA should prompt withholding of methotrexate and specialist advice should be sought [19].

As methotrexate is genotoxic, teratogenic and excreted into breast-milk, one should consider verbally counseling the patient on whether they could already be pregnant, future use of contraception, and washout before planned conception [21]. A pregnancy test may be considered for high-risk uncertain cases. Please refer to local and/or national guidelines for further recommendations.

Sulfasalazine

Pre-treatment FBC, U&Es, creatinine and LFTs should be performed [19].

Monitoring should include FBC and LFTs every 1 month for the first 3 months, and three-monthly thereafter [19]. If following the first year, dose and blood results have been stable, the frequency of monitoring can be reduced to every 6 months for the second year of treatment. After 2 years of therapy, blood monitoring can be discontinued. Consider checking FBC and LFT one month after dose increases.

Leflunomide

Pre-treatment assessment should include FBC, U&Es, creatinine and LFTs [19]. If blood pressure (BP) is >140/90 on two consecutive readings 2 weeks apart, treat hypertension before commencing leflunomide. Baseline weight assessment allows for comparison with future weights to determine if weight loss is attributable to leflunomide.

Monitoring should include FBC and LFTs every 1 month for 6 months, and two-monthly thereafter [19]. Monitoring should be continued long-term and at least once a month if co-prescribed with another immunosuppressant or potentially hepatotoxic agent. Blood pressure and weight should be checked at each monitoring visit.

As leflunomide has shown to be teratogenic and excreted into breast-milk in animal models, one should consider verbally counseling the patient on whether they could already be pregnant, future use of contraception, and washout before planned conception [21]. A pregnancy test may be considered for high-risk uncertain cases. Please refer to local and/or national guidelines for further recommendations.

Baseline Blood Tests and Monitoring During Anti-TNF Therapy

Prior to the initiation of anti-TNF therapy it is recommended to perform several baseline laboratory tests (Table 24.1). FBC and acute phase reactant aid the identification of concomitant infection. Anti-TNF therapy should not be initiated or continued in the presence of serious active infection, but can be recommended once the infection has resolved clinically [22]. Elevated acute-phase reactants help identify patients most likely to benefit from anti-TNF and serve as a reference point for response to anti-TNF. Impairment of renal function (U&Es and creatinine) indicate the patient's likely ability to excrete the anti-TNF agent, and serve as a reference in case of deterioration.

ANA, dsDNA and anti-histone antibodies have value in detecting and monitoring drug-induced lupus due to either synthetic DMARDs (*e.g.* sulfasalazine) or anti-TNF therapy. A full serology profile is therefore worthwhile considering before commencing such agents a unit as a reference when a drug reaction is suspected.

Several registry studies have shown that anti-TNF therapy is associated with an excess risk of acquiring tuberculosis (TB), especially in countries with a high prevalence of latent TB infection. A Spanish registry study demonstrated a 78 % reduction in cases of TB reactivation following the introduction of routine screening prior to anti-TNF initiation [23]. Screening guidelines are often country specific, but in the UK it is recommend that prior to starting anti-TNF therapy, all patients should be screened for mycobacterial infection in accordance with the British Thoracic Society National Guidelines [24], and active mycobacterial infection should be adequately treated before anti-TNF therapy is started [22].

Patients at risk should be screened for human immunodeficiency virus (HIV), hepatitis B virus (HBV) and hepatitis C virus (HCV) prior to anti-TNF initiation [22]. The exact tests to detect these viruses should be sought by consultation with local laboratories.

Research Laboratory Tests and Potential Future Clinical Tests

There is increasing interest and effort to identify biomarkers in PsA as they have potential significant value. Firstly, bionuclears may aid the detection of psoriasis patients with subclinical arthritis, thereby allowing intervention in the pre-clinical phase of PsA. They may identify patients with poor prognosis so they can be prioritised to early intensive therapy before the occurrence of irreversible damage; whilst patients with good prognosis can be spared the toxicity and inconvenience of intensive therapy. Thirdly, bionuclear may facilitate the monitoring of disease activity, thereby informing the clinician of progress and need to alter the regime, rather than waiting for slow endpoints *e.g.* radiographic progression. Bionuclear may facilitate the monitoring of treatment response, so that non- and partial-responders can be identified early and switched to an alternative agent. Lastly, bionuclear may predict treatment response, so that an individual's bio-profile can be used to tailor a therapeutic regime most likely to be efficacious and with minimal toxicity.

Serum-soluble Bone and Cartilage Turnover Biomarkers

A recent systematic review of the literature on serum-soluble bone and cartilage turnover biomarkers in PsA identified several potential candidates (Table 24.2) [25]. Some markers

Table 24.2 Summary of serum-soluble bone and cartilage turnover biomarker associations with PsA

Association of variable with biomarker	MMP-3	DKK-1	M-CSF	CTX-1	TRAIL	OPG	ALP	CPII:C2C	C1-2C	BMP-4	COMP	OC	RANKL
PsA	√	√	√	√	√	?√	?√						
PsA independently of psoriasis	√	√	√			?√		√					
Demographic variables							√						
Clinical variables				√					√	√			
Clinical composite indices							√			√	√	?√	
Laboratory variables			√	√	√	√						√	
Radiographic variables													√

Based on data from Jadon et al. [25]

PsA psoriatic arthritis, *MMP-3* matrix metalloproteinase-3, *DKK-1* Dickkopf-1, *M-CSF* macrophage colony-stimulating factor, *CTX-1* crosslinked telopeptide of collagen-1, *OPG* osteoprotegerin, *TRAIL* tumor necrosis factor-related apoptosis-inducing ligand, *COMP* cartilage oligomeric matrix protein, *RANKL* receptor activator of nuclear factor-κB ligand, *ALP* bone alkaline phosphatase, *OC* osteocalcin, *BMP-4* bone morphogenetic protein-4, *C1-2C* a neoepitope of type 2 cartilage degradation by collagenases, *CPII:C2C* ratio of cartilage degradation *vs.* byproduct formation

directly cause bone or cartilage metabolism by virtue of their enzymatic or cytokine properties, whilst other are byproducts of the process, thereby acting as surrogates of metabolism. The identification and monitoring of these biomarkers in PsA is complicated by the heterogeneity of PsA. Bone loss occurs in PsA: locally in the form of erosion, osteolysis and joint space narrowing; but also systemically as diminished bone mineral density [26]. Conversely, bone formation occurs in both peripheral and axial sites in the form of articular and extra-articular osteoproliferation, ankylosis and syndesmophytosis.

Matrix metalloproteinase (MMP)-3, Dickkopf (DKK)-1, macrophage colony-stimulating factor (M-CSF), crosslinked telopeptide of collagen-1, and tumor necrosis factor-related apoptosis-inducing ligand appear to be associated with PsA. Signals have been identified for an association between PsA and both osteoprotegerin (OPG) and bone alkaline phosphatase (ALP), but needs further clarification. MMP-3, DKK-1, M-CSF, the ratio of a cartilage degradation $vs.$ byproduct formation (CPII:C2C), and possibly OPG appear to be associated with PsA independently of psoriasis. A neoepitope released during collagenase-mediated degradation of type 2 cartilage (C1-2C) has shown association with both tender and swollen joint counts. Bone morphogenetic protein-4 has shown correlation with patient global assessment of disease, pain score and the Bath Ankylosing Spondylitis Disease Activity Index. The bone-related isomer of alkaline phosphatase (ALP) is associated with disease activity. M-CSF and receptor activator of nuclear factor-κB ligand (RANKL) are associated with several plain radiographic features, particularly with the van der Heijde-modified Sharp composite radiographic score, and its subdomains of joint space narrowing, erosions and osteolysis. No association has been demonstrated between RANKL, M-CSF, DKK-1, OPG and osteoproliferation, sacroiliitis, or bone mineral density.

Many studies have had a small sample size, thereby reducing the power to detect a statistically significant association. There has been much heterogeneity in study design, laboratory testing and analytical approaches. No studies have investigated biomarker associations specifically with axial PsA.

Predictors of Response to Anti-TNF Therapy

MMP-3 is one of few metabolic bone markers that has been studied as a potential predictor of anti-TNF response in PsA. In a study of 42 SpA cases (14 PsA, 28 AS), results for the entire cohort showed that anti-TNF responders had higher MMP-3 levels at baseline than non-responders (67 $vs.$ 34 mcg/l; p=0.04) [27]. Anti-TNF responders were also more likely to have higher baseline serum CRP (30 $vs.$ 8 mg/l, respectively; p<0.001) and plasma IL-6 (12 $vs.$ 2.5 ng/ml, respectively; p=0.001) levels than non-responders. CRP is far more available in clinical laboratories than are MMP-3 and IL-6.

These findings were corroborated in an independent cohort of 40 PsA cases, where baseline MMP-3 level was independently associated with responder status (OR 1.067 for each 1-unit increase; p=0.045) [28]. Baseline levels of hsCRP, cartilage oligomeric matrix protein (COMP), RANKL, OPG, TNF superfamily 14 (TNFSF14), aggrecan 846 epitope (CS-846), C-propeptide of type II collagen (CPII) and type II collagen neoepitopes.

Col2-3/4C$_{long\ mono}$ (C2C) were not associated with anti-TNF response. In addition, a reduction in MMP-3 levels with therapy increased the odds of achieving response (OR 1.213 for each 1-unit change; p=0.030). The same was seen for the reduction in COMP levels (OR 0.587, for each 100-unit increase; p=0.039), but not for hsCRP, RANKL, OPG, TNFSF14, CS-846, CPII or C2C.

A randomised placebo-controlled study of golimumab in 100 patients with active PsA tested 92 serum-based biomarkers at baseline, week 4 and week 14, alongside clinical indices [29]. MMP-3 levels at baseline did not predict response to golimumab at week 14, as measured by the American College of Rheumatology 20 % improvement (ACR20) response, 28-joint disease activity score (DAS28) or Psoriasis Area and

Severity Index 75 % improvement (PASI-75). However, the change in CRP level from baseline to week 4 did predict golimumab response at week 14, as measured by ACR20 response, but not DAS28 or PASI-75.

Interleukins

Interleukin-6 (IL-6) has been proposed as a better inflammatory marker than CRP and ESR, based upon a study of 134 PsA and 85 psoriasis-only cases [30]. Of note, plasma IL-6 was significantly higher in PsA cases with active disease plus elevated CRP/ESR, than in PsA cases with active disease plus normal CRP/ESR (p=0.001). In addition, IL-6 levels were higher in both of these PsA groups than in psoriasis-only cases (p<0.001 and p=0.002, respectively). IL-6 levels correlated with the number of arthritic joints (p<0.001; Spearman rank correlation coeficient, r_s=0.248), ESR (p<0.001; r_s=0.459), and CRP (p<0.001; r_s=0.314).

A study comparing 34 PsA cases with ten healthy controls found significantly higher serum levels of IL-6, serum interleukin-2 receptor (sIL-2R), interleukin-1 receptor agonist (IL-1ra), and interleukin-10 (IL-10) in PsA cases [31]. However, IL-6 and IL-10 levels did not correlate with skin or joint severity indices. IL-2R correlated with skin severity (PASI), but not with clinical parameters of joint severity. IL-1ra levels correlated with tender and swollen joint counts.

In a small 2-year study of 15 PsA cases, normal serum-soluble intereukin-2 (IL-2) receptor levels after 6 months of cyclosporin-A therapy had prognostic value for a good outcome, as measured by the non-development of peripheral radiographic erosions [32].

Cellular Blood Biomarkers

Circulating osteoclast precursors (OCPs) have shown signals as diagnostic and prognostic biomarkers in PsA [33]. Their utility is limited by lack of data and few hospitals having the resources to undertake the specialist cell culture. The related dendritic cell-specific transmembrane protein (DC-STAMP) has recently shown potential as an OCP biomarker in inflammatory arthritis [34, 35]. Further research is needed.

Synovial Tissue and Fluid Biomarkers

According to the confidence of the diagnosis of PsA, synovial fluid may be assessed with microscopy (including cell count and differential), Gram-stain, culture, and polarised microscopy for crystals. The synovial fluid cellular repertoire in PsA is not dissimilar to that seen in other non-infectious chronic inflammatory arthritidies: sterile with a modest increase in neutrophils (5000/mm3) and straw-coloured viscous consistency [36]. Polarised crystal microscopy is useful to differentiate mimics of PsA, such osteoarthritis with secondary calcium pyrophosphate disease and mono-/oligoarticular gout.

A study in Toronto, Canada, compared synovial fluid proteins in 10 PsA and ten early-osteoarthritis controls [37]. Of 137 differentially expressed proteins, 12 proteins (EPO, M2BP, DEFA1, H4, H2AFX, ORM1, CD5L, PFN10 C4BP, MMP3, S100A9, and CRP) were up-regulated in PsA cases compared with controls. The authors commented that further investigation is needed to determine if they are linked to PsA pathogenesis, could be used as therapeutic targets, or serve as biomarkers in PsA.

Synovial tissue biopsy is not currently performed in clinical practice, other than for research purposes. The ability to specifically test diseased tissue, rather than circulating markers in a heterogenous disease, in theory seems to offer more promise of finding a robust biomarker. Tissue specific biomarkers have certainly been instrumental in oncology with oestrogen receptors and Ca-125 [38, 39].

Urine Biomarkers

The literature is limited regarding the utility of urine biomarkers in PsA. Al-Awadhi *et al.* tested spot urine samples for type I collagen cross-linked N-telopeptides (NTx) and deoxypyridinoline (DPD) in 35 PsA patients (25 active and 10 inactive disease; median disease duration 2–4 years) and 35 healthy controls (age & sex-matched) [40]. Urine concentrations of NTx (p<0.001) and DPD (p<0.001) were significantly elevated in active (≥ 1 tender and ≥ 1 swollen joints) PsA cases compared with healthy controls, but similar in active compared with inactive PsA cases (both p>0.26). Urine NTx concentrations correlated positively with tender joint count ($r_s = 0.45$; p<0.05), duration of early morning stiffness ($r_s = 0.45$; p<0.05) and physician global assessment of disease ($r_s = 0.43$; p<0.05), but not with swollen joint count, ESR, or patient global assessment of disease activity. Urine DPD concentrations did not correlate with any of the clinical indices.

A German study tested urine pyridinoline and DPD, (markers of bone collagen I and II metabolism), in 99 PsA, 21 psoriasis-only, 154 RA cases and 80 healthy controls [41]. Urine pyridinoline and DPD levels were elevated in PsA, particularly in active PsA. Both correlated with other markers of inflammation, including ESR.

Urine biomarkers warrant further investigation in larger PsA cohorts. However, their utility in metabolic bone diseases has been limited by the need to test the first urine sample of the morning, adjustment for renal function, and potentially being more susceptible to recent diet [42]. Blood biomarkers may not be so prone to these problems.

Genetic Testing

Genetic Associations with PsA
Human leucocyte antigen (HLA)-B27 [43], HLA-Cw*06:02 [44], interleukin 12B (IL12B) [45, 46], interleukin 23 receptor (IL23R) [45, 47], interleukin 23A (IL23A) [48], late cornified envelope gene cluster [49], TRAF3IP2 [50], and TNIP1 [48] genes among others, have shown association with PsA. Unlike other gene polymorphisms, HLA-B27 [51–53] and interleukin 13 (IL13) [54] polymorphisms have shown association with

PsA, independently of psoriasis. Three haplotypes containing HLA-B*27:05 or HLA-B*39:01 were significantly increased in frequency in PsA but not psoriasis cases [53]. A similarly designed study in an independent cohort confirmed several HLA alleles to be significantly associated with PsA compared with psoriasis: HLA-B*08 (OR 1.61), HLA-B*27 (OR 5.17), HLA-B*38 (OR 1.65) and HLA-C*06 (OR 0.58) [55]. Conversely, HLA-C*06:02 is more associated with psoriasis than PsA (frequency 57.5 vs. 28.7 %; p=9.9×10^{-12}) [53].

As in ankylosing spondylitis (AS), the exact mechanism of the association between HLA antigens and PsA has not been established. HLA polymorphisms may result in altered antigen presentation to T-cells, misfolding of the HLA-molecule resulting in altered morphology, be related to altered intracellular peptide handling by aminopeptidases, or simply be in linkage disequilibrium with a pathogenic susceptibility gene at another locus. HLA-B*38:01 and HLA-B*08 may be associated with PsA susceptibility, and allotypes encoding P2 pockets that bind side chains opposite in charge from those encoded by the HLA-B*27 and HLA-B*39 molecules may exert a 'protective' role [53].

Genetic Markers of PsA Phenotypes
Brewerton et al. in 1974 first showed an association between HL-A 27(W27) and PsA (positive in 10/41 cases with peripheral arthropathy, 4/9 with sacroiliitis, and 9/10 with spondylitis) [56]. In a cross-sectional study of 70 PsA cases, 56 % of patients with isolated axial PsA were HLA-B27 positive, compared with 24 % of polyarthritic-axial PsA and 31 % with oligoarthritic-axial PsA (p=0.02) [43]. HLA-B27 positive cases tended to be younger at psoriasis onset (p=0.03) and arthritis onset (p=0.01), and were more likely to be male (p=0.002), have bilateral sacroiliitis (p=0.002), and have uveitis (p=0.03). Surprisingly, no association was demonstrated between HLA-B27 and clinical symptoms of back involvement, syndesmophytes, or functional impairment. An independent study of 282 PsA patients compared HLA-B and HLA-C sequencing data with clinical phenotype in PsA

[57]. *HLA-B*27:05:02* was positively associated with enthesitis, dactylitis and symmetric sacroiliitis (atypical for PsA). The *HLA-B*08:01:01-C*07:01:01* haplotype and its component alleles were positively associated with asymmetrical sacroiliitis (typical for PsA), joint fusion, joint deformities, and dactylitis. *HLA-C*06:02:01* was negatively associated with asymmetrical sacroiliitis. *HLA-B*44* haplotypes were associated with a lower frequency of joint fusion and dactylitis. Signals were present for osteolysis to be associated with *HLA-C*02:02:02* (OR 3.1; p = 0.02), a marker of arthritis mutilans.

Polymorphisms of the *IL23R*, *IL12B* and endoplasmic reticulum aminopeptidase-1 (*ERAP1*) genes have been tested, but not been found to be associated with radiographic axial disease in PsA [46]. Variants of the *TNF-alpha* and *TNF-beta* genes have also been investigated, but similarly did not show association with either a history of inflammatory back pain or radiographic sacroiliitis/spondylitis [58].

HLA-C*06 is associated with more penetrant psoriasis and delayed musculoskeletal phenotype (interval 10 years between skin and articular manifestations) [53]. Whereas *HLA–B* alleles (especially *HLA-B*27*) are associated with coincident skin and musculoskeletal manifestations (interval 1 year), and almost equivalent penetrance of musculoskeletal and cutarevus psoriasis [53]

Genetic Markers of PsA Severity

HLA variants appear to be markers of disease progression in PsA. Multivariate modeling of a cohort of 292 PsA cases followed for 14 years in Canada showed that *HLA-B27* in the presence of *HLA-DR7*, and *HLA-DQw3 in* the absence of *HLA-DR7*, are predictors of disease progression (defined as progression to a higher number of damaged joints) [51]. *HLA-B39* was associated with progression in early disease, whilst *HLA-B22* was associated with a lower risk of disease progression [59]. Examination of an independent cohort of 480 PsA patients in the United Kingdom indicated that PsA cases carrying both *HLA-Cw6* and *HLA-DRB1*07* haplotypes are prone to 41 % fewer damaged and (p = 0.02) and 31 % fewer

involved joints (p = 0.001) compared with those who do not carry these variants [60]. Variants of *HLA-Cw6* and *HLA-DRB1*07* were not independently associated with disease severity; a finding replicated for *HLA-Cw0602* in an independent cohort [61]. *HLA-DRB1*03*, *HLA-DRB1*04* and shared epitope alleles did not predict disease severity. *HLA-B*27:05:02-C*02:02:02*, and *HLA-B*08:01:01-C*07:01:01* have been associated with more severe disease, measured using propensity scores [57].

The presence of peripheral radiographic erosions have been associated with a polymorphism of the *IL23R* gene [46], HLA-C*01:02:01 [57], the *HLA-B*27:05:02-C*01:02:01* haplotype [57], interleukin-4 receptor (*IL4R*) I50V gene [62], *TNF-alpha gene* [58], and *TNF-beta* gene [58]. Frequencies of the *TNF-alpha* and *TNF-beta* genotypes were also significantly different (p = 0.0078 and p = 0.0486, respectively) in progressors (peripheral radiographic erosions over a median 24 months) compared with non-progressors [58]. Conversely, one study showed that patients carrying the *HLA-B27* antigen have less erosive disease than non-carriers (22 *vs.* 46 %; p = 0.05) [61].

Some authors propose that *HLA-B27* status should be obtained in psoriasis-only patients, in order to identify cases likely to develop arthritis, in whom closer monitoring would be prudent [63]. Secondly, *HLA-B27* positivity may identify asymptomatic PsA patients likely to have or develop axial disease [63].

References

1. McHugh NJ. Progression of peripheral joint disease in psoriatic arthritis: a 5-yr prospective study. Rheumatology. 2003;42(6):778–83.
2. Punzi L, Pianon M, Rossini P, Schiavon F, Gambari PF. Clinical and laboratory manifestations of elderly onset psoriatic arthritis: a comparison with younger onset disease. Ann Rheum Dis. 1999;58(4):226–9.
3. Gladman DD, Farewell VT, Nadeau C. Clinical indicators of progression in psoriatic arthritis: multivariate relative risk model. J Rheumatol. 1995;22(4): 675–9.
4. Bond SJ, Farewell VT, Schentag CT, Gladman DD. Predictors for radiological damage in psoriatic

arthritis: results from a single centre. Ann Rheum Dis. 2007;66(3):370–6.

5. Coates LC, Cook R, Lee K-A, Chandran V, Gladman DD. Frequency, predictors, and prognosis of sustained minimal disease activity in an observational psoriatic arthritis cohort. Arthritis Care Res. 2010;62(7): 970–6.

6. Poole CD, Conway P, Currie CJ. An evaluation of the association between C-reactive protein, the change in C-reactive protein over one year, and all-cause mortality in chronic immune-mediated inflammatory disease managed in UK general practice. Rheumatology (Oxford). 2009;48(1):78–82.

7. Tam LS, Tomlinson B, Chu TT, Li M, Leung YY, Kwok LW, et al. Cardiovascular risk profile of patients with psoriatic arthritis compared to controls--the role of inflammation. Rheumatology (Oxford). 2008; 47(5):718–23.

8. Gladman DD, Mease PJ, Choy EH, Ritchlin CT, Perdok RJ, Sasso EH. Risk factors for radiographic progression in psoriatic arthritis: subanalysis of the randomized controlled trial ADEPT. Arthritis Res Ther. 2010;12(3):R113.

9. Ridker PM, Morrow DA. C-reactive protein, inflammation, and coronary risk. Cardiol Clin. 2003;21(3): 315–25.

10. Chandran V, Cook RJ, Edwin J, Shen H, Pellett FJ, Shanmugarajah S, et al. Soluble biomarkers differentiate patients with psoriatic arthritis from those with psoriasis without arthritis. Rheumatology (Oxford). 2010;49(7):1399–405.

11. Gladman DD, Shuckett R, Russell ML, Thorne JC, Schachter RK. Psoriatic arthritis (PSA)--an analysis of 220 patients. Q J Med. 1987;62(238):127–41.

12. Korendowych E, Owen P, Ravindran J, Carmichael C, McHugh NJ. The clinical and genetic associations of anti-cyclic citrullinated peptide antibodies in psoriatic arthritis. Rheumatology (Oxford). 2005;44(8):1056–60.

13. Bogliolo L, Alpini C, Caporali R, Scirè CA, Moratti R, Montecucco C. Antibodies to cyclic citrullinated peptides in psoriatic arthritis. J Rheumatol. 2005;32(3):511–5.

14. Vander Cruyssen B, Hoffman IE, Zmierczak H, Van den Berghe M, Kruithof E, De Rycke L, et al. Anti-citrullinated peptide antibodies may occur in patients with psoriatic arthritis. Ann Rheum Dis. 2005;64(8):1145–9.

15. Johnson SR, Schentag CT, Gladman DD. Autoantibodies in biological agent naive patients with psoriatic arthritis. Ann Rheum Dis. 2005;64(5): 770–2.

16. Tan EM, Feltkamp TE, Smolen JS, Butcher B, Dawkins R, Fritzler MJ, et al. Range of antinuclear antibodies in "healthy" individuals. Arthritis Rheum. 1997;40(9):1601–11.

17. Ogdie A, Schwartzman S, Eder L, Maharaj AB, Zisman D, Raychaudhuri SP, et al. Comprehensive treatment of psoriatic arthritis: managing comorbidities and extraarticular manifestations. J Rheumatol. 2014;41(11):2315–22.

18. Bruce IN, Schentag C, Gladman DD. Hyperuricaemia in psoriatic arthritis does not reflect the extent of skin involvement. J Clin Rheumatol. 2000;6:6–9.

19. Chakravarty K, McDonald H, Pullar T, Taggart A, Chalmers R, Oliver S, et al. BSR/BHPR guideline for Disease-Modifying Anti-Rheumatic Drug (DMARD) therapy in consultation with the British Association of Dermatologists. Rheumatology (Oxford). 2008;47(6): 924–5.

20. Kuijpers AL, van de Kerkhof PC. Risk-benefit assessment of methotrexate in the treatment of severe psoriasis. Am J Clin Dermatol. 2000;1(1):27–39.

21. Joint Formulary Committee. British National Formulary (BNF). 69th ed. British Medical Association and the Royal Pharmaceutical Society; London, 2014.

22. Coates LC, Tillett W, Chandler D, Helliwell PS, Korendowych E, Kyle S, et al. 2012 BSR and BHPR guideline for the treatment of psoriatic arthritis with biologics. Rheumatology (Oxford). 2013;52(10): 1754–7.

23. Carmona L, Gomez-Reino JJ, Rodriguez-Valverde V, Montero D, Pascual-Gomez E, Mola EM, et al. Effectiveness of recommendations to prevent reactivation of latent tuberculosis infection in patients treated with tumor necrosis factor antagonists. Arthritis Rheum. 2005;52(6):1766–72.

24. Ormerod LP. BTS recommendations for assessing risk and for managing mycobacterium tuberculosis infection and disease in patients due to start anti-TNF-alpha treatment. Thorax. 2005;60(10):800–5.

25. Jadon DR, Nightingale AL, McHugh NJ, Lindsay MA, Korendowych E, Sengupta R. Serum soluble bone turnover biomarkers in psoriatic arthritis and psoriatic spondyloarthropathy. J Rheumatol. 2015; 42(1):21–30.

26. Frediani B, Allegri A, Falsetti P, Storri L, Bisogno S, Baldi F, et al. Bone mineral density in patients with psoriatic arthritis. J Rheumatol. 2001;28(1):138–43.

27. Pedersen SJ, Hetland ML, Sorensen IJ, Ostergaard M, Nielsen HJ, Johansen JS. Circulating levels of interleukin-6, vascular endothelial growth factor, YKL-40, matrix metalloproteinase-3, and total aggrecan in spondyloarthritis patients during 3 years of treatment with TNF(alpha) inhibitors. Clin Rheumatol. 2010; 29(11):1301–9.

28. Chandran V, Shen H, Pollock RA, Pellett FJ, Carty A, Cook RJ, et al. Soluble biomarkers associated with response to treatment with tumor necrosis factor inhibitors in psoriatic arthritis. J Rheumatol. 2013; 40(6):866–71.

29. Wagner CL, Visvanathan S, Elashoff M, McInnes IB, Mease PJ, Krueger GG, et al. Markers of inflammation and bone remodelling associated with improvement in clinical response measures in psoriatic arthritis patients treated with golimumab. Ann Rheum Dis. 2013;72(1):83–8.

30. Alenius GM, Eriksson C, Rantapää Dahlqvist S. Interleukin-6 and soluble interleukin-2 receptor alpha-markers of inflammation in patients with psoriatic arthritis? Clin Exp Rheumatol. 2009;27(1): 120–3.

31. Elkayam O, Yaron I, Shirazi I, Yaron M, Caspi D. Serum levels of IL-10, IL-6, IL-1ra, and sIL-2R in patients with psoriatic arthritis. Rheumatol Int. 2000;19(3):101–5.

32. Macchioni P, Boiardi L, Cremonesi T, Battistel B, Casadei-Maldini M, Beltrandi E, et al. The relationship between serum-soluble interleukin-2 receptor and radiological evolution in psoriatic arthritis patients treated with cyclosporin-A. Rheumatol Int. 1998;18(1):27–33.

33. Anandarajah AP, Schwarz EM, Totterman S, Monu J, Feng CY, Shao T, et al. The effect of etanercept on osteoclast precursor frequency and enhancing bone marrow oedema in patients with psoriatic arthritis. Ann Rheum Dis. 2008;67(3):296–301.

34. Chiu YG, Ritchlin CT. Characterization of DC-STAMP+ cells in human bone marrow. J Bone Marrow Res. 2013;19:1.

35. Chiu YH, Mensah KA, Schwarz EM, Ju Y, Takahata M, Feng C, et al. Regulation of human osteoclast development by dendritic cell-specific transmembrane protein (DC-STAMP). J Bone Miner Res Off J Am Soc Bone Miner Res. 2012;27(1):79–92.

36. Jadon DR, McHugh NJ. Other seronegative spondyloarthropathies. Medicine. 2014;42(5):257–61.

37. Cretu D, Prassas I, Saraon P, Batruch I, Gandhi R, Diamandis EP, et al. Identification of psoriatic arthritis mediators in synovial fluid by quantitative mass spectrometry. Clin Proteomics. 2014;11(1):27.

38. Schwab CL, English DP, Roque DM, Pasternak M, Santin AD. Past, present and future targets for immunotherapy in ovarian cancer. Immunotherapy. 2014;6(12):1279–93.

39. Girdler F, Brotherick I. The oestrogen receptors (ER alpha and ER beta) and their role in breast cancer: a review. Breast (Edinburgh, Scotland). 2000;9(4): 194–200.

40. Al-Awadhi AM, Olusi SO, Al-Zaid NS, George S, Sugathan TN. Spot urine concentrations of type I collagen cross-linked N-telopeptides and deoxypyridinoline in psoriatic arthritis. Clin Rheumatol. 1999;18(6): 450–4.

41. Hein G, Schmidt F, Barta U, Muller A. Is there a psoriatic osteopathy? – the activity of bone resorption in psoriatics is related to inflammatory joint process. Eur J Med Res. 1999;4(5):187–92.

42. Clowes JA. Effect of feeding on bone turnover markers and its impact on biological variability of measurements. Bone. 2002.

43. Queiro R, Sarasqueta C, Belzunegui J, Gonzalez C, Figueroa M, Torre-Alonso JC. Psoriatic spondyloarthropathy: a comparative study between HLA-B27 positive and HLA-B27 negative disease. Semin Arthritis Rheum. 2002;31(6):413–8.

44. Ho P, Barton A, Worthington J, Plant D, Griffiths CE, Young HS, et al. Investigating the role of the HLA-Cw*06 and HLA-DRB1 genes in susceptibility to psoriatic arthritis: comparison with psoriasis and undifferentiated inflammatory arthritis. Ann Rheum Dis. 2008;67(5):677–82.

45. Filer C, Ho P, Smith RL, Griffiths C, Young HS, Worthington J, et al. Investigation of association of the IL12B and IL23R genes with psoriatic arthritis. Arthritis Rheum. 2008;58(12):3705–9.

46. Jadon D, Tillett W, Wallis D, Cavill C, Bowes J, Waldron N, et al. Exploring ankylosing spondylitis-associated ERAP1, IL23R and IL12B gene polymorphisms in subphenotypes of psoriatic arthritis. Rheumatology (Oxford). 2013;52(2):261–6.

47. Rahman P, Inman RD, Maksymowych WP, Reeve JP, Peddle L, Gladman DD. Association of interleukin 23 receptor variants with psoriatic arthritis. J Rheumatol. 2009;36:137–40.

48. Bowes J, Orozco G, Flynn E, Ho P, Brier R, Marzo-Ortega H, et al. Confirmation of TNIP1 and IL23A as susceptibility loci for psoriatic arthritis. Ann Rheum Dis. 2011;70(9):1641–4.

49. Bowes J, Flynn E, Ho P, Aly B, Morgan AW, Marzo-Ortega H, et al. Variants in linkage disequilibrium with the late cornified envelope gene cluster deletion are associated with susceptibility to psoriatic arthritis. Ann Rheum Dis. 2010;69(12):2199–203.

50. Huffmeier U, Uebe S, Ekici AB, Bowes J, Giardina E, Korendowych E, et al. Common variants at TRAF3IP2 are associated with susceptibility to psoriatic arthritis and psoriasis. Nat Genet. 2010;42(11):996–9.

51. Gladman DD, Farewell VT. The role of HLA antigens as indicators of disease progression in psoriatic arthritis. Multivariate relative risk model. Arthritis Rheum. 1995;38(6):845–50.

52. Rahman P, Elder JT. Genetic epidemiology of psoriasis and psoriatic arthritis. Ann Rheum Dis. 2005;64 Suppl 2:ii37–9; discussion ii40–1.

53. Winchester R, Minevich G, Steshenko V, Kirby B, Kane D, Greenberg DA, et al. HLA associations reveal genetic heterogeneity in psoriatic arthritis and in the psoriasis phenotype. Arthritis Rheum. 2012;64(4):1134–44.

54. Bowes J, Eyre S, Flynn E, Ho P, Salah S, Warren RB, et al. Evidence to support IL-13 as a risk locus for psoriatic arthritis but not psoriasis vulgaris. Ann Rheum Dis. 2011;70(6):1016–9.

55. Eder L, Chandran V, Pellet F, Shanmugarajah S, Rosen CF, Bull SB, et al. Human leucocyte antigen risk alleles for psoriatic arthritis among patients with psoriasis. Ann Rheum Dis. 2012;71(1):50–5.

56. Brewerton DA, Caffrey M, Nicholls A, Walters D, James DC. HL- A27 and arthropathies associated with ulcerative colitis and psoriasis. Lancet. 1974;1(7864):956–8.

57. Haroon M, Winchester R, Giles JT, Heffernan E, FitzGerald O. Certain class I HLA alleles and haplotypes implicated in susceptibility play a role in

determining specific features of the psoriatic arthritis phenotype. Ann Rheum Dis. 2014.[epub ahead to print].

58. Balding J, Kane D, Livingstone W, Mynett-Johnson L, Bresnihan B, Smith O, et al. Cytokine gene polymorphisms: association with psoriatic arthritis susceptibility and severity. Arthritis Rheum. 2003;48(5): 1408–13.

59. Gladman DD, Farewell VT, Kopciuk KA, Cook RJ. HLA markers and progression in psoriatic arthritis. J Rheumatol. 1998;25(4):730–3.

60. Ho P, Barton A, Worthington J, Thomson W, Silman AJ, Bruce IN. HLA-Cw6 and HLA-DRB1*07 together are associated with less severe joint disease

in psoriatic arthritis. Ann Rheum Dis. 2007;66(6): 807–11.

61. Queiro-Silva R, Torre-Alonso JC, Tinturé-Eguren T, López-Lagunas I. A polyarticular onset predicts erosive and deforming disease in psoriatic arthritis. Ann Rheum Dis. 2003;62(1):68–70.

62. Rahman P, Snelgrove T, Peddle L, Siannis F, Farewell V, Schentag C, et al. A variant of the IL4I50V single-nucleotide polymorphism is associated with erosive joint disease in psoriatic arthritis. Arthritis Rheum. 2008;58(7):2207–8.

63. Gladman DD, Ritchlin C. Clinical manifestations and diagnosis of psoriatic arthritis. In: Romain PL, editor. www.UpToDate.com: UpToDate, Inc.; 2015.

Philip J. Mease

Laura C. Coates and April W. Armstrong

Abstract

Psoriatic arthritis (PsA) is a heterogeneous and multisystem disorder which requires careful collaborative management. In many cases both dermatologists and rheumatologists will be involved in the care of a patient and collaborative working between them can optimise management and patient satisfaction. Recent Group for Research and Assessment of Psoriasis and Psoriatic Arthritis (GRAPPA) treatment recommendations provide an evidence-based review of therapies in PsA across skin, nail and musculoskeletal domains of PsA as well as guidance for management of comorbidities.

Despite increasing evidence for individual therapies in PsA, research into treatment strategies is still lacking. There is mounting evidence for a benefit of early diagnosis within observational cohorts but no randomised trials of early intervention. Most physicians follow a "step-up" regime for PsA and this is supported by the EULAR treatment recommendations. Given the lack of evidence for early combination therapy and the potential toxicity of therapies it seems to be the best option at present. The Tight Control of PsA (TICOPA) study used a step up regime but compared tight control to an objective target (minimal disease activity) to standard care. This study has provided the first evidence of the benefit of treating to a pre-specified target in PsA although further research into treatment strategies are warranted. There is also some early evidence that although treatment withdrawal in PsA often leads to a flare of disease, dose reduction with biologic therapies may be possible in individuals responding well to therapy.

L.C. Coates, MBChB, MCRP, PhD
Leeds Institute of Rheumatic
and Musculoskeletal Medicine,
University of Leeds,
Leeds, UK

Leeds Musculoskeletal Biomedical Research Unit,
Leeds Teaching Hospitals NHS Trust, Chapel
Allerton Hospital, Chapeltown Road, Leeds
LS7 4SA, UK
e-mail: L.C.Coates@leeds.ac.uk

A.W. Armstrong
Department of Dermatology,
University of Colorado,
Denver, USA

© Springer International Publishing Switzerland 2016
A. Adebajo et al. (eds.), *Psoriatic Arthritis and Psoriasis: Pathology and Clinical Aspects*,
DOI 10.1007/978-3-319-19530-8_25

Keywords

Treatment • Strategy • Treatment recommendations • Collaborative working • Combined clinics • Step up DMARD • Early intervention • Treat to target • Tight control • Minimal disease activity • Treatment reduction • Treatment withdrawal

Introduction

Psoriatic arthritis is a heterogeneous condition which can manifest in many different ways. This variability between individual's disease presentation necessitates individualised treatment plans which take all aspects of the disease into account. Indeed many researchers in PsA are now using the term "psoriatic disease" to highlight the significant extra-articular manifestations.

Collaborative Working

The key to optimising medical care for these patients is an integrated approach between different clinical specialities. For most patients, the key clinical teams caring for their psoriatic disease are likely to be from dermatology and rheumatology. The benefits of interdisciplinary collaboration have been recognised in a number of international treatment recommendations including those published by EULAR in 2012 [1] and those recently updated by GRAPPA in 2015 [2]. The EULAR guidelines state that "in the presence of clinically significant skin involvement a rheumatologist and a dermatologist should collaborate in diagnosis and management" but do not make any specific recommendations about shared care for other related SpA conditions or comorbidities [1]. As these recommendations were developed principally by rheumatologists with only one dermatologist on the committee, they concentrate heavily on the articular component of the disease without specific guidance for skin disease or other comorbidities. In contrast, the specific treatment recommendations developed by GRAPPA were drafted by both rheumatologists and dermatolo-

gists and provide specific evidence based recommendations for the therapy of skin, nail and articular components of the disease. The new GRAPPA treatment recommendations also include overarching principles (Table 25.1) and highlight the need for multispeciality approaches in many patients.

With this recognition, a number of combined care clinics have been established at specialist centres to enable collaborative working particularly between dermatologists and rheumatologists. The models for these vary depending on local factors, but the aim of all of them is the same: Collaborative working to improve the outcome for individual patients. Where possible, interested physicians have set up a truly combined dermatology/rheumatology clinics where patients can attend one appointment and will be reviewed by both specialists together. This approach allows contemporaneous discussion about investigations and management of a patient's disease and optimising treatment choices to treat as many manifestations of the disease effectively with the minimum of medications. Clinics such as these have a very high rate of patient satisfaction related to management and convenience [3]. In this situation, both specialists also benefit from discussions on the recent advances in the other specialty. While these combined dermatology-rheumatology clinics represent the optimal approach to a fully integrated multi-disciplinary experience for both patients and providers, in many clinical settings, the cost or logistical challenges in the healthcare system make this particular set up hard to achieve.

Alternative models aiming to maximise collaboration within constraints of the healthcare system also exist. There are dermatology and rheumatology clinics running alongside each

Table 25.1 Overarching principles and agreement by GRAPPA members

No	Principle	Physician agreement (n = 135) (%)	Patient agreement (n = 10) (%)
1.	The ultimate goals of therapy for all patients with psoriatic arthritis (PsA) are: (a) to achieve the lowest possible level of disease activity in all domains of disease. As definitions of remission and low or minimal disease activity become accepted, these will be included in the goal; (b) to optimise functional status, improve quality of life and wellbeing, and prevent structural damage to the greatest extent possible; and (c) to avoid or minimise complications, both from untreated active disease and from therapy	92.6	80
2.	Assessment of patients with PsA requires consideration of all major disease domains, including peripheral arthritis, skin and nail involvement, enthesitis, dactylitis and axial arthritis. The impact of disease on pain, function, quality of life, and structural damage should be examined. In addition, activity in other potential related conditions should be considered, including cardiovascular disease, uveitis and inflammatory bowel disease. Multidisciplinary and multispeciality assessment and management will be most beneficial for individual patients	83.7	80
3.	Clinical assessment ideally includes patient-reported measures with a comprehensive history and physical examination, often supplemented by laboratory tests and imaging techniques (e.g. X-ray, Ultrasound, MRI). The most widely accepted metrics that have been validated for PsA should be utilized whenever possible	88.9	80
4.	A comprehensive assessment of relevant comorbidities (including but not restricted to obesity, metabolic syndrome, gout, diabetes, cardiovascular disease, liver disease, depression and anxiety) should be undertaken and documented	85.2	100
5.	Therapeutic decisions need to be individualized, and are made jointly by the patient and their doctor. Treatment should reflect patient preferences, with the patients provided with the best information and relevant options provided to them. Treatment choices may be affected by various factors, including disease activity, structural damage, comorbid conditions and previous therapies	89.6	80
6.	Ideally, patients should be reviewed promptly, offered regular evaluation by appropriate specialists, and have treatment adjusted as needed in order to achieve the goals of therapy. Early diagnosis and treatment is likely to be of benefit	89.6	80

other allowing patients to be seen in consecutive appointments on the same day. This minimises inconvenience to the patient and still allows for quick management decisions to be made with some immediate feedback from the other specialty. In other areas, this system of parallel clinics may not always manage to combine appointments for each patient on 1 day, but at least the physical and temporal location of the clinics allows for brief discussion and potential review for complex patients where input is required.

Despite best intentions from many specialists, there may be too many barriers that prevent either combined or parallel clinics, particularly where dermatologists and rheumatologists may not work in the same healthcare setting. In this case, communication still remains the key. First, knowing other local specialists with an interest in the condition provides a point of contact and a resource for the management of patients with complex disease. Specifically, it is recommended that dermatologists learn who the local or regional rheumatologists are with a special interest in psoriatic arthritis and reach out to establish a professional relationship with these rheumatologists. Second, establishing a dialogue with the local rheumatologists regarding their expectations of what constitutes proper or optimal referral from dermatologists will help dermatologists triage their referrals of psoriatic patients more efficiently. Third, both dermatologists and rheumatologists need to actively communicate with one another when making therapeutic decisions for a psoriasis patient that could impact both their skin and joints. Finally, regional educational events that involve cross-education of dermatologists and rheumatologists not only enhance learning for both specialists.

Whilst this increased collaborative working is expanding particularly in the fields of dermatology and rheumatology, it should be noted that many other specialties can be involved in the care of patients with psoriatic disease. Related comorbidities such as the metabolic syndrome and other related SpA conditions such as inflammatory bowel disease or iritis mean that other specialties such as ophthalmology, gastroenterology and cardiology can be key to a patient's care. In some settings, collaborative clinics already exist following similar models between rheumatology and gastroenterology, and between rheumatology and ophthalmology.

GRAPPA Treatment Recommendations

As mentioned above, many domains of disease are recognised within psoriatic arthritis or psoriatic disease. The Group for Assessment of Psoriasis and Psoriatic Arthritis (GRAPPA) have developed and recently updated treatment recommendations for psoriatic arthritis particularly addressing seven domains of disease: peripheral arthritis, skin disease, nail disease, enthesitis, dactylitis, axial involvement and related comorbidities.

The process for the development of these GRAPPA treatment recommendations has followed similar methodology on both occasions [2, 4]. Working groups have been convened for each of these domains. In the second iteration of the guidelines in 2013–2014, the skin and nails groups which were combined were separated as the evidence in these domains differs and a new

comorbidities group was convened to research into these related conditions. There has also been increased involvement of patients with a panel of patient research partners within GRAPPA who have contributed to the proceedings.

In both processes, first and foremost a systematic literature review has been conducted by GRAPPA members to identify all of the relevant research for therapy in the different disease domains. Each working group performed a systematic review of the relevant research and in the latest recommendations this was performed up to October 2014. The Grading of Recommendations Assessment, Development and Evaluation (GRADE) approach has been used. Each group wrote appropriate PICO (patient, intervention, control, outcome) questions to assess the evidence for each individual treatment (e.g., drug) or class of drugs within their subgroup. These were all discussed within the domain groups and GRADE recommendations for each of the therapies in each domain were developed.

Whilst this work for the evidence review was ongoing, a number of overarching principles to guide the management of patients with PsA were also developed at GRAPPA meetings. These have been presented to the membership at several meetings and been modified following member (including patient research partner member) feedback. In the final draft, six overarching principles were created and the majority of members (both healthcare professionals and patient research partners) voted to approve these principles (Table 25.1).

Following the production of the GRADE formatted recommendations for different therapies, the groups turned to developing a treatment strategy for their domain. Each group developed a flowchart to guide therapy in their area incorporating the recommended therapies from their literature review. These flowcharts are contained within the GRAPPA schema which aids to guide physician's treatment decisions in patients with PsA (Fig. 25.1). The wording around the schema was also developed during GRAPPA meetings and during teleconference calls with physician and patient research partner members. Both the summary of the GRADE recommendations and

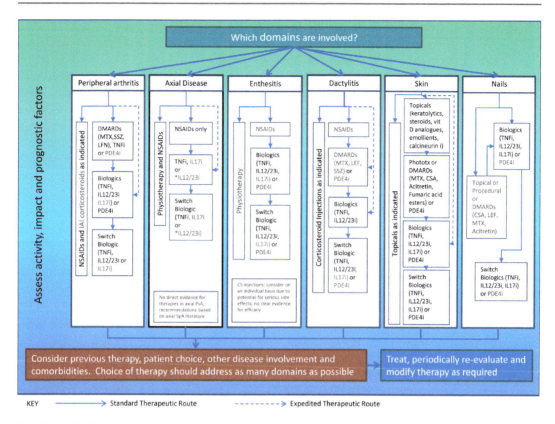

Fig. 25.1 GRAPPA treatment schema for PsA (Adapted from Coates et al. [2])

the GRAPPA schema were supported by the majority of GRAPPA members with any feedback incorporated as far as possible.

The schema highlights the important consideration of comorbidities when making a management plan. The comorbidities group developed their own summary of their GRADE recommendations for inclusion within the GRAPPA recommendations so specific advice is available for patients with comorbid or related SpA conditions.

Treatment Plans – Step Up or Step Down Therapy

The evidence for individual therapies is reviewed in the subsequent chapters (Chaps. 26, 27, 28, and 29). However in addition to establishing the efficacy and potential risk of each therapy, treating physicians ideally need research to establish how best to use these therapies. Unfortunately

the published research in this area in PsA is extremely limited.

The most common differentiation between regimes in rheumatoid arthritis (RA) is a step up vs a step down approach. In a step up approach, one therapy is started and tried initially, before moving onto combined therapies if the initial single therapy is unsuccessful. In contrast, in a step down approach, treatment is started aggressively with combination therapies and if patients achieve their goal then these can be gradually weaned down. In RA, a step down approach with initial intensive therapy has been shown to be beneficial both with combination standard DMARDs and also with early use of biologics. However there is no research in PsA that has investigated the same. The potential benefits of early combination or aggressive treatment strategies need to be examined in an RCT and the associated potential risks of these should be elucidated.

EULAR Guidelines for PsA

The EULAR guidelines for the management of PsA do use a step up approach and were approved by the expert committee consensus [1]. As stated earlier, they include five overarching principles for the management of PsA patients and ten specific recommendations on therapy of PsA with a related algorithm. They recommend initial use of single DMARDs, followed by a second DMARD either in series or in combination or an escalation to biologic therapy dependent on the presence or absence of poor prognostic markers. They performed a comprehensive literature review of therapies in PsA but the lack of evidence on different treatment strategies in PsA means that this unfortunately is not evidence based. Given the lack of evidence for early combination therapy and the potential risk of side effects from therapy, a step up approach probably remains the best option for most patients at this time. They do suggest the use of poor prognostic markers of disease to stratify treatment decisions and these are evidence-based (polyarticular disease, functional impairment, previous joint damage, previous use of corticosteroids). Unfortunately again there is no evidence that using them in a treatment strategy improves care, but currently it seems the best available way to identify those with a poor prognosis for early escalation of treatment. The final key feature of the EULAR guidelines is that they recommend treating patients to a "target" which is assessed every 3–6 months. This is stated to be remission or at least low disease activity but no guidance is given on which outcome should be used and what the cut off should be [1].

Early Intervention

There is evidence that a number of patients suffer a delay in their diagnosis of PsA and studies of cohorts in dermatology often identify undiagnosed PsA within psoriasis clinics. In recent years, observational data from a number of cohorts has shown that this delay in diagnosis, and therefore in starting therapy, has significant impact on patients' outcome. The Swedish early PsA registry looked at predictors of improved disease activity outcomes at 5 year follow up and showed that a shorter duration of symptoms prior to diagnosis was one of the significant factors [5]. In the Bath cohort, Tillett et al. identified that delay in diagnosis of over 12 months was a significant predictor of functional impairment at 10 years [6]. Haroon et al. studied 283 patients with PsA and compared many outcomes for those patients with delayed diagnosis. Patients with over 6 months of symptoms prior to a diagnosis were more likely to have erosive peripheral joint disease, arthritis mutilans, joint deformity, functional impairment and sacroiliitis and were significantly less likely to achieve a drug free remission [7].

Given this strong observational evidence, it seems likely that early intervention with therapies could improve outcome. As with most questions in therapeutic strategies in PsA, this has not been well addressed in research. There is one study addressing this question where patients with recent onset PsA were randomised to immediate treatment with methotrexate or to NSAIDs only for 3 months and then starting methotrexate. The study is small (n = 35) and open label but did not show a significant difference in outcome at 6 months. An improvement in tender and swollen joint counts was seen at 3 months in those patients taking methotrexate, but there was no significant difference in most of the outcome measures between methotrexate or NSAIDs alone at the 3 month timepoint [8]. Therefore this study does not contradict the hypothesis that early intervention can improve outcome as the therapies used (methotrexate 10 mg weekly) were not optimal for treating the disease. The only other indirect evidence of early therapy is the RESPOND trial. This study was an open label study randomising PsA patients to receive methotrexate 15 mg weekly with or without infliximab infusions. The study showed a significant difference between infliximab and methotrexate alone using the ACR20 at 16 weeks, but also showed very high responses in both arms [9]. Part of the reason for this high response rate is likely to be that the study is open label so the patients were aware that all of them were receiving therapy. Obviously one must be cautious when directly comparing these results to other methotrexate or TNF inhibitor studies but they may suggest a better outcome in early, DMARD naïve disease.

Treatment to Target

The concept of tight control or treating to target was developed in rheumatoid arthritis (RA) following studies identifying the link between inflammation and damage in this condition. The pivotal study which showed the benefit of treating to target was the Tight Control of RA (TICORA) study which showed a significant benefit after 18 months of therapy despite only using conventional DMARDs and corticosteroids. Patients in the tight control arm who continued to have a DAS >2.4 at their monthly visits had their DMARD therapy escalated and were given systemic or intra-articular steroids. At the end of the study, 82 % of tight control patients met the EULAR good response compared to 44 % of controls (p<0.0001) [10]. Other studies confirmed the benefit of treating to an objective target [11, 12] and this approach is now being used in the clinic with newly diagnosed RA patients [13].

In PsA, there is also data to support the link between inflammation and damage. Analysis of the Toronto cohort has shown that active inflamed joints predict future joint damage, both clinically [14] and radiographically [15]. Following the success in RA, the concept of treat to target developed in the spondyloarthritides (SpA). A large literature review was performed in 2011 by EULAR to identify research relevant to treat to target in SpA [16]. They were principally looking for "strategic studies that compared a therapy steered towards a prespecified treatment target versus a conventional non-steered approach". However their inclusion criteria included any study where therapy was altered based on the achievement of a pre-specified target. At the time, they identified that there were no studies in any of

Table 25.2 The minimal disease activity criteria for PsA

Patients are classified as being in MDA if they meet ≥5 of the 7 following criteria:

1	Tender joint count	≤1
2	Swollen joint count	≤1
3	Tender enthesitis points	≤1
4	PASI or	≤1
	BSA	≤3 %
5	Patient global VAS	≤20 mm
6	Patient pain VAS	≤15 mm
7	Health assessment questionnaire	≤0.5

the SpA, including PsA, that compared a treat to target to a conventional treatment approach. They did find a small number of studies where treatment was changed based on a pre-specified target, but none of the studies had a comparison. The majority of these were large RCTs of TNF inhibitors in PsA which had "early escape" arms or escalated therapy if an improvement in joint counts was not seen [16].

One of the issues raised by the EULAR literature review and subsequent recommendations on treatment to target in SpA [17] was the difficulty in identifying an appropriate target. The EULAR taskforce recommended remission as the main target for all SpA with low disease activity as an alternative target [17]. Unfortunately at that time, there were no remission criteria validated in PsA and this is still the case at present. The best validated criteria defining low disease activity/remission are the minimal disease activity criteria for PsA [18]. These criteria do not provide a disease activity score, only the definition of a low disease state (Table 25.2). They have been validated in observational cohorts showing responsiveness to change, agreement with treatment decisions and reduced progression of joint damage [19]. In RCT data they have been shown to differentiate between drug and placebo and correlate with other outcome measures. They also show association with radiographic outcome suggesting a prognostic value [20]. Proposed definitions of low disease activity have also now been developed for the new composite measures in PsA:

Table 25.3 Proposed cut offs for disease activity with new composite measures in PsA

	Low	Moderate	High
PASDAS	≤3.2	>3.2 and <5.4	≥5.4
GRACE	≤2.3	>2.3 and <4.7	≥4.7
CPDAI	≤4.0	>4.0 and <8.0	≥8.0

the PASDAS, the GRACE index and the CPDAI [21] as shown in Table 25.3 but these have not yet been validated. The other key consideration for routine clinical use is feasibility. The MDA criteria can be applied in around 5–10 min in the clinic, but the PASDAS, CPDAI and GRACE indices do take longer to do.

The TICOPA Study

Since the EULAR review and recommendations have been published, one study has been published which does fit their primary search: "strategic studies that compared a therapy steered towards a prespecified treatment target versus a conventional non-steered approach". The Tight Control of Psoriatic Arthritis (TICOPA) study recruited 206 patients with recent onset PsA. They were randomized 1:1 to tight control or standard care. Patients in the tight control arm were reviewed 4 weekly by the research rheumatologists and if they did not fulfil the MDA criteria they had their treatment escalated. The study used a treatment algorithm of methotrexate, combination DMARDs and biologics in a step up design. Patients in the standard care arm were reviewed every 12 weeks and were treated by their usual rheumatologist. There were no limitations on their care, except compliance with UK NICE criteria for the use of TNF inhibitors in PsA which was standard across both trial arms [22].

The primary outcome of the trial was ACR20 the odds of achieving ACR20 at 48 weeks were significantly higher in the tight control arm (OR 1.91, p = 0.0392) using intention to treat analysis. The odds of achieving ACR50, ACR70 and PASI75 were all significantly higher for the tight control group. Improvements were also seen in

patient reported outcomes including physical function (HAQ), quality of life (PsQOL) and also BASDAI and BASFI for those with axial disease. No difference in the radiographic progression between the two arms was detected but the mean change in modified van der Heijde-Sharp score was zero in both groups. The tight control arm was associated with increased rates of adverse events and serious adverse events which may be due to the more rapid escalation of DMARD therapy [23].

Reduction or Withdrawal of Therapy

Given the excellent responses seen in PsA with newer biological drugs and the relatively high costs of these therapies, interest has increased in recent years about whether treatments could be reduced or withdrawn in patients whose disease in under control. Cantini et al reported a high proportion of PsA patients achieving remission (just over 50 %) by un-validated but strict criteria modified from the ACR RA criteria. Medication was then suspended once patients had been in continuing remission for at least 4 months and the mean duration of remission after this treatment suspension was 12 months. This compared to a mean duration of remission of 14 months for those continuing on therapy, with no significant difference seen [24]. This encouraged development of treatment withdrawal studies, however two recent studies have shown a high rate of disease relapse with treatment withdrawal. In one study, 20 of 26 patients had disease recurrence after a mean of just 74 days [25]. In a small pilot study in the UK, 17 patients were randomised 2:1 to gradual treatment withdrawal. Six of the 11 withdrawal patients flared within the 3 month trial, with additional patients flaring beyond the follow up time of the trial [26]. In both studies, most patients were able to recapture their disease control after restarting therapies [25, 26], but these experiences caution against treatment withdrawal in PsA.

Other studies have looked at dose reductions with a greater success. A number of clinical practices have tried dose reduction and published their outcomes. In Barcelona, 153 patients on biologics for inflammatory rheumatic diseases were reviewed including 20 with PsA. Half of the PsA patients had reduced the dose of their therapy with no adverse effects [27]. In a later study, 102 PsA patients on treatment with biologics were assessed using clinical outcome measures and musculoskeletal ultrasound. One quarter were receiving tapered doses of biologics following a period of time in remission or MDA. There were no significant differences in any of the outcomes for those on full dose, or those who had reached satisfactory disease control and had their treatment doses reduced [28].

Summary

The key to managing PsA effectively is to tailor treatment to the individual patient depending on their manifestations. Patients are likely to need multidisciplinary and multispecialty care and communication within and between these teams is key to optimal management. Recent international treatment recommendations provide evidence based and expert opinion based therapy options but considerable research is required to establish optimal treatment algorithms for patients with PsA. There is evidence that treating to target using the MDA criteria can improve outcome across multiple measures in patients with recent onset PsA. In those responding well to therapy, treatment withdrawal has often caused recurrence of disease, but there is an increasing observational body of evidence for safe dose reduction after remission or low disease activity has been reached.

References

1. Gossec L, Smolen JS, Gaujoux-Viala C, et al. European league against rheumatism recommendations for the management of psoriatic arthritis with pharmacological therapies. Ann Rheum Dis. 2012; 71:4–12.
2. Coates LC, Kavanaugh A, Mease P, et al. Group for research and assessment of psoriasis and psoriatic arthritis: treatment recommendations for psoriatic arthritis 2015. Arthritis Rheum. 2015 (submitted).
3. Foulkes A, Chinoy H, Warren RB. High degree of patient satisfaction and exceptional feedback in a specialist dermatology and rheumatology clinic. Br J Dermatol. 2012;167(S1):38 (abstract).
4. Ritchlin CT, Kavanaugh A, Gladman DD, et al. Treatment recommendations for psoriatic arthritis. Ann Rheum Dis. 2009;68(9):1387–94.
5. Theander E, Husmark T, Alenius GM, et al. Early psoriatic arthritis: short symptom duration, male gender and preserved physical functioning at presentation predict favourable outcome at 5-year follow-up. Results from the Swedish Early Psoriatic Arthritis Register (SwePsA). Ann Rheum Dis. 2014;73(2): 407–13.
6. Tillett W, Jadon D, Shaddick G, et al. Smoking and delay to diagnosis are associated with poorer functional outcome in psoriatic arthritis. Ann Rheum Dis. 2013;72(8):1358–61.
7. Haroon M, Gallagher P, FitzGerald O. Diagnostic delay of more than 6 months contributes to poor radiographic and functional outcome in psoriatic arthritis. Ann Rheum Dis. 2015;74(6):1045–50.
8. Scarpa R, Peluso R, Atteno M, et al. The effectiveness of a traditional therapeutical approach in early psoriatic arthritis: results of a pilot randomised 6-month trial with methotrexate. Clin Rheumatol. 2008;27(7): 823–6.
9. Baranauskaite A, Raffayova H, Kungurov NV, et al. Infliximab plus methotrexate is superior to methotrexate alone in the treatment of psoriatic arthritis in methotrexate-naive patients: the RESPOND study. Ann Rheum Dis. 2012;71(4):541–8.
10. Grigor C, Capell H, Stirling A, et al. Effect of a treatment strategy of tight control for rheumatoid arthritis (the TICORA study): a single-blind randomised controlled trial. Lancet. 2004;364(9430):263–9.
11. Fransen J, Moens HB, Speyer I, van Riel PL. Effectiveness of systematic monitoring of rheumatoid arthritis disease activity in daily practice: a multicentre, cluster randomised controlled trial. Ann Rheum Dis. 2005;64(9):1294–8.
12. Verstappen SM, Jacobs JW, van der Veen MJ, et al. Intensive treatment with methotrexate in early rheumatoid arthritis: aiming for remission. Computer Assisted Management in Early Rheumatoid Arthritis (CAMERA, an open-label strategy trial). Ann Rheum Dis. 2007;66(11):1443–9.
13. NICE. Rheumatoid arthritis: the management of rheumatoid arthritis in adults. London: National Institute for Health and Clinical Excellence; 2009.
14. Gladman DD, Farewell VT. Progression in psoriatic arthritis: role of time varying clinical indicators. J Rheumatol. 1999;26(11):2409–13.
15. Bond SJ, Farewell VT, Schentag CT, et al. Predictors for radiological damage in psoriatic arthritis: results from a single centre. Ann Rheum Dis. 2007;66(3): 370–6.
16. Schoels MM, Braun J, Dougados M, et al. Treating axial and peripheral spondyloarthritis, including psoriatic arthritis, to target: results of a systematic

literature search to support an international treat-to-target recommendation in spondyloarthritis. Ann Rheum Dis. 2014;73(1):238–42.

17. Smolen JS, Braun J, Dougados M, et al. Treating spondyloarthritis, including ankylosing spondylitis and psoriatic arthritis, to target: recommendations of an international task force. Ann Rheum Dis. 2014;73(1):6–16.

18. Coates LC, Fransen J, Helliwell PS. Defining minimal disease activity in psoriatic arthritis: a proposed objective target for treatment. Ann Rheum Dis. 2010;69(1):48–53.

19. Coates LC, Cook R, Lee KA, Chandran V, Gladman DD. Frequency, predictors, and prognosis of sustained minimal disease activity in an observational psoriatic arthritis cohort. Arthritis Care Res (Hoboken). 2010;62(7):970–6.

20. Coates LC, Helliwell PS. Validation of minimal disease activity for psoriatic arthritis using interventional trial data. Arthritis Care Res. 2010;62(2): 965–9.

21. Helliwell PS, FitzGerald O, Fransen J. Composite disease activity and responder indices for psoriatic arthritis: a report from the GRAPPA 2013 meeting on development of cutoffs for both disease activity states and response. J Rheumatol. 2014;41(6):1212–7.

22. Coates LC, Navarro-Coy N, Brown SR, et al. The TICOPA protocol (TIght COntrol of Psoriatic Arthritis): a randomised controlled trial to compare intensive management versus standard care in early psoriatic arthritis. BMC Musculoskelet Disord. 2013;14:101.

23. Coates LC, Moverley AR, McParland L, Brown S, Navarro-Coy N, O'Dwyer JL, Meads DM, Emery P, Conaghan PG, Helliwell PS. Effect of tight control of inflammation in early psoriatic arthritis (TICOPA): a UK multicentre, open-label, randomised, controlled trial. Lancet. Online 1st Oct 2015.

24. Cantini F, Niccoli L, Nannini C, et al. Frequency and duration of clinical remission in patients with peripheral psoriatic arthritis requiring second-line drugs. Rheumatology (Oxford). 2008;47(6): 872–6.

25. Araujo EG, Finzel S, Englbrecht M, et al. High incidence of disease recurrence after discontinuation of disease-modifying antirheumatic drug treatment in patients with psoriatic arthritis in remission. Ann Rheum Dis. 2015;74(4):655–60.

26. Moverley A, Coates L, Marzo-Ortega H, et al. A feasibility study for a randomised controlled trial of treatment withdrawal in psoriatic arthritis (REmoval of treatment for patients in REmission in psoriatic ArThritis (RETREAT (F)). Clin Rheumatol. 2015.

27. Inciarte-Mundo J, Hernandez MV, Rosario V, et al. Reduction of biological agent dose in rheumatic diseases: descriptive analysis of 153 patients in clinical practice conditions. Reumatol Clin. 2014; 10(1):10–6.

28. Janta I, Martinez-Estupinan L, Valor L, et al. Comparison between full and tapered dosages of biologic therapies in psoriatic arthritis patients: clinical and ultrasound assessment. Clin Rheumatol. 2015; 34(5):935–42.

Topical and Systemic Therapies for Moderate-to-Severe Psoriasis

26

Jason E. Hawkes and Kristina Callis Duffin

Abstract

Topical therapies are the most commonly prescribed agents for psoriasis, owing to their accessibility, relative safety, and rapid onset of action. However, topical therapies, such as corticosteroids, vitamin D analogs, tazarotene, and non-steroidal immunomodulators, have significant limitations. Their use as monotherapy for the treatment of moderate-to-severe psoriasis has largely been replaced by newer, more effective systemic therapies. Nevertheless, topical medications can be highly effective when used appropriately for mild psoriasis or as adjunctive therapy for other systemic treatments. Phototherapy, one of the oldest forms of treatment, remains an important and highly efficacious treatment for psoriasis. Oral systemic medications used in the treatment of moderate-to-severe psoriasis include methotrexate, cyclosporine, and acitretin. Newer oral medications and off-label medications such as apremilast, tofacitinib, and hydroxyurea round out the list of treatments that can be used to manage challenging psoriasis patients.

Keywords

Topical therapy • Systemic therapy • Vitamin D analogs • Phototherapy • Methotrexate • Cyclosporine • Acitretin • Apremilast • Tofacitinib • Hydroxyurea

J.E. Hawkes, MD
Department of Dermatology, University of Utah, Salt Lake City, UT, USA

K.C. Duffin, MD (✉)
Department of Dermatology, University of Utah, 30 N. 1900 E. 4A330 SOM, Salt Lake City, UT 84132, USA
e-mail: Kristina.callis@hsc.utah.edu

Introduction

Prior to 2003, when the first biologic was marketed for the treatment of psoriasis, practitioners relied upon tailored regimens of topical agents, phototherapy, and systemic medications to manage cutaneous psoriasis. Topical therapies have remained the most "most commonly pre-scribed" prescribed agents for psoriasis and can be highly effective when used appropriately for mild psoriasis or as adjunctive therapy to photo-therapy and other systemic medications. Phototherapy, historically the oldest modality used for psoriasis, remains an important and highly efficacious treatment for psoriasis. The "traditional" oral agents (methotrexate, cyclo-sporine, and acitretin) are considered important in the armamentarium for psoriasis. Newer oral drugs, such as apremilast and other chemothera-peutic or immunomodulatory drugs without a formal indication in psoriasis, round out the list of treatments that can be creatively used to man-age challenging psoriasis cases.

Topical Therapies

Topical therapies are the most commonly pre-scribed agents for psoriasis, due to their accessi-bility, relative safety, and rapid onset of action. The most effective therapies include topical cor-ticosteroids, vitamin D analogs, a retinoid (taz-arotene), non-steroidal immunomodulators (tacrolimus and pimecrolimus), and combined corticosteroid-vitamin D preparations. Tar, anthralin, and keratolytics (salicylic acid and urea) have a secondary role in the treatment of psoriasis, but are rarely used as monotherapy or considered first-line agents owing to their lesser efficacy and undesirable properties. Select patients may be able to achieve or maintain ade-quate control of their psoriasis with the proper regimen of topical agents. An approach to treat-ing psoriasis is outlined in Table 26.1.

Topical therapies have significant limitations. Patients are at risk of short and long term cutane-ous and systemic side effects, particular when used continuously over large areas or in difficult-to-treat areas such as the face, body folds, geni-tals, hands, feet, and nails. Topical agents often have limited acceptability to patients due to the look and feel of the vehicle, the frequency of application, and difficulty in applying agents to sites such as the scalp or back.

Corticosteroids

Corticosteroids are the mainstay of topical thera-pies for psoriasis. At the transcriptional level, the proposed mechanism of action is primarily attrib-uted to direct or indirect alteration of transcrip-tion of proteins involved in inflammation [1]. As a result, they exert numerous cutaneous anti-inflammatory, anti-proliferative, and vasocon-strictive effects, permitting potentially rapid improvement and clearance of psoriatic lesions. Corticosteroid potency is ranked 1–7 based on the Stoughton-Cornell vasoconstrictor assays, but is influenced by many other factors including chemical structure modifications, vehicle formu-lation, concentration, hydration of the skin, loca-tion, morphology of the lesions, and method of application [2].

Class I corticosteroids are considered the most effective topical agents for plaque psoriasis on the non-intertriginous areas of the trunk, extremities, and scalp. Halobetasol propionate 0.05 % and clobetasol propionate 0.05 % oint-ments have demonstrated clearance or marked improvement in 96 % and 91 % of patients, respectively, after 4 weeks of therapy [3]. Although class I steroids in an ointment vehicle are generally felt to be more effective, they are often unacceptable to patients. Additionally, the spray preparation of clobetasol has demonstrated excellent efficacy with more than 50 % of patients considered completely clear at 4 weeks in two separate studies [4, 5].

Continuous or inappropriate use of medium to high-potency topical steroids can result in numer-ous adverse cutaneous effects. Atrophy may present as thin-appearing fragile skin, ecchymo-ses, and striae in body folds. Acneiform erup-tions including acne, periorficial dermatitis, and folliculitis can be especially are problematic on the face. Contact dermatitis, tachyphylaxis (decreasing effectiveness associated with chronic use), and steroid withdrawal causing disease flares or changes in psoriasis morphology are less common. Systemic effects of topical corticoste-roids are rarely clinically evident or important, and most are related to excessive or inappropriate use. Hypothalamic–pituitary–adrenal (HPA) axis

Table 26.1 Approach to treatment of psoriasis with topical therapies

Trunk and extremities	**Approach**
	Select appropriate vehicle, e.g. ointment, cream, lotion, foam, gel, tape
	Choose suprapotent topical CS or combined CS/Vitamin D product for initial therapy
	Application of topical product for ~2–4 weeks then use maintenance regimen
	Monitoring for clearance, compliance, and local adverse events
	May select lower potency CS (class II–V) or non-steroid class for maintenance or milder disease
	Initial regimen
	Superpotent topical corticosteroids
	Clobetasol propionate (O, C, L, F, S, Sh, G) BID
	Halobetasol propionate (O, C) BID
	Betamethasone dip. (O, C, L, S, G) BID
	Desoximetasone 0.25 % (O, C, S) BID
	Combined corticosteroid/vitamin D
	Betamethasone dip./calcipotriene (O) daily
	Maintenance regimen
	Vitamin D analogs monotherapy
	Calcipotriene (O, C) BID
	Calcitriol (O) BID
	Alternating vitamin D analog alternating and superpotent topical corticosteroid
	Calcipotriene or calcitriol BID weekdays, superpotent topical corticosteroid BID weekends only
	Calcipotriene or calcitriol BID×1 week, superpotent topical corticosteroid BID×1 week, alternating
	Combined corticosteroid/vitamin D
	Betamethasone dip./calcipotriene (O) daily as needed
	Class II–IV strength topical corticosteroids
	Fluocinonide (II)
	Betamethasone dipropionate (non-augmented) (II–IV)
	Triamcinolone acetonide BID (III–IV)
	Mometasone (O, C) (IV) BID
	Desoximetasone (II–IV)
Lichenified or localized plaques (stubborn localized lesions on trunk, extremities, hands, feet)	**Approach**
	Select superpotent topical CS and utilize under occlusion
	Combine superpotent topical CS with retinoid
	Superpotent topical corticosteroid
	Flurandrenolide tape (apply tape for 12 h)
	Topical retinoid
	Tazarotene 0.1 % gel (with/without short contact method or concomitant corticosteroid)
	Keratolytics
	Salicylic acid
	Ammonium lactate

(continued)

Table 26.1 (continued)

Scalp	**Approach**
	Select appropriate vehicle, e.g. foam, solution, suspension, spray, shampoo, gel, oil
	Choose suprapotent topical CS or combined CS/vitamin D product for initial therapy
	May select lower potency or non-steroid class for maintenance or milder disease
	Monitor for clearance, compliance, and local adverse events
	Superpotent topical corticosteroids
	Clobetasol propionate (L, F, S, Sh, G) BID
	Betamethasone dip. (L, S, G) BID
	Desoximetasone 0.25 % (S) BID
	Combined corticosteroid/vitamin D
	Betamethasone dip./calcipotriene (S, G) daily
	Lower potency topical corticosteroids
	Fluocinolone in oil (e.g. dermasmoothe scalp)
	Fluocinolone shampoo (e.g. capex)
	Betamethasone valerate foam (e.g. luxiq)
	Vitamin D analogs
	Calcipotriene (S)
	Calcitriol (S)
	Topical retinoid
	Tazarotene 0.1 % gel
	Shampoos, tar, and keratolytics (usually inadequate as monotherapy)
	Tar, salicyclic acid-containing shampoo
	Tar-based foam (Scytera)
Inverse psoriasis (intertriginous/body folds or genitals) face	**Approach**
	Choose class V–VII topical CS, vitamin D analog, or non-steroidal immunomodulator as initial therapy
	Monitor for clearance, compliance, and local adverse events
	Class V–VII topical corticosteroids
	Hydrocortisone butyrate 0.1 % (O, C, L) (V)
	Hydrocortisone valerate 0.2 % (O, C, L) (V)
	Desonide (O, C, L, F) (VI)
	Hydrocortisone hydrochloride 2.5 % (VI)
	Hydrocortisone hydrochloride 1 % (VII)
	Vitamin D analogs
	Calcipotriene (O, C)
	Calcitriol (O)
	Non-steroid immunomodulators
	Pimecrolimus 1 % C
	Tacrolimus 0.03 %, 0.1 % O

suppression can be demonstrated on laboratory testing after only 1–2 weeks of using moderate to ultrapotent corticosteroids, but is associated with continuous use over large skin areas [6].

Vitamin D Analogs

Topical vitamin D analogs, including calcipotriene, calcitriol, and tacalcitol, are commonly used agents for the treatment of psoriasis due to their safety profile and proven efficacy. Vitamin D analogs exert their effects by binding to the vitamin D receptor, but when applied locally may also impact cell growth, differentiation, and immune function without negatively impacting systemic calcium metabolism. When used as monotherapy, Vitamin D analogs have been shown in clinical trials to be equivalent in efficacy to the class II corticosteroid agent, fluocinonide 0.05 % [7].

A successful approach to treating plaque psoriasis requires choosing the correct strength, vehicle, and application frequency based on the location and severity of lesions. For the extremities, scalp, and non-intertriginous trunk, many dermatologists employ "sequential therapy", where a potent topical corticosteroid in the desired vehicle is applied to lesions twice daily to clear lesions for 2–4 weeks, then a vitamin D agent is used twice daily as maintenance with corticosteroids used only on weekends or alternating weeks [8, 9]. Alternatively, a combination corticosteroid/vitamin D preparation (e.g. betamethasone/calcipotriol) can be used once daily. Solution, spray, foam, and shampoo preparations are preferred vehicles for scalp disease. For the face and intertriginous areas, low potency (class V–VII) corticosteroids can be used safely, but treated skin should still be monitored closely for signs of atrophy. Vitamin D agents and immunomodulators, such as tacrolimus and pimecrolimus, are also efficacious in these areas. Calcitriol has been shown to be more efficacious and less irritating than calcipotriene when used on the face, axillae, and groin [10].

Tazarotene

Tazarotene is a topical retinoid that is approved in the United States and other countries for plaque psoriasis. It is a vitamin A derivative that selectively binds to the γ and β retinoic acid receptors. Tazarotene may exert its anti-psoriatic effect by decreasing dermal lymphocytes, decreasing expression of intracellular adhesion molecules, and altering keratinocyte differentiation and proliferation [11]. Although clinical trials demonstrated that 70 % of patients had "treatment success" and was equivalent to twice daily fluocinonide 0.05 %, tazarotene is limited by its cost and tendency to cause irritation, redness, and discomfort. Strategies such as the "short contact method" [12] or using tazarotene in combination with topical corticosteroids may improve the tolerability and the efficacy of treatment [12, 13]. Tazarotene is most commonly utilized on thick plaques to help reduce scaling and increase the effectiveness of topical corticosteroids and phototherapy. It is also felt to reduce the risk of steroid-induced atrophy [14]. Patients must be counseled regarding irritation and advised to not use this medication during pregnancy.

Methotrexate

Methotrexate is a dihydrofolate reductase (DHFR) inhibitor that was discovered to be effective for psoriasis in the 1950s. It is one of the most widely and commonly used systemic agents for psoriasis due to its relatively low cost, availability, and effectiveness for most forms of psoriasis and psoriatic arthritis. The mechanism of action of methotrexate in psoriasis is not fully elucidated. When ingested, methotrexate is taken up by various cell types, including erythrocytes and T cells, and undergoes polyglutamation and retention within the cell. By inhibiting DHFR, it can inhibit de novo purine and pyrimidine synthesis, which historically was believed to inhibit epidermal proliferation. When psoriasis was discovered to be a T cell-mediated disorder, it was proposed that methotrexate exerted its anti-inflammatory effects by inducing T cell apoptosis. More recent studies have demonstrated that methotrexate causes suppression of T cell activation and adhesion molecule expression, likely due to its effects on both adenosine and folic acid [15].

Methotrexate is a commonly used first-line systemic agent for patients with moderate-to-severe psoriasis. Although early trials of methotrexate monotherapy for psoriasis showed that it was highly effective, many were not placebo controlled and did not use PASI as a trial endpoint. The CHAMPION study, a placebo-controlled comparator study to the biologic agent adalimumab showed that 35.5 % of patients in the methotrexate arm achieved PASI 75 at week 16, compared to 18.9 % of placebo and 79.6 % on adalimumab [16]. However, this study was criticized for its relatively low baseline dosing, slow upward dose titration, and high placebo rates. A head-to-head trial of briakinumab and methotrexate revealed similar efficacy (PASI 75 achieved in 39.9 % on methotrexate at week 24) [17].

Methotrexate is frequently used in combination with other therapies to improve efficacy for psoriasis. When added to adalimumab, methotrexate has been shown to reduce the presence of neutralizing antibodies in rheumatoid arthritis and PsA populations, thus improving the persistence of biologic therapies. Etanercept in combination with methotrexate has been shown to be superior to etanercept monotherapy [18]. In a randomized controlled trial, 478 patients with moderate-to-severe psoriasis were given etanercept 50 mg twice weekly for 12 weeks, then randomized 1:1 to etanercept 50 mg weekly plus methotrexate (7.5–15 mg/week) or etanercept 50 mg weekly as monotherapy. In the group receiving methotrexate, 77.3 % of patients reached PASI 75 compared to 60.3 % (P < 0.0001) in the etanercept monotherapy group [18].

Methotrexate for psoriasis is typically administered orally or by subcutaneous or intramuscular injection at weekly intervals in a dose range of 7.5–30 mg/week [19]. Most guidelines recommend starting at a low dose (5–15 mg per week) and titrating up to 20–25 mg/week unless adverse effects are observed. There are differences in the guidelines regarding test dose, starting doses, and dose escalation protocols. The rationale for a test dose is to determine if a patient will have hematologic abnormalities or other adverse events within 1–2 weeks of the dose. Anecdotal reports suggest using this regimen in older patients who are at more risk for hematologic effects, presumably those with impaired renal function or pre-existing liver disease. Regardless, all patients should be monitored closely in the first few weeks.

Patients on methotrexate should be monitored for a variety of common and uncommon adverse effects, including laboratory tests for bone marrow toxicity, hepatotoxicity, and renal function abnormalities. Nausea and other gastrointestinal effects, fatigue, and malaise commonly occur within the first 24 h of taking the medication, but can be persistent. Gastrointestinal effects can sometimes be mitigated with injectable administration or oral folic acid supplementation. A 2013 Cochrane Review supports the protective effects of either folic or folinic acid for reduction of gastrointestinal side effects and transaminitis; although there was a trend toward reduction of stomatitis, the effect was not statistically significant [20]. There are conflicting data regarding the effect of folic acid on efficacy. Even though many physicians do not observe an effect on efficacy [21], a randomized placebo-controlled trial of folate supplementation with long-term methotrexate use for psoriasis showed a reduction of mean PASI score at 12 weeks compared to no effect on efficacy in the placebo group [22]. This data conflicts with other data showing that folic acid supplementation is associated with methotrexate survival [23].

Transaminitis is the most common hepatic effect and is typically asymptomatic. Long-term use of methotrexate has been associated with fibrosis and cirrhosis, particularly in patients who have additional risk factors such as alcohol consumption, diabetes, persistent transaminitis, obesity, hyperlipidemia, personal or family history of underlying liver disease, concomitant hepatotoxic drug use, and the absence of folate supplementation. Early consensus guidelines recommended that all patients undergo liver biopsy after 1–1.5 G cumulative dose [24]. However, due to the potential risks of this procedure in low risk patients, revisions based on consensus conferences have been suggested [25]. Guidelines now suggest considering a liver biopsy after a cumulative dose of 3.5–4 G in low risk individuals. If five of nine serum AST levels are elevated over the course of 12 months, or if the serum albumin level is decreased in the context of normal nutritional status and well-controlled psoriasis, a liver biopsy should be performed. Once patients have reached this dose, options include consultation with hepatology, proceeding with a liver biopsy, or discontinuing methotrexate therapy.

Other serious adverse events, such as pneumonitis, bone marrow suppression with pancytopenia, and nephritis, are uncommon but warrant close monitoring of all patients regardless of dose. Methotrexate is also highly teratogenic and is absolutely contraindicated in women of childbearing potential who are pregnant or desire pregnancy.

Cyclosporine

Cyclosporine is a highly effective, systemic agent used in the treatment of psoriasis. Discovered in 1970, this agent is most commonly used to prevent organ rejection in transplant patients [26].

By binding cyclophillin, cyclosporine inhibits intracellular calcineurin resulting in reduced T lymphocyte activity and reduced pro-inflammatory cytokines such as IL-2 and IFN-γ [27]. Cyclosporine is approved by the FDA for the treatment of psoriasis and has been shown to be effective in all subtypes of this chronic inflammatory disorder. Unlike other calcineurin inhibitors (e.g. tacrolimus and pimecrolimus), cyclosporine has no topical absorption and is available as an oral systemic therapy. Dosing of cyclosporine is usually 3–5 mg/kg/day divided in two or three doses to mitigate toxicity.

Multiple randomized clinical trials and long-term studies have demonstrated the clinical efficacy and safety of cyclosporine as a monotherapy and adjuvant therapy for other topical or systemic agents [28–31]. In a placebo double-blinded study, as many as 80 % of psoriasis patients treated with cyclosporine were assessed as "clear" or "almost clear" after 8 weeks of therapy [28]. The high-percentage (50–70 %) of patients achieving PASI 75 after 12–16 weeks of cyclosporine treatment is also documented [31]. Finally, a prospective, randomized, head-to-head, assessor-blind analysis evaluating the efficacy of cyclosporine versus methotrexate found no significant difference between the two treatment groups, though responses were observed earlier for cyclosporine [32].

Despite cyclosporine's rapid onset and clinical efficacy, its long-term use is limited by a number of important adverse effects, including nephrotoxicity. The nephrotoxicity associated with cyclosporine is dose-dependent and correlates strongly with the duration of therapy [31, 33]. Prior to the use of cyclosporine, kidney function should be determined in all patients, checked weekly during dose escalation, and monthly thereafter during treatment. In order to avoid permanent renal impairment, it is generally recommended that cyclosporine therapy not exceed 1 year [31]. Additionally, cyclosporine should be discontinued after 3–4 months in patients where no clinical improvement is observed with at least 5 mg/kg/day dosing.

Cyclosporine is also associated with hypertension and is, therefore, contraindicated in patients with vascular-related medical conditions such as stroke. Elevated blood pressure may occur in patients with or without a prior history of hypertension and is more commonly seen in elderly patients [34]. Blood pressure measurements should be taken in all patients prior to the use of cyclosporine, checked weekly during dose escalation, and monitored closely throughout the treatment period. Cyclosporine-associated hypertension should initially be managed by decreasing the treatment dose by 25–50 %. For persistent hypertension, it may be appropriate to initiate anti-hypertensive medications or make adjustments to existing medications in patients who already on treatment. Calcium channel blockers are preferred for the treatment of cyclosporine-induced hypertension [31].

Other adverse reactions associated with cyclosporine include headaches, gastrointestinal symptoms, hypertrichosis, gingival hyperplasia, hypercholesterolemia, and decreased magnesium levels. Due to its effect on the immune system, cyclosporine should not be given to immunocompromised patients or those with active infections (e.g. tuberculosis, hepatitis, or HIV). Live vaccines should also be avoided. Finally, cyclosporine is metabolized by the cytochrome P450 3A4 system, and co-administration with medications that interfere with its metabolism may increase cyclosporine levels and potentiate drug-related toxicities [31].

Cyclosporine safety has not yet been established in the pediatric and adolescent populations, but is generally considered safe when used for short periods of time for the treatment of moderate-to-severe psoriasis [31]. However, cyclosporine is considered category C for pregnancy and should be avoided in nursing females or pregnancy unless the benefits clearly outweigh the risks. The FDA has also issued a "black-box warning" for cyclosporine due to its association with lymphoma and other malignancies, particularly non-melanoma skin cancer. While there is no clear causal relationship between cyclosporine and lymphoma, the association is stronger for the increased risk of non-melanoma skin cancers [33]. The increased skin cancer risk associated with this medication is primarily in patients who are immunocompromised or have a history of 200 or more PUVA treatments [35].

In summary, cyclosporine is a highly effective, fast-acting systemic therapy approved for the treatment of moderate-to-severe psoriasis. Its use is generally well tolerated by psoriasis patients with minimal adverse effects when used for short periods of time. Unfortunately, longer treatment periods are associated with significant adverse effects, namely nephrotoxicity and hypertension. For this reason, cyclosporine in psoriasis is considered a short-term, bridging, or adjuvant therapy reserved for the treatment of acute flares, moderate-to-severe psoriasis, or refractory disease.

Phototherapy

Phototherapy is one of the oldest modalities used to treat psoriasis. Phototherapy modalities used today include narrowband ultraviolet B (NBUVB), but broadband UVB (BBUVB), targeted NBUVB with the 308 nm excimer laser, and psoralen with ultraviolet A (oral, paint, or soak PUVA). The mechanism of action of phototherapy is not completely understood but appears to have myriad effects on the immunologic pathways involved in psoriasis. UV exposure decreases expression of co-stimulatory modules and HLA-DR expression on antigen presenting cells (APCs) making them unable to effectively interact with T lymphocytes; exposure of T regulatory (Treg) cells can induce platelet activating factor, increasing interleukin-10 and TGB-beta, which also decreases co-stimulatory molecule and HLA-DR expression on APCs [36]. UV also may trigger migration of APC's from the skin to lymph nodes [36].

Psoralen, a furocoumarin found in many plants, combined with UVA therapy is a highly effective form of phototherapy for many skin diseases including psoriasis. Psoralen is an intercalating agent which, when combined with UVA radiation, leads to cross-linkage of psoralen to pyrimidine bases thereby inhibiting DNA synthesis. This, combined with UV-triggered generation of reactive oxygen species, leads to diminished epidermal proliferation and apoptosis of lymphocytes and keratinocytes with overall reductions in cytokine production and adhesion molecule expression [36].

UVB

Ultraviolet B, which includes ultraviolet rays in the 290–320 nm ranges, penetrates the skin to the level of the upper dermis. Narrowband UVB (311–314 nm) is preferred over broadband UVB as it is more efficacious with more rapid clearance and can be administered less frequently (2–3 times per week); therefore BBUVB will not be discussed here. NBUVB is considered first-line therapy after topical agents for many patients with psoriasis [37] and is particularly ideal for patients with widespread and relative thin plaques of psoriasis on the trunk and extremities.

NBUVB

The efficacy of NBUVB is well established. Two separate randomized trials comparing NBUVB to PUVA for plaque psoriasis in patients with Fitzpatrick type I–IV skin showed 63 and 65 % of patients achieved PASI 75, respectively, when used twice weekly for (x) weeks [38, 39]. Initiating treatment first requires a determination of initial dose by either using a formal minimal erythema dose (MED testing) or empirically choosing dose based upon Fitzpatrick skin type and published algorithms. [40] Typically patients will treat 2–3 times per week. Once patients clear, frequency and/or dose can be reduced. Typically, patients will enjoy a short remission with NBUVB but often require a maintenance treatment regimen of once weekly.

NBUVB has essentially no systemic adverse effects. The most common side effects include sunburn, photosensitivity, pruritus, xerosis, hyperpigmentation, risk of herpes simplex infection reactivation, and long-term photoaging. It is ideal for patients who wish to avoid or cannot safely use oral or biologic medications. Populations where NBUVB is particularly useful include children, pregnant women, patients with guttate psoriasis, and patients with HIV. NBUVB is not highly effective for patients with thick indurated plaques as the UVB cannot penetrate deeply enough and is relatively contraindicated in patients with pustular psoriasis, erythrodermic psoriasis, or a strong history of skin cancer. Contraindications also include history of intolerance to UV (i.e. worsening of psoriasis or underlying photosensitivity due to skin disorders such as lupus or polymorphous light eruption). Caution must be used if patients are taking photosensitizing medications such as thiazide diuretics or tetracycline antibiotics like doxycycline.

Patients who have more recalcitrant or more indurated plaques may require topical or systemic agents to enhance the efficacy of UV. Simple use of emollients and application of mineral oil prior to therapy is helpful. Keratolytics, with or without occlusion, such as salicylic acid, salicylic acid in liquor carbonis detergens, or coal tar can reduce psoriatic scales that scatter the light and improve UV absorption. Addition of Vitamin D analogs and topical tazarotene can increase efficacy. Addition of oral acitretin 10–25 mg daily (known as re-NBUVB or re-UVB) in appropriate patients is effective; acitretin with UVB cleared 89 % of patients compared to 23 % of patients with acitretin alone and 62.5 % with UVB alone [41, 42]. Combination of NBUVB with methotrexate and biologics also has demonstrated short-term improved efficacy over either treatment alone.

PUVA

Psoralen with UVA (PUVA) is historically one of the most effective treatments for moderate-to-severe psoriasis [43]. However, the risk of skin cancer, particularly squamous cell carcinoma with increasing cumulative dose, systemic side effects such as nausea, accessibility to biologic therapies, and the unavailability of psoralen internationally have led to reduced use of PUVA. Systemic PUVA ("photochemotherapy") is typically administered by having the patient ingest of methoxsalen (0.4 mg/kg) followed by exposure to UVA (320–400 nm) radiation approximately 1–1.5 h later, twice weekly. Patients who may benefit from PUVA include those with thick plaques, those who have failed to respond to UVB, darker skin types (Fitzpatrick III and higher) and who cannot use systemic or biologic agents.

Compared to NBUVB, systemic PUVA is highly efficacious with 84 % of patients achieving PASI 75 in (x) weeks vs. 63–65 % of patients treated with NBUVB twice weekly [38, 39]. Patients are more likely to achieve a remission at 6 months with PUVA [44] and may be able to use a maintenance regimen of one exposure every 1–4 weeks. Like NBUVB, addition of acitretin or methotrexate can improve efficacy. Topical PUVA, where methoxsalen is directly applied to the skin by either by soaking in a diluted solution or applying it in a compounded cream or lotion, is effective for patients who require localized treatment (e.g. to hands and feet) or who wish to reduce risks of systemic exposure to psoralen. Topical PUVA tends to be less efficacious and the most common adverse effect is phototoxicity.

Acitretin

Acitretin is a systemic retinoid used in the treatment of plaque, pustular, palmoplantar, and erythrodermic forms of psoriasis. Actretin is the active metabolite of the prodrug, etretinate. Although etretinate was a more efficacious drug for psoriasis [45], acitretin is less lipophilic and has a shorter half-life. Therefore, etretinate was withdrawn from the market in favor of acitretin in 1997. Acitretin binds to all three subtypes of retinoic acid receptors and has been shown to reduce stratum corneum thickness and alter cellular differentiation and inflammation of the epidermis and dermis.

Monotherapy with acitretin for plaque psoriasis is relatively slow and has limited efficacy. Early studies were small, did not use standardized efficacy endpoints [46], and examined doses that are higher than what are typically tolerated in regular practice. A 2013 study of 61 patients randomized to 25, 35, and 50 mg/day found that 47 %, 69 % and 53 % of patients achieved PASI 75 at 12 weeks, respectively [47]. In a randomized trial against etanercept or combination etanercept and acitretin, PASI 75 was achieved by 10 of 22 patients (45 %) in the etanercept 25 mg twice weekly group, 6 of 20 in the acitretin group (30 %), and 8 of 18 (44 %) in the group treated with etanercept plus acitretin [48]. This study supports the limited efficacy of acitretin monotherapy and does not provide much additional efficacy to non-phototherapy based concomitant therapies.

Phototherapy with UVB or PUVA combined with acitretin, as discussed previously, is a highly efficacious regimen for plaque and for palmoplantar plaque psoriasis [41, 42]. Acitretin can be used as monotherapy for generalized pustular psoriasis or erythrodermic psoriasis at doses of 25–50 mg/day or even higher, although combination with methotrexate or other agents like cyclosporine or biologics may be required if more rapid efficacy is required.

Acitretin, like other systemic retinoids, is highly teratogenic. It is contraindicated in women of childbearing potential who are pregnant or may become pregnant for up to 3 years after taking the medication. Pseudotumor cerebri is another rare but serious side effect most commonly seen when acitretin is used concomitantly with tetracycline antibiotics. The most common adverse effects of acitretin are mucocutaneous and musculoskeletal, with cheilitis, xerosis, skin peeling, dermatitis, xerophthalmia, and myalgia being most common. Alopecia is disturbing to patients, but is usually reversible 6–8 weeks after discontinuing the drug. Laboratory abnormalities, including primarily hyperlipidemia and transaminitis are common. Severe hypertriglyceridemia (5–8 times the normal value) is rare but can be associated with pancreatitis, thus warranting close monitoring with dietary and pharmacologic management should it occur.

Apremilast

Apremilast is a novel, oral phosphodiesterase-4 (PDE4) inhibitor with anti-inflammatory properties [49]. The anti-inflammatory effects of PDE4 inhibitors have been demonstrated in a number of chronic inflammatory conditions, including psoriasis, rheumatoid arthritis, inflammatory bowel disease, asthma, and multiple sclerosis [49]. In 2014, apremilast received approval by the FDA for the treatment or plaque psoriasis. The molecular mechanism by which this class of medication mitigates inflammation has been described elsewhere. In short, apremilast inhibits the degradation of cyclic adenosine monophosphate (cAMP), resulting in increased cAMP and subsequent protein kinase A (PKA) activity. PKA phosphorylates the transcription factor CREB, which induces the transcription of anti-inflammatory cytokines such as IL-10. Activated CREB also inhibits the transcription of pro-inflammatory cytokines such as TNF-α, IFN-γ, and IL-12/23 by competing with NF-kB p65 subunit for binding of the coactivator CREB binding protein [50]. The overall anti-inflammatory effect of apremilast have been observed in a broad range of cell types (e.g. keratinocyte, dendritic, T, and NK cells) and validated with *in vitro, in vivo*, and human studies [51, 52]. In this way, apremilast plays a central role in maintaining immune homeostasis in the skin and other tissues.

Several Phase III, multicenter, randomized, double-blind, placebo-controlled studies, including the ESTEEM trials, have demonstrated the clinical efficacy and tolerability of apremilast (30 mg twice daily) for plaque psoriasis. At week 16, the percentage of patients with moderate-to-severe plaque psoriasis achieving PASI 75 ranged from 29 to 41 % [53–55]. Early, unpublished results from the LIBERATE phase III trial comparing apremilast to etanercept were released at the 73rd American Academy of Dermatology (San Francisco, CA) and reported that PASI 75 was achieved in 40 % and 48 % of apremilast patients at 16 and 32 weeks, respectively. However, a high percentage (54–83 %) of patients experience at least one mild-to-moderate side effect during treatment [53–55]. Weight loss, nausea, vomiting, and diarrhea were the most common adverse effects reported [53–55]. These side effects are minimized when the dosing regimen is slowly ramped up to target doses. The modest clinical efficacy, common gastrointestinal side effects, and high cost make apremilast less preferable than alternative therapies approved for moderate-to-severe psoriasis.

Tofacitinib

Tofacitinib citrate is a novel, oral inhibitor of the Janus kinase (JAK) family that acts by interfering with the intracellular JAK-STAT signaling pathway. Following cytokine-mediated cell stimulation, JAK family kinases form intracytoplasmic heterodimers and phosphorylate cytokine receptors allowing for subsequent STAT binding and activation of the STAT signaling pathway [56].

The JAK-STAT signaling pathway is involved in a variety of cellular processes, including hematopoiesis and the regulation of inflammatory and immune responses [57, 58]. Tofacitinib selectively inhibits JAK1 and JAK3, thus interfering with the production of pro-inflammatory cytokines such as IL-15, IL-17, IL-22, IL-12/23, and IFN-γ [56, 57, 59].

Three phase III clinical trials evaluating tofacitinib for moderate-to-severe psoriasis support efficacy that is comparable to that of etanercept. In a combined analysis of two III placebo-controlled trials (OPT Pivotal 1 and OPT Pivotal 2), 39.9 and 46 % of patients receiving tofacitinib 5 mg BID, 59.2 and 59.6 % receiving tofacitinib 10 mg BID, and 6.2 and 11.4 % receiving placebo achieved PASI 75 at 16 weeks (all $p < 0.0001$ vs placebo) [60]. A third trial evaluating tofacitinib 5 and 10 mg BID doses, etanercept 50 mg twice weekly versus placebo demonstrated that PASI 75 was achieved in 39.5 % of the tofacitinib 5 mg group, 63.6 % of the tofacitinib 10 mg group, compared to 58.8 % of the etanercept group, meeting the non-inferiority endpoint for the higher tofacitinib dose [61].

The most common reported adverse side effects of oral tofacitinib were upper respiratory infections, nasopharyngitis, headache, and nausea. [62] A subset of patients treated with tofacitinib also developed hypercholesterolemia and serious infections, thus highlighting the need for continued investigation into the long-term risks associated with this oral immunosuppressive medication. Of note, the clinical efficacy for a topical formulation of tofacitinib has been described and may have a role in the treatment of mild plaque psoriasis [59].

Unconventional, Off-Label Therapies for Psoriasis

Tacrolimus

Tacrolimus, previously known as FK506, is a macrolide immunosuppressive medication commonly used in patients with organ transplants. Its mechanism of action is similar to that of cyclosporine described above. Tacrolimus is available as oral and topical formulations, and both have been tried in patients with psoriasis. There are limited randomized controlled trials or long-term studies looking at the use of tacrolimus in psoriasis, but its efficacy has been suggested in a number of small cohort studies [31, 63]. Specifically, one randomized controlled double-blind trial showed the efficacy of tacrolimus ointment twice daily for patients with intertriginous psoriasis or thin plaque psoriasis involving the face [31, 33, 63]. Nevertheless, studies have failed to demonstrate a clear benefit in adult patients with typical plaque psoriasis. As with cyclosporine, a patient's willingness to use topical tacrolimus may be reduced due to the FDA's "black-box warning" for its possible link to lymphoma and other malignancies, including non-melanoma skin cancers.

Hydroxyurea

Hydroxyurea is an antimetabolite medication that is primarily used in patients with myeloproliferative disorders. Its mechanism of action is due primarily to inhibition of DNA replication in rapidly dividing cells, including cells within the basal layer of the epidermis [63].

The effect of this medication on rapidly dividing cells generated interest in its potential use as a systemic therapy for psoriasis. While there are no randomized psoriasis trials for this medication, the clinical efficacy of hydroxyurea in psoriasis has been described [64]. The efficacy rates observed in these studies was highly variable and demonstrated limited benefit for hydroxyurea as a monotherapy [31, 64]. Hydroxyurea appears to be more useful as an adjuvant to other systemic therapies, such as cyclosporine, or an enhancer of phototherapy when methotrexate or acitretin are contraindicated [33]. Additionally, hydroxyurea has been shown to improve psoriasis control and reduce viral loads in HIV patients with severe, recalcitrant psoriatic disease [63, 65]. The use of hydroxyurea is most often limited by its slow onset of action (maximum benefit seen at 6–8 weeks), associated bone marrow toxicity, and undesirable gastrointestinal side effects [66].

Thioguanine

Thioguanine (6-thioguanine) is an oral purine analog used in treatment of leukemia. It is a natural metabolite of azathioprine and has an effect that is greater than its parent compound [31]. Like hydroxyurea, its primary mechanism of action is inhibition of DNA replication and cytotoxicity to rapidly dividing cells [67]. There are no randomized controlled trials for the use of thioguanine in psoriasis. Its clinical efficacy in psoriasis has been described in small cohorts, but the dosing of thioguanine was highly variable [31]. Its off-label status, lack of carefully designed psoriasis studies, and high rates (~50 %) of myelosuppression makes thioguanine a less preferable systemic therapy for psoriasis.

References

1. Norris DA. Mechanisms of action of topical therapies and the rationale for combination therapy. J Am Acad Dermatol. 2005;53:S17–25.
2. Cornell RC, Stoughton RB. Correlation of the vasoconstriction assay and clinical activity in psoriasis. Arch Dermatol. 1985;121:63–7.
3. Goldberg B, Hartdegen R, Presbury D, et al. A double-blind, multicenter comparison of 0.05 % halobetasol propionate ointment and 0.05 % clobetasol propionate ointment in patients with chronic, localized plaque psoriasis. J Am Acad Dermatol. 1991;25:1145–8.
4. Beutner K, Chakrabarty A, Lemke S, et al. An intraindividual randomized safety and efficacy comparison of clobetasol propionate 0.05 % spray and its vehicle in the treatment of plaque psoriasis. J Drugs Dermatol JDD. 2006;5:357–60.
5. Sofen H, Hudson CP, Cook-Bolden FE, et al. Clobetasol propionate 0.05 % spray for the management of moderate-to-severe plaque psoriasis of the scalp: results from a randomized controlled trial. J Drugs Dermatol JDD. 2011;10:885–92.
6. Levin E, Gupta R, Butler D, et al. Topical steroid risk analysis: differentiating between physiologic and pathologic adrenal suppression. J Dermatolog Treat. 2014;25:501–6.
7. Ashcroft DM, Po AL, Williams HC, et al. Systematic review of comparative efficacy and tolerability of calcipotriol in treating chronic plaque psoriasis. BMJ. 2000;320:963–7.
8. Brodell RT, Bruce S, Hudson CP, et al. A multi-center, open-label study to evaluate the safety and efficacy of a sequential treatment regimen of clobetasol propionate 0.05 % spray followed by Calcitriol 3 mg/g

ointment in the management of plaque psoriasis. J Drugs Dermatol JDD. 2011;10:158–64.

9. Lebwohl M, Yoles A, Lombardi K, et al. Calcipotriene ointment and halobetasol ointment in the long-term treatment of psoriasis: effects on the duration of improvement. J Am Acad Dermatol. 1998;39:447–50.

10. Ortonne JP, Humbert P, Nicolas JF, et al. Intra-individual comparison of the cutaneous safety and efficacy of calcitriol 3 microg g(−1) ointment and calcipotriol 50 microg g(−1) ointment on chronic plaque psoriasis localized in facial, hairline, retroauricular or flexural areas. Br J Dermatol. 2003;148:326–33.

11. Duvic M, Asano AT, Hager C, et al. The pathogenesis of psoriasis and the mechanism of action of tazarotene. J Am Acad Dermatol. 1998;39:S129–33.

12. Veraldi S, Caputo R, Pacifico A, et al. Short contact therapy with tazarotene in psoriasis vulgaris. Dermatology. 2006;212:235–7.

13. Lebwohl M, Poulin Y. Tazarotene in combination with topical corticosteroids. J Am Acad Dermatol. 1998;39:S139–43.

14. Lesnik RH, Mezick JA, Capetola R, et al. Topical all-trans-retinoic acid prevents corticosteroid-induced skin atrophy without abrogating the anti-inflammatory effect. J Am Acad Dermatol. 1989;21:186–90.

15. Johnston A, Gudjonsson JE, Sigmundsdottir H, et al. The anti-inflammatory action of methotrexate is not mediated by lymphocyte apoptosis, but by the suppression of activation and adhesion molecules. Clin Immunol. 2005;114:154–63.

16. Saurat JH, Stingl G, Dubertret L, et al. Efficacy and safety results from the randomized controlled comparative study of adalimumab vs. methotrexate vs. placebo in patients with psoriasis (CHAMPION). Br J Dermatol. 2008;158:558–66.

17. Reich K, Langley RG, Papp KA, et al. A 52-week trial comparing briakinumab with methotrexate in patients with psoriasis. N Engl J Med. 2011;365:1586–96.

18. Gottlieb AB, Langley RG, Strober BE, et al. A randomized, double-blind, placebo-controlled study to evaluate the addition of methotrexate to etanercept in patients with moderate to severe plaque psoriasis. Br J Dermatol. 2012;167:649–57.

19. Menting SP, Dekker PM, Limpens J, et al. Methotrexate dosing regimen for plaque-type psoriasis: a systematic review of the use of test-dose, start-dose, dosing scheme, dose adjustments, maximum dose and folic acid supplementation. Acta Derm Venereol. 2015 [Epub ahead of print].

20. Shea B, Swinden MV, Tanjong Ghogomu E, et al. Folic acid and folinic acid for reducing side effects in patients receiving methotrexate for rheumatoid arthritis. Cochrane Database Syst Rev. 2013; (5):CD000951.

21. Kirby B, Lyon CC, Griffiths CE, et al. The use of folic acid supplementation in psoriasis patients receiving methotrexate: a survey in the United Kingdom. Clin Exp Dermatol. 2000;25:265–8.

22. Salim A, Tan E, Ilchyshyn A, et al. Folic acid supplementation during treatment of psoriasis with methotrexate: a randomized, double-blind, placebo-controlled trial. Br J Dermatol. 2006;154:1169–74.

23. Shalom G, Zisman D, Harman-Boehm I, et al. Factors associated with drug survival of methotrexate and acitretin in patients with psoriasis. Acta Derm Venereol. 2015 [Epub ahead of print].

24. Roenigk Jr HH, Auerbach R, Maibach HI, et al. Methotrexate in psoriasis: revised guidelines. J Am Acad Dermatol. 1988;19:145–56.

25. Kalb RE, Strober B, Weinstein G, et al. Methotrexate and psoriasis: 2009 National Psoriasis Foundation Consensus Conference. J Am Acad Dermatol. 2009;60:824–37.

26. Mueller W, Herrmann B. Cyclosporin A for psoriasis. N Engl J Med. 1979;301:555.

27. Prens EP, van Joost T, Hegmans JP, et al. Effects of cyclosporine on cytokines and cytokine receptors in psoriasis. J Am Acad Dermatol. 1995;33:947–53.

28. Ellis CN, Fradin MS, Messana JM, et al. Cyclosporine for plaque-type psoriasis. Results of a multidose, double-blind trial. N Engl J Med. 1991;324:277–84.

29. Faerber L, Braeutigam M, Weidinger G, et al. Cyclosporine in severe psoriasis. Results of a meta-analysis in 579 patients. Am J Clin Dermatol. 2001;2:41–7.

30. Flytstrom I, Stenberg B, Svensson A, et al. Methotrexate vs. ciclosporin in psoriasis: effectiveness, quality of life and safety. A randomized controlled trial. Br J Dermatol. 2008;158:116–21.

31. Menter A, Korman NJ, Elmets CA, et al. Guidelines of care for the management of psoriasis and psoriatic arthritis: section 4. Guidelines of care for the management and treatment of psoriasis with traditional systemic agents. J Am Acad Dermatol. 2009; 61:451–85.

32. Heydendael VM, Spuls PI, Opmeer BC, et al. Methotrexate versus cyclosporine in moderate-to-severe chronic plaque psoriasis. N Engl J Med. 2003;349:658–65.

33. Lebwohl M, Menter A, Koo J, et al. Combination therapy to treat moderate to severe psoriasis. J Am Acad Dermatol. 2004;50:416–30.

34. Lowe NJ, Wieder JM, Rosenbach A, et al. Long-term low-dose cyclosporine therapy for severe psoriasis: effects on renal function and structure. J Am Acad Dermatol. 1996;35:710–9.

35. Marcil I, Stern RS. Squamous-cell cancer of the skin in patients given PUVA and ciclosporin: nested cohort crossover study. Lancet. 2001;358:1042–5.

36. Tartar D, Bhutani T, Huynh M, et al. Update on the immunological mechanism of action behind phototherapy. J Drugs Dermatol JDD. 2014;13:564–8.

37. Wan J, Abuabara K, Troxel AB, et al. Dermatologist preferences for first-line therapy of moderate to severe psoriasis in healthy adult patients. J Am Acad Dermatol. 2012;66:376–86.

38. Gordon PM, Diffey BL, Matthews JN, et al. A randomized comparison of narrow-band TL-01 phototherapy and PUVA photochemotherapy for psoriasis. J Am Acad Dermatol. 1999;41:728–32.

39. Yones SS, Palmer RA, Garibaldinos TT, et al. Randomized double-blind trial of the treatment of chronic plaque psoriasis: efficacy of psoralen-UV-A therapy vs narrowband UV-B therapy. Arch Dermatol. 2006;142:836–42.

40. Anderson KL, Feldman SR. A guide to prescribing home phototherapy for patients with psoriasis: the appropriate patient, the type of unit, the treatment regimen, and the potential obstacles. J Am Acad Dermatol. 2015;72:868–78. e1.

41. Iest J, Boer J. Combined treatment of psoriasis with acitretin and UVB phototherapy compared with acitretin alone and UVB alone. Br J Dermatol. 1989;120:665–70.

42. Tanew A, Guggenbichler A, Honigsmann H, et al. Photochemotherapy for severe psoriasis without or in combination with acitretin: a randomized, double-blind comparison study. J Am Acad Dermatol. 1991;25:682–4.

43. Stern RS. Psoralen and ultraviolet a light therapy for psoriasis. N Engl J Med. 2007;357:682–90.

44. Archier E, Devaux S, Castela E, et al. Efficacy of psoralen UV-A therapy vs. narrowband UV-B therapy in chronic plaque psoriasis: a systematic literature review. J Eur Acad Dermatol Venereol JEADV. 2012;26 Suppl 3:11–21.

45. Kragballe K, Jansen CT, Geiger JM, et al. A double-blind comparison of acitretin and etretinate in the treatment of severe psoriasis. results of a nordic multicentre study. Acta Derm Venereol. 1989;69:35–40.

46. Olsen EA, Weed WW, Meyer CJ, et al. A double-blind, placebo-controlled trial of acitretin for the treatment of psoriasis. J Am Acad Dermatol. 1989;21:681–6.

47. Dogra S, Jain A, Kanwar AJ. Efficacy and safety of acitretin in three fixed doses of 25, 35 and 50 mg in adult patients with severe plaque type psoriasis: a randomized, double blind, parallel group, dose ranging study. J Eur Acad Dermatol Venereol JEADV. 2013;27:e305–11.

48. Gisondi P, Del Giglio M, Cotena C, et al. Combining etanercept and acitretin in the therapy of chronic plaque psoriasis: a 24-week, randomized, controlled, investigator-blinded pilot trial. Br J Dermatol. 2008;158:1345–9.

49. Schafer PH, Parton A, Gandhi AK, et al. Apremilast, a cAMP phosphodiesterase-4 inhibitor, demonstrates anti-inflammatory activity in vitro and in a model of psoriasis. Br J Pharmacol. 2010;159:842–55.

50. Parry GC, Mackman N. Role of cyclic AMP response element-binding protein in cyclic AMP inhibition of NF-kappaB-mediated transcription. J Immunol (Baltimore, Md: 1950). 1997;159:5450–6.

51. Schafer PH, Day RM. Novel systemic drugs for psoriasis: mechanism of action for apremilast, a specific inhibitor of PDE4. J Am Acad Dermatol. 2013;68:1041–2.

52. Schafer PH, Parton A, Capone L, et al. Apremilast is a selective PDE4 inhibitor with regulatory effects on innate immunity. Cell Signal. 2014;26:2016–29.

53. Gottlieb AB, Matheson RT, Menter A, et al. Efficacy, tolerability, and pharmacodynamics of apremilast in recalcitrant plaque psoriasis: a phase II open-label study. J Drugs Dermatol JDD. 2013;12:888–97.

54. Papp K, Cather JC, Rosoph L, et al. Efficacy of apremilast in the treatment of moderate to severe psoriasis: a randomised controlled trial. Lancet. 2012;380:738–46.

55. Papp KA, Kaufmann R, Thaci D, et al. Efficacy and safety of apremilast in subjects with moderate to severe plaque psoriasis: results from a phase II, multicenter, randomized, double-blind, placebo-controlled, parallel-group, dose-comparison study. J Eur Acad Dermatol Venereol JEADV. 2013;27:e376–83.

56. Meyer DM, Jesson MI, Li X, et al. Anti-inflammatory activity and neutrophil reductions mediated by the JAK1/JAK3 inhibitor, CP-690,550, in rat adjuvant-induced arthritis. J Inflamm. 2010;7:41.

57. Hsu L, Armstrong AW. JAK inhibitors: treatment efficacy and safety profile in patients with psoriasis. J Immunol Res. 2014;2014:283617.

58. O'Shea JJ. Targeting the Jak/STAT pathway for immunosuppression. Ann Rheum Dis. 2004;63 Suppl 2:ii67–71.

59. Ports WC, Khan S, Lan S, et al. A randomized phase 2a efficacy and safety trial of the topical Janus kinase inhibitor tofacitinib in the treatment of chronic plaque psoriasis. Br J Dermatol. 2013;169:137–45.

60. Papp KA, Menter MA, Abe M, et al. Tofacitinib, an oral Janus kinase inhibitor, for the treatment of chronic plaque psoriasis: results from two, randomised, placebo-controlled, Phase 3 trials. Br J Dermatol. 2015 [Epub ahead of print].

61. Bachelez H, van de Kerkhof PC, Strohal R, et al. Tofacitinib versus etanercept or placebo in moderate-to-severe chronic plaque psoriasis: a phase 3 randomised non-inferiority trial. Lancet. 2015;386(9993):552–61.

62. Papp KA, Menter A, Strober B, et al. Efficacy and safety of tofacitinib, an oral Janus kinase inhibitor, in the treatment of psoriasis: a Phase 2b randomized placebo-controlled dose-ranging study. Br J Dermatol. 2012;167:668–77.

63. Halverstam CP, Lebwohl M. Nonstandard and off-label therapies for psoriasis. Clin Dermatol. 2008;26:546–53.

64. Strober BE, Siu K, Menon K. Conventional systemic agents for psoriasis. A systematic review. J Rheumatol. 2006;33:1442–6.

65. Menon K, Van Voorhees AS, Bebo Jr BF, et al. Psoriasis in patients with HIV infection: from the medical board of the National Psoriasis Foundation. J Am Acad Dermatol. 2010;62:291–9.

66. Layton AM, Sheehan-Dare RA, Goodfield MJ, et al. Hydroxyurea in the management of therapy resistant psoriasis. Br J Dermatol. 1989;121:647–53.

67. Nelson JA, Carpenter JW, Rose LM, et al. Mechanisms of action of 6-thioguanine, 6-mercaptopurine, and 8-azaguanine. Cancer Res. 1975;35:2872–8.

Oral Non-biologic Therapies and Non-pharmacological Therapies in PsA

Enrique Roberto Soriano
and María Laura Acosta Felquer

Abstract

Traditional disease-modifying antirheumatic drugs (DMARD) are the first line for the treatment of psoriatic arthritis (PsA) globally, in spite of the lack of evidence from randomized control trials. Most of the evidence comes from observational studies that will be reviewed in this chapter. Rehabilitation in rheumatology focuses on prevention of functional disorders of the musculoskeletal system, maintenance of working ability and prevention of care dependency. Rehabilitation and physical therapy is part of non-pharmacological treatment in patients with rheumatic disease. Few studies have been identified in PsA, related to this issue, and are included in this review. Finally, surgery is preferably preventable, but necessary in some cases. Evidence suggests that results of orthopedic surgery in PsA are similar to those reported in other inflammatory diseases.

Keywords

Traditional disease-modifying antirheumatic drugs • Treatment psoriatic arthritis • Psoriatic arthritis

Introduction

Traditional disease-modifying antirheumatic drugs (DMARD) are the first line for the treatment of psoriatic arthritis (PsA) globally [1, 2]. In spite of the fact that several reviews and meta-ananalyses have demonstrated lack of evidence of the efficacy of these drugs in PsA [3–6], they are still recommended as first choice for peripheral arthritis in all published guidelines and recommendations [7, 8]. There are several reasons that explain this paradox between

E.R. Soriano, MD, MSC (✉)
Department of Rheumatology, Instituto Universitario
Hospital Italiano de Buenos Aires,
Peron 4190 (1181), CABA, Buenos Aires, Argentina
e-mail: enrique.soriano@hospitalitaliano.org.ar

M.L. Acosta Felquer, MD
Rheumatology Unit, Internal Medical Service,
Hospital Italiano de Buenos Aires,
Capital Federal, Buenos Aires, Argentina

© Springer International Publishing Switzerland 2016
A. Adebajo et al. (eds.), *Psoriatic Arthritis and Psoriasis: Pathology and Clinical Aspects*,
DOI 10.1007/978-3-319-19530-8_27

evidence and clinical use, and are: the general feeling of most rheumatologists that DMARDs work, at least in some patients; their good efficacy/toxicity balance strengthened by many years of experience; their low cost and high accessibility in most countries; and the lack of evidence that a short delay in starting more effective treatments will produces a significant impact on long term outcomes such as disability and quality of life.

Traditional Disease Modifying Rheumatic Agents

Traditional DMARDs used in PsA include: methotrexate, sulfasalazine, leflunomide, and cyclosporine.

As described in several recent reviews that give support to treatment recommendations [5, 6] the evidence of effectiveness of this drugs is scarce. The major support for the use of these drugs comes from observational studies and clinical practice. Observational studies are summarized in Table 27.1.

Methotrexate (MTX)

In the last years two new randomized control trials (RCT) have been published [10, 11]. Scarpa et al. randomized patients with early oligoarthritis (less than 12 weeks' disease duration) to NSAID alone or NSAID plus MTX for 3 months; thereafter all patients continued with the combination [10]. While there was a significant improvement at 3 and 6 months compared with baseline in both groups, at 3 months patients on MTX/NSAID combination had significantly better joint count response than patients with NSAID alone. However at 6 months when both groups were taking MTX/NSAID there was no differences between groups. This study shows that in patients with early oligoarthritis MTX is better than NSAIDs, however it also shows that a short delay (3 months) in the administration of MTX was not harmful at 6 months related to symptom control. Differences on radiographic

progression could not be excluded as x-rays were not performed.

In the MIPA (Methotrexate In Psoriatic Arthritis) trial, 221 patients were randomized to MTX (target dose 15 mg/week) or placebo and outcomes assessed at 6 months with the PsA response criteria (PsARC) as the primary endpoint [11]. At 6 months, there were no significant differences in any of the individual outcomes except for patient global and physician global assessments between placebo and MTX groups [11]. The MIPA trial however has some features that should be taken into account before deriving definitive conclusions. In spite of the study's short duration, only 65 and 69 % of patients in the active and placebo groups, respectively, completed the trial, which might bias results towards a null effect; patient recruitment lasted 5 years, which might reflect some selection bias.; and in addition, approximately 35 % of the patients included had oligoarticular disease and the maximum dose of MTX was 15 mg/week and achieved by only 78 % of patients.

As previously mentioned, most of the evidence comes from observational studies [22]. In the reevaluation of the efficacy of MTX in the University of Toronto PsA registry it was found that patients in the 1994–2004 cohort received higher MTX doses (16.2 vs 10.8 mg/week) compared with the 1978–1993 cohort, and showed less radiographic progression, suggesting that higher doses might be more effective [14]. Cantini et al. reported a remission rate (using very strict remission criteria) of 19 %, and ACR 20/50/70 responses in 34 %, 23 % and 10 % respectively in 121 patients with peripheral PsA treated with MTX monotherapy [15, 23]. In another study, the same authors found a remission rate of 30 % at 6 years in patients treated with MTX [15]. In the Norwegian DMARD registry, after 6 months of MTX treatment both PsA (430) and RA (1280) patients improved in most disease activity measures and patient-reported outcomes [24]. MTX retention rates at 2 years were 65 and 66 % in PsA and RA patients respectively [24]. This study provides indirect evidence of similar efficacy and tolerance of MTX for PsA

Table 27.1 Summary of randomized control trials and observational studies, with traditional and new DMARDs

Study or first author	Type of study	Population	Intervention	Comparator	Patients (n) on active treatment/controls	Primary outcome	Outcome reached at 12 weeks	Outcome reached at 24 weeks
Willkens et al. [9]	RCT	Active (>3 SWJ) PsA DMARD naïve	MTX (7.5–15 mg)	Placebo	16/21	Swollen joint score	No	–
Scarpa et al. [10]	RCT	Active Oligoarthritis	MTX 10 mg wIM	NSAID	16/19	Swollen joint count	–	No
MIPA [11]	RCT	Active (>1 SWJ) PsA MTX naïve	MTX up to 15 mg/w	Placebo	109/112	PsARC	No	No
TOPAS [12]	RCT	Active (>3 SWJ) PsA DMARD naïve or I-R	Leflunamide 20 mg/day	Placebo	98/92	PsARC		Yes
Clegg et al. [13]	RCT	Active (>3 SWJ) PsA DMARD naïve	Sulfasalazine 2 g/day	Placebo	109/112	PsARC		Yes
Chandran [14]	OS	PsA patients treated with MTX for at least 2 years	MTX 16.2 vs 10.8 mg/week	Cohort 1978–1993	59/19	Radiographic damage		Yes
Cantini et al. [15]	OS	PsA with MTX monotherapy	MTX (NA)	Cohort RA	121	Remission		Yes
Norwegian DMARD registry	OS	PsA with MTX monotherapy	MTX 13.7 mg/week	Cohort RA	430/1218	DAS28 Remission		Yes
RESPOND study [16]	OLS	Active (>5 SWJ) PsA MTX naïve	MTX 15 mg/week	MTX + Infliximab	58/59	ACR20	Yes[a]	
PALACE 1 [17]	RCT	Active (>3 SWJ) PsA DMARDs or TNFi I-R	Apremilast 20 mg or 30 mg bid	Placebo	324/165	ACR 20	Yes[a]	–
PALACE 2 [18]	RCT	Active (>3 SWJ) PsA DMARDs or TNFi I-R	Apremilast 20 mg or 30 mg bid	Placebo	325/159	ACR20	Yes[a]	
PALACE 3 [19]	RCT	Active (>3 SWJ) PsA DMARDs or TNFi I-R	Apremilast 20 mg or 30 mg bid	Placebo	322/164	ACR20	Yes[a]	

(continued)

Table 27.1 (continued)

Study or first author	Type of study	Population	Intervention	Comparator	Patients (n) on active treatment/controls	Primary outcome	Outcome reached at 12 weeks	Outcome reached at 24 weeks
PALACE 4 [20]	RCT	Active (>3 SWJ) PsA DMARDs naïve	Apremilast 20 mg or 30 mg bid	Placebo	271/NA	ACR20	Yes[a]	
Tofacitinib [21]	RT	Active (>3 SWJ) PsA DMARDS naïve or DMARDS I-R	Tofacitinib 5 mg bid or 10 mg bid	No controls	12	ACR20	NA	NA

SWJ swollen joint count, *DMARD* disease modifying drug, *PsA* psoriatic arthritis, *MTX* metothrexate, *bid* twice daily, *w* week, *IM* intramuscular, *NA* not applicable/not available, *OS* observational study, *RCT* randomized control trial, *OLS* open label study, *RT* randomized trial, *RA* rheumatoid arthritis

[a]16 weeks

than for RA, this later disease in which MTX efficacy is well established.

In an open-label study 115 patients with mild PsA were randomized to MTX or MTX plus infliximab [16] . Although patients on combination therapy achieved significantly better response, ACR 20/50/70 responses were obtained in 67 %, 40 % and 19 % respectively in patients treated with MTX monotherapy, showing some apparent effect [16] . Recently a study in Japanese patients was published [25]. Fifty one patients with PsA treated with TNFi plus MTX, or MTX alone were retrospectively investigated. Both treatments were equally effective in achieving reduction of clinical measurements [25].

Differences in MTX toxicities have been observed between patients with rheumatoid arthritis (RA) compared to patients with psoriasis or PsA [26]. It was recently found that pulmonary toxicity was more common in RA patients compared to patients with PsA, and that hepatotoxicity was more common in PsA patients [2]. A meta-analysis of long-term MTX treatment studies in RA and psoriatic disease showed a threefold greater risk of hepatic fibrosis in patients with psoriatic disease [27]. The reasons for such differences are unclear, but there may be justification for different toxicity monitoring for patients with psoriatic disease [26]. At the 2007 GRAPPA meeting the following statements were agreed related to MTX toxicity [26]: Insufficient data exist to recommend or not recommend serial liver biopsies, but presence of other risk factors may help guide decision-making. Although there are insufficient data upon which to base a recommendation, in practice small amounts of alcohol are probably safe; 3 months off treatment, prior to conception for both female and male partner is appropriate; the combination of MTX with sulfasalazine or with an anti-TNF agent is safe. Much less consensus existed regarding the combination of MTX with leflunomide or with cyclosporine [26].

Leflunomide

Leflunomide was significantly superior to placebo in a 24 week RCT on 186 patients with improvements in PsARC, tender and swollen joint scores, HAQ and Dermatology Life Quality Index [12]. More recently the results of a multi-national observational study in 440 patients with active PsA treated with leflunomide were reported [28]. At 24 weeks 86 % of patients achieved a PsARC response with significant improvements also seen in tender and swollen joint count, patient and physician global assessments, fatigue, skin disease, dactylitis and nail lesions [28]. Of 85 patients followed at the University of Toronto PsA Clinic who received leflunomide (43 patients) alone or in combination with methotrexate (42 patients) 55 patients continued the drug, and 38 %, 48 % and 56 % achieved a $\geq$40 % reduction of actively inflamed joint count at 3, 6 and 12 months, respectively [29]. Patients taking MTX in combination with leflunomide were more likely to achieve a PASI50 response than patients taking leflunomide alone [29].

Related to tolerability and safety, withdrawal due to toxicity was almost four times more frequent with leflunomide than with placebo in a published meta-analysis [4]. In the European study, 13 % of patients experienced adverse events, (ARD) being the more frequent ones: diarrhea (16.3 % of all ADR), alopecia (9.2 %), hypertension (8.2), and pruritus (5.1 %). Only three adverse events were serious, affecting two patients, and none of the unexpected ADR was considered as serious by the investigator. It was shown that the add-on of leflunomide to concomitant DMARDs did not lead to an increase in adverse events [28].

Sulfasalazine

In a systematic review of sulfasalazine in PsA, 6 RCT comparing SSZ with placebo showed efficacy of SSZ in articular manifestations but not the skin [3]. SSZ does not appear to halt radiographic progression in PsA. In a case-control study, in whom 20 patients who received SSZ for more than 3 months were compared with 20 control patients there was not statistically significant differences in the mean change in radiographic score at 24 months [30]. A trend has been observed in most of the RCT towards higher withdrawal rates in the SSZ group compared with the placebo group, mostly related to adverse events such as gastrointestinal intolerance, dizziness, and liver toxicity, which have been observed in up to one-third of the patients receiving SSZ [13].

Traditional DMARDs in Combination with TNFi

In rheumatoid arthritis it is clear that the combination of TNFi with traditional DMARDs improves efficacy, however whether combining methotrexate with a TNFi benefits patients with PsA remains controversial. The randomized placebo-controlled trials of the five commercially available TNF antagonists involved stratification on whether methotrexate was used concomitantly and showed no significant differences regarding the effect on PsA manifestations [31]. However, it must be kept in mind that subjects enrolling in these trials were considered to have an inadequate response to MTX prior to study entry, so this represents a skewed population against MTX efficacy. Data from registries also showed no differences of efficacy between TNFi monotherapy or combined with MTX, although some of them showed better TNFi survival with the combination. The Swedish registry (SSATG) showed that concomitant methotrexate (MTX) (hazard ratio (HR) 0.64, 95 % CI 0.39–0.95, p=0.03), at treatment initiation was associated with higher TNFi survival [32].

In the Danish (DANBIO) registry except for the subgroup of infliximab-treated patients, in which concomitant methotrexate therapy improved biotherapy continuation, drug continuation rates were not significantly different with and without methotrexate [33]. In the Norwegian (NOR-DMARD) registry drug continuation rates at 1 and 2 years were higher with combination therapy, with the difference being greatest in the infliximab-treated subgroup while EULAR response rates to TNFi with and without methotrexate were similar at 6 months [34]. In summary neither RCTs, nor registries have provided

conclusive evidence that MTX should be combined with TNFi to improve efficacy. Some data from registries suggests that the combination might improve drug survival, especially with infliximab, possibly due to the ability of MTX to lower immunogenicity. There is no evidence that adding a traditional DMARD to a patient that failed TNFi monotherapy would improve efficacy [31].

Two other important issues when traditional DMARDs are considered are that none of the studies have shown inhibition on radiographic progression, and there is no evidence that they have efficacy in other domains involved such as enthesitis, dactylitis, or axial disease.

At the time of this writing, a large trial has initiated to study PsA patients naïve to MTX who will be randomized to TNFi monotherapy, MTX monotherapy, and combination of the two, evaluating all clinical domains of PsA including structural damage. It is hoped that this study will provide more definitive evidence for the effect of MTX, both as monotherapy as well as in combination with TNFi.

New Synthetic DMARDs

Phosphodiesterase Four Inhibitor: Apremilast

Apremilast, is a small molecule that specifically inhibits phosphodiesterase 4, increasing cyclic AMP in immune cells, which down-regulates the inflammatory responses through partially inhibition the expression of inflammatory cytokines and increasing expression of anti-inflammatory mediators such as interleukin-10 [35]. This agent has been approved by the FDA for the treatment of adults with active psoriatic arthritis. In PALACE 1, 2 and 3, the pivotal phase III studies, approximately 1,500 patients were randomized 1:1:1 to receive either apremilast 20 mg twice daily, apremilast 30 mg twice daily, or placebo, with primary endpoint at 16 weeks. PALACE 1 (504 patients), 2 (484 patients), 3 (505 patients) compared the efficacy and safety of apremilast with placebo in PsA patients previously treated with DMARDs and/or biologic therapy, PALACE 4 (527 patients) evaluated apremilast in DMARD-naïve PsA patients [17, 36, 37]. Patients in the PALACE-1, -2, and -3 trials were stratified by prior DMARD use and were allowed to continue receiving stable DMARD therapy in addition to study medication. The primary endpoint of the PALACE studies was the proportion of patients achieving ACR20 response at week 16 [17, 36, 37]. In the PALACE-1, -2, and -3 trials, significantly higher proportion of patients receiving apremilast achieved ACR20 response rate than placebo at week 16 (Table 27.1). Secondary end-points including swollen and tender joint counts, Maastricht Ankylosing Spondylitis Enthesitis Score (MASES), dactylitis count, Short Form-36 (SF-36) physical function and Physical Component Summary scores, Health assessment Questionnaire Disability Index (HAQ-DI), Disease Activity Score (DAS28), and PASI scores also demonstrated significant improvement [17, 18, 38]. ACR20 responses were maintained through week 52 in all three studies. Patients who had been switched to apremilast from placebo at week 16 or week 24 had response rates similar with patients who had been treated with apremilast throughout the study in all three trials. In PALACE -1 study 119 (23.6 %) had prior biologic exposure, and 47 (9.3 %) were considered biologic therapeutic failures [17]. Whereas significantly, more patients receiving apremilast 20 mg BID (31 %) and 30 mg BID (28 %) achieved an ACR-20 response versus placebo (5 %) in the group of patients with prior biologic exposure, statistically significant improvement was not found among the small number of patients classified as biologic therapeutic failures [17].

Apremilast was effective in DMARD-naive patients in the PALACE-4 study [20]. ACR20 response rates at week 16 were 29.2 %, 32.3 % and 16.9 % for apremilast 20, apremilast 30 mg bid and placebo respectively.

Apremilast was generally well tolerated in phase III trials. A total of 1,493 patients received study medication and were included in the safety analysis of pooled data from the PALACE-1, -2, and -3 trials [39].

The most common adverse events were gastrointestinal, such as nausea and diarrhea, and generally occurred early, were self-limiting and infrequently led to discontinuation. [39]. Nausea and headache, upper respiratory tract infection (3.9 vs 1.8 % for placebo), vomiting, nasopharyngitis, and upper abdominal pain were also reported. During clinical trials, 1.0 % of patients treated with apremilast reported depression or depressed mood compared to 0.8 % treated with placebo. Body weight loss of 5–10 % was reported in 10 % of patients taking apremilast [39].

Janus Kinase Inhibitor

Janus kinase (JAK) inhibitors are agents which inhibit intracellular signaling from cytokines which signal through the JAK signaling pathway. The JAK family consists of four members: JAK1, JAK2, JAK3, and tyrosine-protein kinase 2 (TYK2). These molecules interact with various members of the signal transducers and activators of transcription (STAT) family to modulate gene transcription downstream of a variety of cell surface cytokine and growth factor receptors [40]. JAKs are associated with different cytokine receptors, briefly: JAK1 and 3 associate with the IL-2Rg chain (IL-2, -4, -7, -9, -15 and -21), JAK1 and 2 associate with the gp130 subunit (IL-6, -11, -33, LIF, OSM, CT-1, CNTF, CLC) and interferon receptors; JAK2 also associates with receptors of erythropoietin, growth hormone, prolactin, thrombopoietin, whereas TYK2 has been implicated in interferon-a, IL-6, -10, and -12 signalling [41].

Tofacitinib

Tofacitinib is an oral inhibitor of JAK3, JAK1, and, to a lesser degree, JAK2, now approved for the treatment of rheumatoid arthritis in a dose of 5 mg bid. Studies in psoriasis have demonstrated efficacy in both 5 and 10 mg bid dosing [42, 43]. There are 3 unpublished studies looking at the efficacy of tofacitinib in PsA: two of them (including the open label extension), are still recruiting and one has been completed, and some information is available through www.clinicaltrials.gov. This last study is an a phase 3, multi-site, randomized, double blind study of the long-term safety, tolerability and efficacy of 2 oral doses of tofacitinib in subjects with moderate to severe plaque psoriasis and/or psoriatic arthritis in Japanese population [21]. No controls were included and both doses were not compared among them. Only 12 patients with psoriatic arthritis were included (4 in the 5 mg bid dose and 8 in the 10 mg bid dose). By week 16 (primary outcome), 100 %, 83 % and 58 % achieved ACR20/50/70 response respectively. This response was achieved by week 52 (open label) in 83 %, 75 % and 73 % of patients respectively. Due to the small number of patients and the fact that there was no control group, conclusions about efficacy awaits results of larger controlled trials.

Rehabilitation and Physical Therapy

Rehabilitation in rheumatology focuses on prevention of functional disorders of the musculoskeletal system, maintenance of working ability and prevention of care dependency. Rehabilitative therapy in rheumatology includes physiotherapy, patient education and occupational therapy [44]. Inflammation in rheumatic diseases leads to muscle weakness and joint stiffness; Physical therapy is important to prevent muscle weakness and to preserve range of motion. It is also one of the most useful ways to restore function and health status.

Physical therapy is part of non-pharmacological treatment in patients with rheumatic disease and part of the integral management of ankylosing spondylitis.

In 2009 Lubrano et al. after a systematic literature review on PsA and rehabilitation [45], found only minor studies on the role of physical therapies [45] such as interferential current [46], effects of climatic therapy at Tiberias Hot Springs [47], and effect of balneotherapy in the Dead Sea area for patients with PsA and concomitant fibromyalgia [48]. Exercise was considered as an important part of the treatment plan and a good approach to reduce the chance of joint deformity by patients that completed a self-administered questionnaires [49]. That study showed that in general, physical therapy and exercise have good acceptance among patients. Lubrano et al. proposed a rehabilitation program for patients with PsA with predominant peripheral or axial involvement (Table 27.2) [45].

In PsA patients with axial involvement (ax PsA), rehabilitation plays an important role in the management of the disease. Due to very little evidence available for PsA, data has been borrowed from studies on rehabilitation in ankylosing spondylitis; and was considered by the GRAPPA Group (Group for Research and Assessment of Psoriasis and Psoriatic Arthritis), as a surrogate for evidence for treatment of axial PsA [50]

Most of the techniques and methods could only be implemented once inflammation and pain are under medical control, so in general some degree of disease control is needed before physical therapy can be started [51]. Each patient should receive a properly designed program of physical activity planned for each patient's needs, combining flexibility (ROM), strengthening or aerobic exercises.

The main results on rehabilitation in PsA could be summarized as follows: (1) very little evidence is available to evaluate the efficacy of rehabilitation; (2) most data have been borrowed from studies on AS; and (3) covering aspects of the disease by the standard measures

Table 27.2 Proposal for a rehabilitation program for patients with psoriatic arthritis (PsA)

Predominant peripheral disease	Predominant axial involvement
Muscle-strengthening exercises	Muscle-strengthening exercises
General fitness exercises	General fitness exercises
Stretching exercises	Stretching exercises
Physical therapy (when necessary)	Physical therapy (when necessary)
Occupational therapy	Occupational therapy
Patient education	Patient education
	Postural exercises
	Breathing exercises

Reprinted from Lubrano et al. [45]. With permission from *The Journal of Rheumatology*

of functioning presents difficulties [45]. At the OMERACT 8 meeting consensus was obtained to measure physical function as a core domain, which could be considered an important achievement for future studies on the role of rehabilitation in PsA [52].

Surgical Management

There are a limited number of studies in the literature related to surgical procedures in patients with PsA. Most of them included small number of patients or are retrospectives studies.

In a cohort study of patients with PsA in Rochester, Minnesota, 66 patients were newly diagnosed with PsA between 1982 and 1991. After a mean period of follow up of 7.2 years, six orthopedic procedures were performed: three synovectomies, one arthroplasty, and two reconstructive surgeries [53].

Seven percent of 444 PsA patients were subjected to surgical management after an average of 14 years of disease onset in another retrospective study [54]. Other reports indicate that 23.8 % of PsA patients required hand surgery, 1.8 % required hip arthroplasty, 1.4 % underwent total knee replacement, and 1.2 % needed foot or ankle surgery [55]. Extended radiological damage and a high active joint count at initial assessment were predictors of the need of future surgical treatment [54]. The surgical management is dependent on the pattern and severity of joint involvement and the most frequent surgical procedures are total joint arthroplasty, arthrodesis and arthroscopic synovectomy [55].

Zangger et al. described 10-year results of 71 orthopedic surgical procedures performed in 43 PsA patients [56]. Patients were categorized as having either distal PsA (involving DIP and PIP joints), oligoarticular PsA, or polyarticular disease. Those with distal disease (10 %) underwent PIP and DIP fusions. Patients with oligoarticular disease (25 %) were treated with such large joint surgery as hip replacement, knee replacement, or knee synovectomy. Those with polyarticular disease (65 %) underwent a variety of upper and lower extremity surgeries, most

of them being reconstructive procedures. The authors concluded that outcomes were similar to those of surgical management of other forms of arthritis [56].

Joint replacement is an uncommon procedure in PsA patients. In a cohort study in 504 PsA patients only 32 (6 %) developed symptomatic hip disease [57]. After a mean follow up of 5,7 years (range 1–45 years) data were available for 17 of these 32 patients. Nine (53 %) underwent hip arthroplasty within 5 years after onset of hip pain [57].

In a prospective study of surgical treatment in PsA and RA, arthroscopic knee synovectomy was performed in 32 patients (17 with PsA, 15 with RA) [58]. Patients who underwent synovectomy had 73 % possibility of definite improvement and 61 % of clinical remission, which was higher in PsA than RA knees (86.3 % versus 45.7 %, respectively), after 36 months of follow up [58].

Hand and wrist surgery procedures include total wrist fusion, distal ulna resection, arthroplasty, manipulation, arthrodesis and synovectomy. A retrospective study reviewed 25 PsA patients who underwent hand and wrist surgery [59]. Eight patients received wrist surgery because of persistent wrist pain, joint erosion, and /or deformity at that level. Three were managed with arthroplasty, 3 with distal ulna resections, and 2 with fusions. Although all eight patients reported improvement in relief of wrist pain, range of motion (ROM) in the arthroplasty cases was limited. Seventeen of the 25 patients in that cohort underwent surgical intervention for PIP joint disease [59]. Fifty PIP fusions, 11 arthroplasties, and 10 joint manipulations were performed during the study period. Every arthrodesis case achieved union without incident. Overall range of motion, after PIP arthroplasty was limited to 20°. Malposition of spontaneous DIP joint ankylosis was treated with realignment and arthrodesis in eight patients, each of whom experienced pain relief and improved function [59, 60].

Buryanov et al, analyzed 14 metacarpophalangeal joint silicone arthroplasty in nine PsA patients during 3–6 years, they concluded that is an effective method because patients experienced improvement in pain and ROM [61].

Before surgery procedures in this patients, special considerations should be given to the prevention of site infections, and awareness of the chance of a Koebner phenomenon (exacerbation of psoriatic skin lesions in the surgical site) occurring at the surgical site [62].

Future Considerations/Summary

Traditional DMARDs remain first-line agents for PsA despite a paucity of randomized controlled trial evidence. As psoriatic arthritis is a heterogeneous disease with involvement of many different domains, when the major involvement is not peripheral arthritis, the first treatment choice should change to therapies proved to be effective in that manifestation. One new oral DMARAD (apremilast) has been very recently approved for use in PsA, and has evidence for efficacy on different disease domains, and different PsA populations, so would be another option for the treatment of the disease. Rehabilitation remains as an important part of non-pharmacological treatment in patients with PsA, and each patient should receive a properly designed program of physical activity planned for their needs, combining flexibility (ROM), strengthening or aerobic exercises. Surgical management in PsA is dependent on the pattern and severity of joint involvement and the most frequent surgical procedures are, total joint arthroplasty, arthrodesis and arthroscopic synovectomy. Results are similar to those reported in other arthritis.

Psoriatic arthritis is still well behind rheumatoid arthritis in the number of alternative agents available to treat the condition, and on the evidence for efficacy of the most frequently used agents. More research on the physiopathology, and more drugs based on that knowledge are being developed and experimented. The future looks promising and is probably a good time for young rheumatologist, and investigators to choose psoriatic arthritis as their main academic focus.

References

1. Soriano ER. The actual role of therapy with traditional disease-modifying antirheumatic drugs in psoriatic arthritis. J Rheumatol Suppl. 2012;89:67–70. doi:10.3899/jrheum.120248.
2. Helliwell PS, Taylor WJ, Group CS. Treatment of psoriatic arthritis and rheumatoid arthritis with disease modifying drugs – comparison of drugs and adverse reactions. J Rheumatol. 2008;35(3):472–6.
3. Soriano ER, McHugh NJ. Therapies for peripheral joint disease in psoriatic arthritis. A systematic review. J Rheumatol. 2006;33(7):1422–30.
4. Ravindran V, Scott DL, Choy EH. A systematic review and meta-analysis of efficacy and toxicity of disease modifying anti-rheumatic drugs and biological agents for psoriatic arthritis. Ann Rheum Dis. 2008;67(6):855–9. doi:10.1136/ard.2007.072652.
5. Ash Z, Gaujoux-Viala C, Gossec L, Hensor EM, FitzGerald O, Winthrop K, van der Heijde D, Emery P, Smolen JS, Marzo-Ortega H. A systematic literature review of drug therapies for the treatment of psoriatic arthritis: current evidence and meta-analysis informing the EULAR recommendations for the management of psoriatic arthritis. Ann Rheum Dis. 2012;71(3):319–26. doi:10.1136/ard.2011.150995.
6. Acosta Felquer ML, Coates LC, Soriano ER, Ranza R, Espinoza LR, Helliwell PS, FitzGerald O, McHugh N, Roussou E, Mease PJ. Drug therapies for peripheral joint disease in psoriatic arthritis: a systematic review. J Rheumatol. 2014;41(11):2277–85. doi:10.3899/jrheum.140876.
7. Soriano ER. Treatment guidelines for psoriatic arthritis. Int J Clin Rheumatol. 2009;4:329–42.
8. Gossec L, Smolen JS, Gaujoux-Viala C, Ash Z, Marzo-Ortega H, van der Heijde D, FitzGerald O, Aletaha D, Balint P, Boumpas D, Braun J, Breedveld FC, Burmester G, Canete JD, de Wit M, Dagfinrud H, de Vlam K, Dougados M, Helliwell P, Kavanaugh A, Kvien TK, Landewe R, Luger T, Maccarone M, McGonagle D, McHugh N, McInnes IB, Ritchlin C, Sieper J, Tak PP, Valesini G, Vencovsky J, Winthrop KL, Zink A, Emery P, European League Against R. European League Against Rheumatism recommendations for the management of psoriatic arthritis with pharmacological therapies. Ann Rheum Dis. 2012;71(1):4–12. doi:10.1136/annrheumdis-2011-200350.
9. Willkens RF, Williams HJ, Ward JR, Egger MJ, Reading JC, Clements PJ, Cathcart ES, Samuelson Jr CO, Solsky MA, Kaplan SB, et al. Randomized, double-blind, placebo controlled trial of low-dose pulse methotrexate in psoriatic arthritis. Arthritis Rheum. 1984;27(4):376–81.
10. Scarpa R, Peluso R, Atteno M, Manguso F, Spano A, Iervolino S, Di Minno MN, Costa L, Del Puente A. The effectiveness of a traditional therapeutical approach in early psoriatic arthritis: results of a pilot randomised 6-month trial with methotrexate. Clin Rheumatol. 2008;27(7):823–6. doi:10.1007/s10067-007-0787-7.

11. Kingsley GH, Kowalczyk A, Taylor H, Ibrahim F, Packham JC, McHugh NJ, Mulherin DM, Kitas GD, Chakravarty K, Tom BD, O'Keeffe AG, Maddison PJ, Scott DL. A randomized placebo-controlled trial of methotrexate in psoriatic arthritis. Rheumatology. 2012;51(8):1368–77. doi:10.1093/rheumatology/kes001.

12. Kaltwasser JP, Nash P, Gladman D, Rosen CF, Behrens F, Jones P, Wollenhaupt J, Falk FG, Mease P, Treatment of Psoriatic Arthritis Study G. Efficacy and safety of leflunomide in the treatment of psoriatic arthritis and psoriasis: a multinational, double-blind, randomized, placebo-controlled clinical trial. Arthritis Rheum. 2004;50(6):1939–50. doi:10.1002/art.20253.

13. Clegg DO, Reda DJ, Mejias E, Cannon GW, Weisman MH, Taylor T, Budiman-Mak E, Blackburn WD, Vasey FB, Mahowald ML, Cush JJ, Schumacher Jr HR, Silverman SL, Alepa FP, Luggen ME, Cohen MR, Makkena R, Haakenson CM, Ward RH, Manaster BJ, Anderson RJ, Ward JR, Henderson WG. Comparison of sulfasalazine and placebo in the treatment of psoriatic arthritis. A Department of Veterans Affairs Cooperative Study. Arthritis Rheum. 1996;39(12):2013–20.

14. Chandran V, Schentag CT, Gladman DD. Reappraisal of the effectiveness of methotrexate in psoriatic arthritis: results from a longitudinal observational cohort. J Rheumatol. 2008;35(3):469–71.

15. Cantini F, Niccoli L, Nannini C, Cassara E, Pasquetti P, Olivieri I, Salvarani C. Criteria, frequency, and duration of clinical remission in psoriatic arthritis patients with peripheral involvement requiring second-line drugs. J Rheumatol Suppl. 2009;83:78–80. doi:10.3899/jrheum.090234.

16. Baranauskaite A, Raffayova H, Kungurov NV, Kubanova A, Venalis A, Helmle L, Srinivasan S, Nasonov E, Vastesaeger N, investigators R. Infliximab plus methotrexate is superior to methotrexate alone in the treatment of psoriatic arthritis in methotrexate-naive patients: the RESPOND study. Ann Rheum Dis. 2012;71(4):541–8. doi:10.1136/ard.2011.152223.

17. Kavanaugh A, Mease PJ, Gomez-Reino JJ, Adebajo AO, Wollenhaupt J, Gladman DD, Lespessailles E, Hall S, Hochfeld M, Hu C, Hough D, Stevens RM, Schett G. Treatment of psoriatic arthritis in a phase 3 randomised, placebo-controlled trial with apremilast, an oral phosphodiesterase 4 inhibitor. Ann Rheum Dis. 2014;73(6):1020–6. doi:10.1136/annrheumdis-2013-205056.

18. Cutolo M, Myerson G, Fleischmann R, Liote F, Diaz-Gonzalez F, Van den Bosch F, et al. Long-term (52-week) results of a phase 3, randomized, controlled trial of apremilast, an oral phosphodiesterase 4 inhibitor, in patients with psoriatic arthritis (PALACE 2). Arthritis Rheum. 2013;65(Suppl):S346.

19. Schett G, Wollenhaupt J, Papp K, Joos R, Rodrigues JF, Vessey AR, Hu C, Stevens R, de Vlam KL. Oral apremilast in the treatment of active psoriatic arthritis: results of a multicenter, randomized, double-blind, placebo-controlled study. Arthritis Rheum. 2012;64(10):3156–67. doi:10.1002/art.34627.

20. Wells A, Edwards C, Aea A. Apremilast in the treatment of DMARD-naive psoriatic arthritis patients: results of a phase 3 randomized, controlled trial (PALACE 4). Arthritis Rheum. 2013;65(12):3320–1.

21. A Phase 3, Multi Site, Randomized, Double Blind Study of the Long-Term Safety, Tolerability and Efficacy of 2 Oral Doses of CP 690,550 in Subjects with Moderate to Severe Plaque Psoriasis and/or Psoriatic Arthritis. https://clinicaltrials.gov/ct2/show/NCT01519089?term=A3921137&rank=1. Last accessed on 10 July 2015.

22. Ceponis A, Kavanaugh A. Use of methotrexate in patients with psoriatic arthritis. Clin Exp Rheumatol. 2010;28(5 Suppl 61):S132–7.

23. Cantini F, Niccoli L, Nannini C, Cassara E, Pasquetti P, Olivieri I, Salvarani C. Frequency and duration of clinical remission in patients with peripheral psoriatic arthritis requiring second-line drugs. Rheumatology. 2008;47(6):872–6. doi:10.1093/rheumatology/ken059.

24. Lie E, van der Heijde D, Uhlig T, Heiberg MS, Koldingsnes W, Rodevand E, Kaufmann C, Mikkelsen K, Kvien TK. Effectiveness and retention rates of methotrexate in psoriatic arthritis in comparison with methotrexate-treated patients with rheumatoid arthritis. Ann Rheum Dis. 2010;69(4):671–6. doi:10.1136/ard.2009.113308.

25. Mori Y, Kuwahara Y, Chiba S, Itoi E. Efficacy of methotrexate and tumor necrosis factor inhibitors in Japanese patients with active psoriatic arthritis. Mod Rheumatol. 2014;25(3):431–4. doi:10.3109/14397595.2014.958891.

26. Taylor WJ, Korendowych E, Nash P, Helliwell PS, Choy E, Krueger GG, Soriano ER, McHugh NJ, Rosen CF. Drug use and toxicity in psoriatic disease: focus on methotrexate. J Rheumatol. 2008;35(7):1454–7.

27. Whiting-O'Keefe QE, Fye KH, Sack KD. Methotrexate and histologic hepatic abnormalities: a meta-analysis. Am J Med. 1991;90(6):711–6.

28. Behrens F, Finkenwirth C, Pavelka K, Stolfa J, Sipek-Dolnicar A, Thaci D, Burkhardt H. Leflunomide in psoriatic arthritis: results from a large European prospective observational study. Arthritis Care Res. 2013;65(3):464–70. doi:10.1002/acr.21848.

29. Asiri A, Thavaneswaran A, Kalman-Lamb G, Chandran V, Gladman DD. The effectiveness of leflunomide in psoriatic arthritis. Clin Exp Rheumatol. 2014;32(5):728–31.

30. Rahman P, Gladman DD, Cook RJ, Zhou Y, Young G. The use of sulfasalazine in psoriatic arthritis: a clinic experience. J Rheumatol. 1998;25(10):1957–61.

31. Paccou J, Wendling D. Current treatment of psoriatic arthritis: update based on a systematic literature review to establish French Society for Rheumatology (SFR) recommendations for managing spondyloarthritis. Joint Bone Spine. 2014. doi:10.1016/j.jbspin.2014.05.003.

32. Kristensen LE, Gulfe A, Saxne T, Geborek P. Efficacy and tolerability of anti-tumour necrosis factor

therapy in psoriatic arthritis patients: results from the South Swedish Arthritis Treatment Group register. Ann Rheum Dis. 2008;67(3):364–9. doi:10.1136/ard.2007.073544.

33. Glintborg B, Ostergaard M, Dreyer L, Krogh NS, Tarp U, Hansen MS, Rifbjerg-Madsen S, Lorenzen T, Hetland ML. Treatment response, drug survival, and predictors thereof in 764 patients with psoriatic arthritis treated with anti-tumor necrosis factor alpha therapy: results from the nationwide Danish DANBIO registry. Arthritis Rheum. 2011;63(2):382–90. doi:10.1002/art.30117.

34. Fagerli KM, Lie E, van der Heijde D, Heiberg MS, Lexberg AS, Rodevand E, Kalstad S, Mikkelsen K, Kvien TK. The role of methotrexate co-medication in TNF-inhibitor treatment in patients with psoriatic arthritis: results from 440 patients included in the NOR-DMARD study. Ann Rheum Dis. 2013. doi:10.1136/annrheumdis-2012-202347.

35. Schafer P. Apremilast mechanism of action and application to psoriasis and psoriatic arthritis. Biochem Pharmacol. 2012;83(12):1583–90. doi:10.1016/j.bcp.2012.01.001.

36. Schett G, Mease P, Gladman D. Apremilast, an oral phosphodiesterase 4 inhibitor, is associated with long-term (52-week) improvement in physical function in patients with psoriatic arthritis: results from three phase 3, randomized, controlled trials [abstract]. Arthritis Rheum. 2013;65(Suppl):143.

37. Cutolo M, Mease P, Gladman D. Apremilast, an oral phosphodiesterase 4 inhibitor, is associated with long-term (52-week) improvement in tender and swollen joint counts in patients with psoriatic arthritis: results from three phase 3, randomized, controlled trials [abstract]. Arthritis Rheum. 2013;65(Suppl):135–6.

38. Edwards C, Blanco F, Crowley J, C-C H, Stevens R, Birbara CL-t-wroap, randomized, controlled trial of apremilast, an oral phosphodiesterase 4 inhibitor, in patients with psoriatic arthritis and current skin involvement (PALACE 3) [abstract]. Arthritis Rheum. 2013;65(Suppl):S132. Long-term (52-week) results of a phase 3, randomized, controlled trial of apremilast, an oral phosphodiesterase 4 inhibitor, in patients with psoriatic arthritis and current skin involvement (PALACE 3) [abstract]. Arthritis Rheum. 2013;65(Suppl):S132.

39. Mease PJ, Kavanaugh A, Adebajo AO, et al. Laboratory abnormalities in patients with psoriatic arthritis receiving apremilast, an oral phosphodiesterase 4 inhibitor: pooled safety analysis of three phase 3, randomized, controlled trials. Arthritis Rheum. 2013;65:S151.

40. Hansen RB, Kavanaugh A. Novel treatments with small molecules in psoriatic arthritis. Curr Rheumatol Rep. 2014;16(9):443. doi:10.1007/s11926-014-0443-6.

41. Meier FM, McInnes IB. Small-molecule therapeutics in rheumatoid arthritis: scientific rationale, efficacy and safety. Best Pract Res Clin Rheumatol. 2014;28(4):605–24. doi:10.1016/j.berh.2014.10.017.

42. Papp KA, Menter A, Strober B, Langley RG, Buonanno M, Wolk R, Gupta P, Krishnaswami S, Tan H, Harness JA. Efficacy and safety of tofacitinib, an oral Janus kinase inhibitor, in the treatment of psoriasis: a Phase 2b randomized placebo-controlled dose-ranging study. Br J Dermatol. 2012;167(3):668–77. doi:10.1111/j.1365-2133.2012.11168.x.

43. Mamolo C, Harness J, Tan H, Menter A. Tofacitinib (CP-690,550), an oral Janus kinase inhibitor, improves patient-reported outcomes in a phase 2b, randomized, double-blind, placebo-controlled study in patients with moderate-to-severe psoriasis. J Eur Acad Dermatol Venereol. 2013;28(2):192–203. doi:10.1111/jdv.12081.

44. Luttosch F, Baerwald C. Rehabilitation in rheumatology. Internist (Berl). 2010;51(10):1239–45. doi:10.1007/s00108-010-2626-1.

45. Lubrano E, Spadaro A, Parsons WJ, Atteno M, Ferrara N. Rehabilitation in psoriatic arthritis. J Rheumatol Suppl. 2009;83:81–2. doi:10.3899/jrheum.09235.

46. Walker UA, Uhl M, Weiner SM, Warnatz K, Lange-Nolde A, Dertinger H, Peter HH, Jurenz SA. Analgesic and disease modifying effects of interferential current in psoriatic arthritis. Rheumatol Int. 2006;26(10):904–7. doi:10.1007/s00296-006-0102-y.

47. Hashkes PJ. Beneficial effect of climatic therapy on inflammatory arthritis at Tiberias Hot Springs. Scand J Rheumatol. 2002;31(3):172–7.

48. Sukenik S, Baradin R, Codish S, Neumann L, Flusser D, Abu-Shakra M, Buskila D. Balneotherapy at the Dead Sea area for patients with psoriatic arthritis and concomitant fibromyalgia. Isr Med Assoc J. 2001;3(2):147–50.

49. Lubrano E, Helliwell P, Parsons W, Emery P, Veale D. Patient education in psoriatic arthritis: a cross sectional study on knowledge by a validated self-administered questionnaire. J Rheumatol. 1998;25(8):1560–5.

50. Nash P. Therapies for axial disease in psoriatic arthritis. A systematic review. J Rheumatol. 2006;33(7):1431–4.

51. Dougados M, Revel M, Khan MA. Spondylarthropathy treatment: progress in medical treatment, physical therapy and rehabilitation. Baillieres Clin Rheumatol. 1998;12(4):717–36.

52. Gladman DD, Mease PJ, Strand V, Healy P, Helliwell PS, Fitzgerald O, Gottlieb AB, Krueger GG, Nash P, Ritchlin CT, Taylor W, Adebajo A, Braun J, Cauli A, Carneiro S, Choy E, Dijkmans B, Espinoza L, van der Heijde D, Husni E, Lubrano E, McGonagle D, Qureshi A, Soriano ER, Zochling J. Consensus on a core set of domains for psoriatic arthritis. J Rheumatol. 2007;34(5):1167–70.

53. Shbeeb M, Uramoto KM, Gibson LE, O'Fallon WM, Gabriel SE. The epidemiology of psoriatic arthritis in Olmsted County, Minnesota, USA, 1982–1991. J Rheumatol. 2000;27(5):1247–50.

54. Zangger P, Gladman DD, Bogoch ER. Musculoskeletal surgery in psoriatic arthritis. J Rheumatol. 1998;25(4):725–9.

55. Day MS, Nam D, Goodman S, Su EP, Figgie M. Psoriatic arthritis. J Am Acad Orthop Surg. 2012;20(1):28–37. doi:10.5435/JAAOS-20-01-028.
56. Zangger P, Esufali ZH, Gladman DD, Bogoch ER. Type and outcome of reconstructive surgery for different patterns of psoriatic arthritis. J Rheumatol. 2000;27(4):967–74.
57. Michet CJ, Mason TG, Mazlumzadeh M. Hip joint disease in psoriatic arthritis: risk factors and natural history. Ann Rheum Dis. 2005;64(7):1068–70. doi:10.1136/ard.2004.022228.
58. Fiocco U, Cozzi L, Rigon C, Chieco-Bianchi F, Baldovin M, Cassisi GA, Gallo C, Doria A, Favaro MA, Piccoli A, de Candia A, Rubaltelli L, Todesco S. Arthroscopic synovectomy in rheumatoid and psoriatic knee joint synovitis: long-term outcome. Br J Rheumatol. 1996;35(5):463–70.
59. Belsky MR, Feldon P, Millender LH, Nalebuff EA, Phillips C. Hand involvement in psoriatic arthritis. J Hand Surg Am. 1982;7(2):203–7.
60. Rose JH, Belsky MR. Psoriatic arthritis in the hand. Hand Clin. 1989;5(2):137–44.
61. Buryanov A, Kotiuk V, Kvasha V, Samokhin A. Three- to six-year results of metacarpophalangeal joints arthroplasty in psoriatic arthritis. J Long Term Eff Med Implants. 2013;23(4):285–92.
62. Lofin I, Levine B, Badlani N, Klein GR, Jaffe WL. Psoriatic arthritis and arthroplasty: a review of the literature. Bull NYU Hosp Jt Dis. 2008;66(1):41–8.

Biologic Therapy for Psoriasis

28

Jacqueline Moreau, Erica Bromberg,
and Laura Korb Ferris

Abstract

Biologic therapies have revolutionized the treatment of psoriasis due to their effectiveness and relatively safe side effect profile. Biologic drugs used to treat psoriasis are generally monoclonal antibodies, or derivatives of these molecules, that target specific proteins involved in the pathogenesis of psoriasis. Unlike traditional systemic agents like cyclosporine and methotrexate, biologics specifically target only one or two cytokines or cellular receptors central to psoriasis pathophysiology. Furthermore, biologics generally have very few drug-drug interactions and can usually be used in patients with comorbid conditions such as renal insufficiency or liver disease, a population that is otherwise challenging to treat with conventional systemic agents.

Keywords

Psoriasis • Biologic • TNF-α • IL-12 • IL-23 • IL-17

Introduction

Biologic therapies have revolutionized the treatment of psoriasis due to their effectiveness and relatively safe side effect profile. Biologic drugs used to treat psoriasis are generally monoclonal antibodies, or derivatives of these molecules, that target specific proteins involved in the pathogenesis of psoriasis. Unlike traditional systemic agents like cyclosporine and methotrexate, biologics specifically target only one or two cytokines or cellular receptors central to psoriasis pathophysiology. Furthermore, biologics generally have very few drug-drug interactions and can

J. Moreau, MD, MS
Department of Internal Medicine, University of Pittsburgh Medical Center, Pittsburgh, PA, USA

E. Bromberg, BA
Department of Dermatology, Psoriasis Clinical Trials, University of Pittsburgh Medical Center, Pittsburgh, PA, USA

L.K. Ferris, MD, PhD (✉)
Department of Dermatology, University of Pittsburgh, 3601 Fifth Avenue, 5th Floor, Pittsburgh, PA, USA
e-mail: ferrislk@upmc.edu

© Springer International Publishing Switzerland 2016
A. Adebajo et al. (eds.), *Psoriatic Arthritis and Psoriasis: Pathology and Clinical Aspects*,
DOI 10.1007/978-3-319-19530-8_28

usually be used in patients with comorbid conditions such as renal insufficiency or liver disease, a population that is otherwise challenging to treat with conventional systemic agents.

Classification and Efficacy of Biologics

Currently, there are five drugs that are approved by the United States Food and Drug Administration (FDA) for the treatment of plaque-type psoriasis (Table 28.1). Several additional drugs are currently under development as well.

TNF-α Antagonists

TNF-α antagonists were initially approved for the treatment of Crohn's disease and were among the first biologics the Food and Drug Administration (FDA) approved for the treatment of psoriasis and psoriatic arthritis. As they have been used as a class for the longest among the biologic therapies, and have more patient-

years of exposure than any other class of biologic therapy for psoriasis, there are significant long-term safety and efficacy data for this class of drugs. As TNF-α drives the proliferation of both T cells and keratinocytes, as well as the production of vascular endothelial growth factor, blocking this cytokine improves psoriasis severity in most patients [14]. Currently there are three TNF-α antagonists approved by the FDA for the treatment of psoriasis; two are monoclonal antibodies, and one is a fusion protein. In addition, there are two TNF-α antagonists approved for the treatment of psoriatic arthritis that also have some efficacy in treating cutaneous psoriasis.

Infliximab

Infliximab is a chimeric antibody that is 75 % human and 25 % murine in composition which is of the human IgG1 subtype. Infliximab was first considered as a therapy for psoriasis when it was noted that a patient with both Crohn's disease and psoriasis had dramatic clearance of her psoriasis after initiating therapy with infliximab [15]. In fact, this observation sparked interest in TNF-α antagonists as a class as a therapy for psoriasis.

Table 28.1 Biologics currently FDA approved for the treatment of psoriasis

Drug	Structure	Molecular target	Dosing for psoriasis	Key references
Infliximab	Chimeric antibody (25 % mouse, 75 % human, IgG1 subtype)	TNF-α	5 mg/kg IV at weeks 0, 2, 6 then every 8 weeks	[1–3]
Etanercept	Recombinant protein, fusion of p75 TNF-α receptor and human Fc of IgG1	TNF-α	50 mg sc twice weekly for 12 weeks, then 50 mg sc once weekly	[4–7]
Adalimumab	Fully human monoclonal antibody, IgG1 subtype	TNF-α	80 mg sc at week 0, then at week 1 start 40 mg sc every other week	[8–10]
Ustekinumab	Fully human monoclonal antibody, IgG1 subtype	Common p40 subunit of IL-12 and IL-23	For patients <100 kg, 45 mg per dose. For patients ≥100 kg, 90 mg per dose. Dosed at month 0 and 1 then every 3 months	[11, 12]
Secukimumab	Fully human monoclonal antibody, IgG1 subtype	IL-17A	300 mg sc at weeks 0, 1, 2, 3 and 4 then every 4 weeks	[13]

Infliximab is dosed at 5 mg/kg IV at weeks 0, 2, and 6 and then once every subsequent 8 weeks. In EXPRESS, a double-blind, randomized, placebo-controlled phase III trial of infliximab, 378 patients with moderate to severe plaque psoriasis were treated with infliximab or placebo (4:1 ratio) using this dosing schedule. At 10 weeks, 80 % of infliximab-treated individuals had a 75 % or greater reduction in Psoriasis Area and Severity Index (PASI) score from baseline (PASI 75 response), vs. 3 % in the placebo group. A PASI 90 response was achieved by 57 % of infliximab-treated patients and 1 % of placebo-treated patients. At 50 weeks, 61 % maintained a PASI 75 response and 45 % had a PASI 90 response [16]. Infliximab is also effective for nail psoriasis. In a Cochrane meta-analysis, there was a 57.2 % improvement in nail disease severity over 6–12 months in patients treated with infliximab [17].

Optimally, once therapy with infliximab is started it should be given continuously as opposed to given in response to disease recurrence because patients who are continuously treated with infliximab tend to have better overall clinical outcomes, likely at least in part because they are less likely to develop antibodies to infliximab and infusion reactions than those patients who are dosed intermittently [18]. In one study, the prevalence of infusion reactions in patients treated for psoriasis with infliximab alone was significantly higher than in patients who received concomitant methotrexate, presumably due to lower immunogenicity (27 % vs. 4 %, $P = 0.05$) [1].

Etanercept

Etanercept is a soluble fusion protein, created by joining the TNF-α receptor encoded by *TNFR-2* (p75, weighing 75 kDa) with the Fc portion of human IgG1. The resultant fusion protein binds to and thus decreases the free concentration of TNF-α in the serum. Because etanercept contains the binding region of the p75 TNF-α receptor, it also binds to the other natural ligand of the p75 receptor, lymphotoxin B. For psoriasis, etanercept is dosed subcutaneously at a dose of 50 mg twice a week for 12 weeks and then at 50 mg

weekly thereafter for maintenance. In a double-blind, randomized, placebo-controlled phase III trial of etanercept at this dosing, 49 % of subjects reached a PASI 75 response at week 12, and 59 % of subjects reached a PASI 75 response at week 24 [4]. Additional studies found that at this dosing, after 24 weeks of treatment, patients with scalp psoriasis, the mean severity of scalp decreased by over 90 % at week 24 [19], and in patients with nail psoriasis, an improvement of greater than 70 % in severity of disease achieved [20]. Although no biologics are currently FDA-approved for the treatment of pediatric psoriasis, in a study of 211 patients age 4–17 with psoriasis, a PASI75 response was achieved by 57 % of patients receiving etanercept, compared with 11 % of those receiving placebo [5].

Adalimumab

Adalimumab is a fully human monoclonal antibody that binds to both cell-bound and soluble TNF-α. For psoriasis, it is dosed subcutaneously at 80 mg the first week, 40 mg the following week, and 40 mg every 2 weeks thereafter. In REVEAL, a 52 week double-blind, randomized, placebo-controlled phase III trial of adalimumab at this dosing, 71 % of adalimumab-treated patients reached a PASI 75 response; by 52 weeks of continuous treatment, 5 % of patients lost this response to adalimumab [8]. In the CHAMPION study, a head-to-head study with methotrexate, more patients achieved clearance with adalimumab than with methotrexate [9]. Additionally, adalimumab has been shown to be effective in the treatment of scalp and nail psoriasis with median reductions in disease severity of 100 and 39.5 %, respectively, after 16 weeks of treatment [21].

Efficacy in Skin of TNF-α Antagonists Approved for Psoriatic Arthritis

Golimumab is a fully human monoclonal antibody to TNF-α which is currently FDA approved for the treatment of psoriatic arthritis at a dose of 50 mg subcutaneously every 4 weeks. As a secondary endpoint in one study, PASI75 responses was assessed in subjects with psoriatic arthritis who also had ≥ 3 % body surface area (BSA) involvement with psoriasis. After 14 weeks of treatment, PASI75 response was reached by 40 % of subjects who received the 50 mg dose of golimumab. However, it is important to note that PASI scores are less accurate in patients with low BSA involvement. Furthermore, patients in this study could also have been concomitantly taking methotrexate. In the same study, after 24 weeks of treatment with 50 mg of golimumab monthly, patients with nail psoriasis at baseline had a median improvement of 33 % in NAPSI scores [22].

Certolizumab pegol is a pegylated antibody fragment (fragment antigen binding [Fab]) that is FDA-approved for the treatment of psoriatic arthritis at a dose of 400 mg initially and at week 2 and 4, followed by 200 mg every other week; for maintenance dosing, 400 mg every 4 weeks can be considered. Although not currently approved for the treatment of psoriasis, in a phase II study of certolizumab pegol for the treatment of psoriasis, PASI75 responses at week 12 in subjects receiving certolizumab 200 mg, 400 mg, or placebo every 2 weeks were 75 %, 83 %, and 7 %, respectively [23]. Phase III studies investigating certolizumab pegol for psoriasis are ongoing

IL-12/IL-23 Antagonists

Ustekinumab

Ustekinumab is a fully human monoclonal antibody to the common p40 subunit shared by the cytokines IL-12 and IL-23. Human IL-23 is primarily produced by antigen-presenting cells and induces differentiation of T_H17 cells and T_H22 cells. Like infliximab, dosing of ustekinumab is weight-based. Patients who weigh less than 100 kg receive 45 mg per dose, and those who weigh 100 kg or greater receive 90 mg per dose. Ustekinumab is dosed subcutaneously at weeks 0 and 4, and then once every subsequent 12 weeks. Ustekinumab was found to be effective in two double-blind, randomized, placebo-controlled phase III trials (PHOENIX 1 AND PHOENIX 2). In PHOENIX 1, 766 patients with chronic plaque psoriasis and a PASI of 12 or greater were randomized to receive ustekinumab 45 mg, 90 mg,

or placebo at 0 and 4 weeks. At week 16 week, subjects taking ustekinumab continued on their current dose every 12 weeks. Subjects who started on placebo were crossed over to either 45 mg or 90 mg of ustekinumab at week 12 [24]. Those who achieved at least PASI 75 at weeks 28 and 40 were re-randomized at week 40 to either receive maintenance ustekinumab or placebo to assess the impact of maintenance therapy. At week 12, a PASI 75 response was achieved by 67.1 % of participants initially in the 45 mg group, 66.4 % in the 90 mg group, and 3.1 % in the placebo group. At week 28, PASI 75 was achieved in 71.2 % in the 45 mg group, 78.2 % in the 90 mg group, 65.9 % in the placebo to 45 mg group, and 84.9 % in the placebo to 90 mg group. Subsequently, maintenance of PASI 75 was better in those who received maintenance therapy than placebo [11]. In PHOENIX 2, which was very similar to PHOENIX 1, partial (less than PASI 75) responders were re-randomized at week 28 to continue therapy every 12 weeks or escalate their dose to 90 mg every 8 weeks [12]. More partial responders who received 90 mg of ustekinumab every 8 weeks ultimately achieved PASI 75 than did those who continued to receive the same dose every 12 weeks (68.8 % vs. 33.3 %) [12]. PHOENIX 1 also showed that at week 24, patients with nail psoriasis who received ustekinumab had NAPSI score improvements of 46.5 % (ustekinumab 45 mg) and 48.7 % (ustekinumab 90 mg) from baseline [24].

IL-17 Antagonists

Secukinumab

Secukinumab is a monoclonal antibody to IL-17A. It is dosed at 300 mg or 150 mg subcutaneously given at weeks 0,1,2,3, and 4, and then once every 4 weeks for maintenance. Two phase III double-blind, placebo-controlled studies of secukinumab (ERASURE and FIXTURE) showed efficacy of this drug for the treatment of psoriasis. In ERASURE, subjects were assigned 1:1:1 to 300 mg secukinumab, 150 mg secukinumab, or placebo according to the aforementioned dosing schedule. In FIXTURE, participants were assigned 1:1:1:1, as with the first three groups in ERASURE and a fourth group who received etanercept twice 50 mg weekly until week 12, then once weekly was added. In ERASURE and FIXTURE respectively, PASI 75 responses were achieved at week 12 by 81.6 % and 77.1 % of subjects who received 300 mg, 71.6 % and 67.0 % who received 150 mg, and in 4.5 % and 4.9 % of those received placebo. PASI 75 responses were achieved by 44.0 % of subjects in the etanercept treatment arm of FIXTURE. In addition, maintenance of a PASI75 response was seen in the majority of patients in both studies, with a higher proportion of subjects with maintained response seen among those treated with the 300 mg dose of secukinumab than those treated with 150 mg or etanercept [13].

Emerging Therapies

Two other biologics targeting the IL-17 pathway (ixekizumab and brodalumab) are currently under investigation as well. Ixekizumab is a humanized IgG4 monoclonal antibody to IL-17 A. In a phase II double-blind, placebo-controlled study in which subjects were dosed subcutaneously at weeks 0, 2, 4, 8, 12, and 16, at a dose of 75 mg or 150 mg, a PASI 75 response was achieved in 82.8 and 82.1 % of subjects, respectively, who received ixekizumab and in 7.7 % of those who received placebo. Results were sustained out to week 20, and differences in efficacy were observed as early as 1 week after the first dose [25]. In an open-label extension, among those who initially responded to ixekizumab with a PASI 75 response, this response was maintained in 95 % of subjects at 52 weeks of treatment [26]. Brodalumab is a human monoclonal antibody that binds to the IL-17 receptor, thereby inhibiting signaling in the IL-17 pathway. In a phase II double-blind, placebo-controlled study, in which subjects were dosed subcutaneously with brodalumab or placebo at baseline and weeks 1, 2, 4, 6, 8,10, a PASI 75 response was achieved at week 12 by 77 and 82 % of subjects in the 140 and 210 mg dosing groups, respectively, and by 0 % of subjects in the placebo arm [27]. However, ongoing clinical trials of brodalumab were recently halted due to an unanticipated increase in suicidal ideation and suicides among patients taking brodalumab, although the known relationship between psoriasis and depression make establishing causality challenging [28].

Three drugs that specifically target IL-23 but not IL-12 (guselkumab, BI 655066, and tildrakizumab) are currently under investigation for the treatment of psoriasis. These monoclonal antibodies selectively bind to the p19 subunit that is unique to IL-23. In a double-blind, randomized, placebo-controlled trial of guselkumab in 24 patients, 50 % (10 mg), 60 % (30 and 100 mg), and 100 % (300 mg) of guselkumab-treated patients, but 0 % of placebo-treated patients, achieved a PASI 75 response at week 12 after a single dose of drug, and responses were maintained in most patients out to week 24 [29]. In a double-blind, randomized, placebo-controlled trial of 39 subjects dosed with BI 655066, given as a single intravenous or subcutaneous dose, PASI 75 responses were seen in 87 % of those patients who received active drug, but in none who received placebo, Doses ranged from 0.01 to 5 mg/kg IV, and 0.25 to 1 mg/kg subcutaneously, and clinical improvement was observed up to 66 weeks following treatment [30]. For both drugs, adverse event rates were similar among the placebo and drug-treated groups [29, 30]. In a 77-subject phase I, dose-escalation study, 13/14 subjects treated with 10 mg/kg tildrakizumab intravenously at days 1, 28, and 56 achieved a PASI75 response by day 112 [31].

Comparing Efficacy Among the Biologics

Until recently, few head-to-studies existed that compared new psoriasis therapies to existing treatments. However, this has begun to change in recent years. The CHAMPION study showed that the efficacy of adalimumab was superior to that of methotrexate [9]. In the ACCEPT study, a head-to-head study comparing the efficacy of ustekinumab and etanercept, a PASI75 response was achieved at week 12 by 67.5 % of patients who received 45 mg of ustekinumab, 73.8 % of patients who received 90 mg, and 56.8 % of those who received etanercept. The response to both doses of usekinumab was statistically superior to the response to etanercept [32]. In the FIXTURE study, the efficacy of secukinumab was shown to be statistically superior to that of etanercept [13]. In two studies, UNCOVER-2 and UNCOVER-3, patients were randomized to receive either placebo, etanercept (at a dose of 50 mg twice weekly), or ixekizumab (at an initial dose of 160 mg followed by a dose of 80 mg either every 2 or 4 week). At week 12 PASI 75 responses in UNCOVER-2 and UNCOVER-3 for placebo were 2.4 % and 7.3 %, respectively; for etanercept were 41.6 % and 53.4 %, respectively; for ixekizumab every 4 weeks were 77.5 % and 84.2 %, respectively; and for ixekizumab every 2 weeks were 89.7 % and 87.3 %, respectively.

In the absence of head-to-head comparisons, meta-analyses can provide useful information. In one such study of biologics which adjusted for cross-trial differences and placebo response rates, the estimated probability of a PASI75 response was highest for infliximab 5 mg/kg at 80.5 % (95 % CI 74.8–85.7). It was 72.5 % (95 % CI 66.1–78.3) with ustekinumab 90 mg; 67.5 % (95 % CI 60.7–73.9) with ustekinumab 45 mg; 66.2 % (95 % CI 57.3–73.3) with adalimumab 40 mg; and 51.9 % (95 % CI 45.7–58.4) with etanercept 50 mg (all at FDA- and EMA-approved doses) [33].

Combining Biologic and Other Psoriasis Therapies

Often, patients will require a combination of two or more psoriasis treatments. Topical therapies, including topical steroids and vitamin D3 analogs, can generally be combined with any biologic therapy and are a good option for the treatment of recalcitrant plaques. Methotrexate is frequently used in combination with biologics, particularly TNF-α antagonists. In one study, the combination of methotrexate and etanercept was found to be superior to treatment with etanercept alone [34]. Few studies have examined the efficacy of using phototherapy together with biologics. In two randomized studies of etanercept as monotherapy vs. with concomitant narrow band UVB (NB-UVB), there was not a significant benefit to adding phototherapy in terms of patients reaching PASI75 responses [35]. In a split body study in which patients were given ustekinumab and NB-UVB for half of their body, the half of the body treated with NB-UVB saw an 82 % mean PASI reduction compared with a 54 % mean PASI reduction in the other half of the body at week 6 [36]. It should be noted, however, that the ustekinumab prescribing information recommends against the concurrent use of phototherapy due to a theoretical increase in risk of skin cancer. There are no randomized studies to support the concurrent use of biologics with acitretin or cyclosporine, although limited case reports and series suggest these combinations may be beneficial in some patients [37].

Safety Issues for Specific Agents

TNF-α Antagonists

One of the risks of treatment with TNF-α antagonists is an increased risk of infection. Of particular concern is reactivation of latent tuberculosis, so it is standard to screen for latent tuberculosis in all patients prior to initiating therapy with any of the biologic agents. One review of the biologics found that the risk of serious infections per 100 patient-years of treatment was 0.9–1.6 for etanercept, 1.5–2.0 for adalimumab, and 1.8–2.4 for infliximab [38]. Data from patients with psoriasis enrolled in one registry shows that serious infections are more common with infliximab use than with other TNF-α inhibitor (adalimumab, etanercept) use (2.73/100 person years), and that TNF-α inhibitor use is a risk factor for major infection (1.80/100 person years) compared to no TNF-α inhibitor use. Data from the British Society of Rheumatology Biologics Register (BSRBR) showed that there was a small but significant increase in risk of infection in those who took TNF antagonists vs. standard disease modifying agents of rheumatic diseases (DMARDs), with an adjusted hazard ration of 1.2 (95 % CI 1.1, 1.5), and that this risk is greatest in the first

6 month after initiating treatment [39]. Patients on TNF antagonists area also at increased risk of zoster, with a hazard ratio, compared to treatment with standard DMARDs alone, of 1.8 (95 % CI 1.2–2.8) [40]. While suppression of the immune response with biologic therapy raises the concern of increased risk of malignancy, experience in the rheumatoid arthritis (RA) population found no increased risk of solid organ malignancy among patients treated with TNF antagonists vs. those treated with standard DMARDs [41]. Other uncommon serious potential complications of TNF-α use include worsening of congestive heart failure, central and peripheral demyelinating disease, and drug-induced lupus [42].

One side effect of TNF-α therapy is the paradoxical induction of psoriatic skin lesions in patients treated with these drugs for other indications such as inflammatory bowel disease, rheumatoid arthritis, or ankylosing spondylitis. The incidence of TNF antagonist-induced psoriasiform disease in these patients is unknown, but it is relatively rare. Skin lesions generally develop several months to years after starting therapy and may clinically be eczematous, plaque-like, or primarily palmoplantar in presentation. Treatment of TNF-antagonist induced therapy can be challenging, particularly if the patient is seeing other benefits from the medication due to improvement in their rheumatologic or gastrointestinal disease. Cessation of the TNF-antagonist usually, but not always, will result in improvement in skin disease. In some cases, switching medications within the class is helpful. In many cases skin disease is improved with the addition of topical steroids and/or methotrexate [43–45]. The mechanism by which this paradoxical induction of psoriasis occurs is not well-defined, however there is some evidence that other cytokines that are known to be involved in the pathogenesis of psoriasis, such as interferon alpha, IL-17, and IL-23, are increased in the skin of patients exposed to TNF antagonists [43, 46].

IL-12/23 Antagonists

The most concerning potential risk of IL-12/23 inhibitors is increased risk of major adverse cardiovascular events (MACEs). Despite impressive efficacy, the IL-12/23 p40 antagonist briakinumab was ultimately withdrawn from further investigation due to an observed increase in MACEs in treated subjects in early clinical trials. A meta-analysis pooling the data from published studies of briakinumab and ustekinumab showed that 10 of 3179 patients receiving anti-IL-12/23 therapies experienced MACEs; no events were seen in 1474 patients receiving placebo. Notably, however, this difference did not reach statistical significance [47]. Analysis of a large registry of over 12,095 psoriasis patients, of whom 3,308 had ever received ustekinimab, did not show an increased risk of MACE events relative to patients who received other psoriasis therapy. However, this was not a randomized study, reported results were not age-adjusted, and patients on ustekinumab were younger than those on non-biologic therapy [48].

Risk of infection is another major consideration with these agents. There are a few individuals who lack p40 entirely due to mutations in the *IL12B* gene, and these individuals have increased susceptibility to infection with Salmonella species, bacteria Calmette–Guérin (BCG), and other non-tuberculous mycobacteria. Although no cases of these infections have been observed in clinical studies, they are still considered theoretical risks, and patients taking ustekinumab are advised to avoid vaccination with BCG.

IL-17 Antagonists

Cases of mucocutaneous candidiasis and neutropenia have been reported in patients taking IL-17 pathway antagonists, although none were serious or required systemic therapy [13, 25, 27]. Deficiency of IL-17RA and IL-17 F is associated with the development of chronic mucocutaneous candidiasis, warranting concern about the risk of candida infection when the IL-17 pathway is blocked in the treatment of psoriasis [49]. In one clinical trial studying the efficacy of secukinumab as a treatment for Crohn's disease, there was a trend toward worsening disease in those patients randomized to receive secukinumab [50]. Thus, secukinumab carries a warning that it should be used with caution in patients with active Crohn's disease. Although clinical trials of the IL-17 receptor antagonist brodalumab have been halted due to a noted increase in suicidality and suicides among treated patients, similar findings have not been noted to date with other antagonists of the IL-17 pathway.

Immunogenicity of Biologics

Immunogenicity refers to the ability of a substance (i.e. antigen, epitope) to cause a humoral or cell-mediated immune response. Biologic therapies are immunogenic because they are foreign proteins, and the development of anti-drug antibodies (ADAs) can reduce the therapeutic response to these medications. There are two primary mechanisms through which this can occur: neutralization of drug activity through the formation of antibodies that bind to the antigen binding portion of the biologic, thus directly interfering with the drug's therapeutic activity (e.g., the majority of biologics, which are antibodies), or non-neutralizing antibodies that increase drug clearance by binding to a portion of the drug that is not essential for its therapeutic activity (e.g., to a new epitope like the fusion portion of etanercept). The most immunogenic biologic therapy for psoriasis is infliximab, a result of being 25 % of murine origin. The EXPRESS II study showed that anti-infliximab antibodies had formed in 35.8 % of patients treated with the currently FDA approved dose of infliximab (5 mg/kg) and in 51.5 % of those received a lower dose, 3 mg/kg. Additionally, ADAs were more common in the group treated with infliximab as needed as opposed to continuously (41.5 % vs. 35.8 %) [18]. Humanized monoclonal antibodies also induce ADAs, albeit less frequently. In the PHOENIX I AND II studies, anti-ustekinumab antibodies had formed in 13.6 % of patients treated with ustekinumab 90 mg and in 18.4 % of those who received a lower dose, 45 mg [51]. It is also important to note that immunogenicity can be dynamic. In one study, 28 % of patients treated with adalimumab had anti-adalimumab antibod-

ies at 3 years, but only 67 % of them had these antibodies at 28 weeks [52].

ADAs not only have the ability to decrease drug activity against psoriasis, but also may result in serious or even life-threatening infusion reactions or anaphylaxis. Prevention would be the best way to manage this problem, but the question of who is likely to develop ADAs remains unclear. Outside the rare case of an infusion reaction, it is difficult for the dermatologist to know which patients have developed ADAs. ADAs usually develop within the first 6 months of treatment and are more common with lower doses of drug. Methotrexate may decrease the production of antidrug antibodies in patients taking biologics which may help to diminish loss of response to these drugs over time [52].

Extracutaneous Effects of Biologics

There are several potential health benefits of biologics, beyond their impact on skin disease severity. Several studies have demonstrated an association between psoriasis and metabolic syndrome (including obesity, hypertension, and hyperlipidemia), and treatment with biologics, as well as methotrexate, may decrease the risk of cardiovascular adverse events [53]. In patients with rheumatoid arthritis or psoriasis, starting a TNF-antagonist decreases the risk of subsequently developing type II diabetes (hazard ratio: 0.62 (95 % CI, 0.42–0.91) compared to those patients not treated with a TNF-antagonist) [54]. Another study found that patients with psoriasis treated with a TNF inhibitor had 50 % less risk of cardiovascular disease than those treated with topical medicines [55].

Psoriasis patients are also more likely than members of the general population to suffer from depression. One study found that using validated questionnaires, the prevalence of depressive symptoms among patients with psoriasis is 28 % [28]. Population-based studies show that psoriasis patients are at least one and a half times more likely to experience depression and over four time more likely to use antidepressants than are control patients [28]. In clinical trials of adalimumab, there were significant reductions in depression symptom scores at follow-up compared with baseline and no significant reduction in the placebo groups [56]. In one study comparing etanercept with placebo, subjects treated with etanercept had statistically significantly greater improvement in scores measuring depression and fatigue than did those subjects treated with placebo [57]. In a study comparing ustekinumab with placebo, there was a significantly lower proportion of people meeting the Hospital and Anxiety Depression Scale criteria for depression in the ustekinumab group vs. the placebo group after 12 weeks [56].

Patients with psoriasis frequently complain of pruritus. Use of etanercept is associated with a significant decrease in itch scores at week 12 and week 24, which also correlated with an improvement in quality of life [58]. Results of a phase III study showed a statistically significant reduction in psoriasis-related pruritus with adalimumab, but not placebo [59]. In one small open-label study, treatment with infliximab was also associated with a reduction in pruritus [2]. Ixikizumab has also been shown to reduce itching, with the degree of reduction in pruritus correlating with improvement life quality as measured by the DLQI.

serology (for hepatitis B surface antigen, surface antibody, and core antibody) [60], a complete blood count (CBC), and liver transaminases. Most guidelines recommend that the CBC and liver transaminases be repeated every 6 months [61]. For patients who have evidence of past, acute, or chronic hepatitis B, a biologic should only be started in collaboration with the patient's hepatologist [60].

It is recommended that, if possible, patients receive updated vaccinations, preferably with a lead time of at least 1 month, prior to starting a biologic. The reasons for this are three-fold. First, the immune response to vaccines may be diminished in patients taking biologics. Second, patients may be at increased risk of some infections, particularly zoster, while taking biologics. Finally, there is a theoretical risk of infection with a vaccine strain pathogen associated with giving a live vaccine to a patient who is on a biologic. The two live vaccines most likely to be offered to psoriasis patients are the intranasal influenza vaccine and the zoster vaccine (for patients 60 years and older). Given the increased risk of developing zoster associated with use of TNF-α antagonists, vaccination against this in patients 60 or older prior to starting a biologic is strongly recommended [61].

Monitoring Patients on Biologics

While biologics are generally safe, the risk of infection, particularly reactivation of latent tuberculosis, is well-documented. In addition, patients with chronic hepatitis B are at risk of developing fulminant infection when treated with TNF-antagonists. Further, lab abnormalities are rare but can occur and the use of biologics has been associated with isolated pancytopenias as well as elevated transaminases. Prior to starting any biologic, patients should be screened for latent tuberculosis, generally with a tuberculin skin test (TST) or interferon gamma release assay (IGRA). It is recommended that this testing be repeated annually while the patient is taking a biologic. Additional testing appropriate prior to starting a biologic appropriate includes baseline hepatitis B

Special Patient Populations and Consideration in the Use of Biologics for Psoriasis

Use of Biologics in Pregnancy

There is relatively little data on the impact on the mother or fetus of biologic use during pregnancy, though they are currently pregnancy FDA category B drugs based on animal data. A review of the FDA database of spontaneously reported adverse events associated with etanercept, infliximab, and adalimumab during pregnancy during a 7 year period found that 41 children born to mothers who took one of these medications had a birth defect that can be associated with a syndrome of vertebral abnormalities, anal atresia, cardiac defect, tracheoesophageal, renal, and limp abnormalities (VACTERL) [62]. This study gained a lot of interest, but these finding were not confirmed in a controlled study using a population based congenital anomalies database [63]. Results from the British Society of Rheumatology Biologics Register show that among patients with rheumatic disease who because pregnant, 24 % 12 of women exposed to anti-TNF therapy only at the time of conception, 17 % 10 of those formerly exposed to anti-TNF therapy, and 10 % 1 of those with no history of exposure to anti-TNF therapy had spontaneous abortion. Statistical significance was not reported due to small sample size [64]. Other considerations for the use of biologics in pregnancy are that most biologics have an IgG1-based Fc structure. Because IgG1 can cross the placenta, fetal exposure to drug is likely. Data from patients taking TNF-α antagonists for inflammatory bowel disease (IBD) showed that there is high trans-placental transmission of infliximab and [65] adalimumab, but not of certolizumab which contains the Fab, but not the Fc portion, of the molecule [66]. One systematic review found no association between administration of TNF inhibitors for IBD during pregnancy and adverse pregnancy outcome or congenital abnormalities as well as no increased relative risk of infections in the first year of life in offspring of mothers who received biologics [67]. However, there is one case report of fatal disseminated BCG in an infant who was born to a mother taking infliximab and subsequently vaccinated with BCG at 3 months of age [68]. Thus, caution should be exercised in using live attenuated vaccines in infants with *in utero* exposure to biologics.

Use of Biologics in Patients with Viral Hepatitis

Patients with psoriasis who are also infected with hepatitis B and / or C often have limited systemic treatment options given the hepatotoxicity associated with many oral systemic therapies. While biologic therapies are appealing because of the limited hepatotoxicity associated with their use, there is concern about the potential risks associated with suppression of anti-viral immunity that may be associated by these drugs. However, no prospective studies have been performed to evaluate the safety of biologic therapy in patients with viral hepatitis. There is a small, although not negligible risk, or reactivation of hepatitis B in patients who have occult or inactive disease. Thus, it is recommended that individuals are screened for anti-hepatitis B core antibody, hepatitis B surface antigen, and anti-hepatitis B surface antibody (HBcAb, HBSAg, and HBsAb, respectively). Patients with acute hepatitis B (HBsAg+, HBcAb+, HBSAb-) should not be treated with TNF antagonists. Patients with resolved, chronic, or occult disease should be tested for hepatitis B e antigen and antibody and should have HBV DNA levels quantified and consultation with a hepatologist should occur prior to treatment. Very little is known about the safety of ustekinumab and other biologics in patients with hepatitis B [60]. Retrospective data suggest that TNF antagonists, particularly etanercept and adalimumab, are relatively safe in patients with hepatitis C and these are commonly used in this patient population; little is known about the safety of others biologics in patients with hepatitis C [69].

Use of Biologics in Patients Who Travel Internationally

For the patient who travels who internationally, several factors should be taken into consideration. Because biologics require refrigeration, this should be taken into consideration and the frequent traveler may find use of a biologic that is dosed less frequently, such as ustekinumab, more convenient as it would not need to be transported and stored if the trip were under 3 months in duration. For travel to certain locations, vaccination against yellow fever, which is a live attenuated vaccine, is recommended. In general, it is recommended that biologic therapy be stopped for a period of time before and after such vaccines, although there are not clear guidelines on the duration for which therapy should be held. Vaccination against hepatitis B is also particularly important for patients treated with biologics. Traveler to areas in which tuberculosis is endemic should exercise caution and should be screened for symptoms of new onset tuberculosis. Finally, given the risk of food-borne illnesses such as salmonella and listeria in patients taking biologics, particularly TNF antagonists, it is important that these patients avoid undercooked food in general, but particularly in areas in which food safety practices may be questionable [70].

Conclusions

Biologic therapy has revolutionized the treatment of psoriasis. These drugs are generally highly effective and relatively safe, with the major risk being an increased rate of infection among treated patients. It is important to note that these drugs are very expensive and thus their use is generally limited to patients who have failed or have a contraindication to other systemic therapies for psoriasis. However, they fill an important therapeutic niche and are an option for those patients who have failed or have contraindications to other systemic therapies.

References

1. Wee JS, Petrof G, Jackson K, et al. Infliximab for the treatment of psoriasis in the U.K.: 9 years' experience of infusion reactions at a single centre. Br J Dermatol. 2012;167:411–6. doi:10.1111/j.1365-2133.2012.10931.x.
2. Schopf RE, Aust H, Knop J. Treatment of psoriasis with the chimeric monoclonal antibody against tumor necrosis factor alpha, infliximab. J Am Acad Dermatol. 2002;46:886–91.
3. Chaudhari U, Romano P, Mulcahy LD, et al. Efficacy and safety of infliximab monotherapy for plaque-type psoriasis: a randomised trial. Lancet. 2001;357:1842–7.
4. Leonardi CL, Powers JL, Matheson RT, et al. Etanercept as monotherapy in patients with psoriasis. N Engl J Med. 2003;349:2014–22. doi:10.1056/NEJMoa030409.
5. Paller AS, Siegfried EC, Langley RG, et al. Etanercept treatment for children and adolescents with plaque psoriasis. N Engl J Med. 2008;358:241–51. doi:10.1056/NEJMoa066886.
6. Mease PJ, Goffe BS, Metz J, et al. Etanercept in the treatment of psoriatic arthritis and psoriasis: a randomised trial. Lancet. 2000;356:385–90. doi:10.1016/S0140-6736(00)02530-7.
7. Papp KA, Tyring S, Lahfa M, et al. A global phase III randomized controlled trial of etanercept in psoriasis: safety, efficacy, and effect of dose reduction. Br J Dermatol. 2005;152:1304–12. doi:10.1111/j.1365-2133.2005.06688.x.
8. Menter A, Tyring SK, Gordon K, et al. Adalimumab therapy for moderate to severe psoriasis: a randomized, controlled phase III trial. J Am Acad Dermatol. 2008;58:106–15. doi:10.1016/j.jaad.2007.09.010.
9. Saurat J-H, Stingl G, Dubertret L, et al. Efficacy and safety results from the randomized controlled comparative study of adalimumab vs. methotrexate vs. placebo in patients with psoriasis (CHAMPION). Br J Dermatol. 2008;158:558–66. doi:10.1111/j.1365-2133.2007.08315.x.
10. Mrowietz U, Kragballe K, Reich K, et al. An assessment of adalimumab efficacy in three Phase III clinical trials using the European Consensus Programme criteria for psoriasis treatment goals. Br J Dermatol. 2013;168:374–80. doi:10.1111/j.1365-2133.2012.11214.x.
11. Leonardi CL, Kimball AB, Papp KA, et al. Efficacy and safety of ustekinumab, a human interleukin-12/23 monoclonal antibody, in patients with psoriasis: 76-week results from a randomised, double-blind, placebo-controlled trial (PHOENIX 1). Lancet. 2008;371:1665–74. doi:10.1016/S0140-6736(08)60725-4.
12. Papp KA, Langley RG, Lebwohl M, et al. Efficacy and safety of ustekinumab, a human interleukin-12/23 monoclonal antibody, in patients with psoriasis: 52-week results from a randomised, double-blind, placebo-controlled trial (PHOENIX 2). Lancet. 2008;371:1675–84. doi:10.1016/S0140-6736(08)60726-6.
13. Langley RG, Elewski BE, Lebwohl M, et al. Secukinumab in plaque psoriasis – results of two phase 3 trials. N Engl J Med. 2014;371:326–38. doi:10.1056/NEJMoa1314258.
14. Baliwag J, Barnes DH, Johnston A. Cytokines in psoriasis. Cytokine. 2015. doi:10.1016/j.cyto.2014.12.014.
15. Oh CJ, Das KM, Gottlieb AB. Treatment with anti-tumor necrosis factor alpha (TNF-alpha) monoclonal antibody dramatically decreases the clinical activity of psoriasis lesions. J Am Acad Dermatol. 2000;42:829–30.
16. Reich K, Nestle FO, Papp K, et al. Infliximab induction and maintenance therapy for moderate-to-severe psoriasis: a phase III, multicentre, double-blind trial. Lancet. 2005;366:1367–74. doi:10.1016/S0140-6736(05)67566-6.
17. De Vries ACQ, Bogaards NA, Hooft L, et al. Interventions for nail psoriasis. Cochrane Database Syst Rev. 2013;1:CD007633. doi:10.1002/14651858.CD007633.pub2.
18. Menter A, Feldman SR, Weinstein GD, et al. A randomized comparison of continuous vs. intermittent infliximab maintenance regimens over 1 year in the treatment of moderate-to-severe plaque psoriasis. J Am Acad Dermatol. 2007;56:31.e1. doi:10.1016/j.jaad.2006.07.017.

19. Bagel J, Lynde C, Tyring S, et al. Moderate to severe plaque psoriasis with scalp involvement: a randomized, double-blind, placebo-controlled study of etanercept. J Am Acad Dermatol. 2012;67:86–92. doi:10.1016/j.jaad.2011.07.034.

20. Ortonne JP, Paul C, Berardesca E, et al. A 24-week randomized clinical trial investigating the efficacy and safety of two doses of etanercept in nail psoriasis. Br J Dermatol. 2013;168:1080–7. doi:10.1111/bjd.12060.

21. Thaçi D, Unnebrink K, Sundaram M, et al. Adalimumab for the treatment of moderate to severe psoriasis: subanalysis of effects on scalp and nails in the BELIEVE study. J Eur Acad Dermatol Venereol. 2015;29:353–60. doi:10.1111/jdv.12553.

22. Kavanaugh A, McInnes I, Mease P, et al. Golimumab, a new human tumor necrosis factor alpha antibody, administered every four weeks as a subcutaneous injection in psoriatic arthritis: twenty-four-week efficacy and safety results of a randomized, placebo-controlled study. Arthritis Rheum. 2009;60:976–86. doi:10.1002/art.24403.

23. Reich K, Ortonne J-P, Gottlieb AB, et al. Successful treatment of moderate to severe plaque psoriasis with the PEGylated Fab' certolizumab pegol: results of a phase II randomized, placebo-controlled trial with a re-treatment extension. Br J Dermatol. 2012;167:180–90. doi:10.1111/j.1365-2133.2012.10941.x.

24. Rich P, Bourcier M, Sofen H, et al. Ustekinumab improves nail disease in patients with moderate-to-severe psoriasis: results from PHOENIX 1. Br J Dermatol. 2014;170:398–407. doi:10.1111/bjd.12632.

25. Leonardi C, Matheson R, Zachariae C, et al. Anti-interleukin-17 monoclonal antibody ixekizumab in chronic plaque psoriasis. N Engl J Med. 2012;366:1190–9. doi:10.1056/NEJMoa1109997.

26. Gordon KB, Leonardi CL, Lebwohl M, et al. A 52-week, open-label study of the efficacy and safety of ixekizumab, an anti-interleukin-17A monoclonal antibody, in patients with chronic plaque psoriasis. J Am Acad Dermatol. 2014;71:1176–82. doi:10.1016/j.jaad.2014.07.048.

27. Papp KA, Leonardi C, Menter A, et al. Brodalumab, an anti-interleukin-17-receptor antibody for psoriasis. N Engl J Med. 2012;366:1181–9. doi:10.1056/NEJMoa1109017.

28. Dowlatshahi EA, Wakkee M, Arends LR, Nijsten T. The prevalence and odds of depressive symptoms and clinical depression in psoriasis patients: a systematic review and meta-analysis. J Invest Dermatol. 2014;134:1542–51. doi:10.1038/jid.2013.508.

29. Sofen H, Smith S, Matheson RT, et al. Guselkumab (an IL-23-specific mAb) demonstrates clinical and molecular response in patients with moderate-to-severe psoriasis. J Allergy Clin Immunol. 2014;133:1032–40. doi:10.1016/j.jaci.2014.01.025.

30. Krueger JG, Ferris LK, Menter A, et al. Anti-IL-23A mAb BI 655066 for treatment of moderate-to-severe psoriasis: safety, efficacy, pharmacokinetics, and biomarker results of a single-rising-dose, randomized, double-blind, placebo-controlled trial. J Allergy Clin Immunol. 2015. doi:10.1016/j.jaci.2015.01.018.

31. Kopp T, Riedl E, Bangert C, et al. Clinical improvement in psoriasis with specific targeting of interleukin-23. Nature. 2015. doi:10.1038/nature14175.

32. Griffiths CEM, Strober BE, van de Kerkhof P, et al. Comparison of ustekinumab and etanercept for moderate-to-severe psoriasis. N Engl J Med. 2010;362:118–28. doi:10.1056/NEJMoa0810652.

33. Signorovitch JE, Betts KA, Yan YS, et al. Comparative efficacy of biological treatments for moderate-to-severe psoriasis: a network meta-analysis adjusting for cross-trial differences in reference arm response. Br J Dermatol. 2015;172:504–12. doi:10.1111/bjd.13437.

34. Gottlieb AB, Langley RG, Strober BE, et al. A randomized, double-blind, placebo-controlled study to evaluate the addition of methotrexate to etanercept in patients with moderate to severe plaque psoriasis. Br J Dermatol. 2012;167:649–57. doi:10.1111/j.1365-2133.2012.11015.x.

35. Lynde CW, Gupta AK, Guenther L, et al. A randomized study comparing the combination of nbUVB and etanercept to etanercept monotherapy in patients with psoriasis who do not exhibit an excellent response after 12 weeks of etanercept. J Dermatolog Treat. 2012;23:261–7. doi:10.3109/09546634.2011.607795.

36. Wolf P, Weger W, Legat FJ, et al. Treatment with 311-nm ultraviolet B enhanced response of psoriatic lesions in ustekinumab-treated patients: a randomized intraindividual trial. Br J Dermatol. 2012;166:147–53. doi:10.1111/j.1365-2133.2011.10616.x.

37. Armstrong AW, Bagel J, Van Voorhees AS, et al. Combining biologic therapies with other systemic treatments in psoriasis: evidence-based, best-practice recommendations from the medical board of the national psoriasis foundation. JAMA Dermatol. 2014. doi:10.1001/jamadermatol.2014.3456.

38. Mansouri Y, Goldenberg G. Biologic safety in psoriasis: review of long-term safety data. J Clin Aesthet Dermatol. 2015;8:30–42.

39. Galloway JB, Hyrich KL, Mercer LK, et al. Anti-TNF therapy is associated with an increased risk of serious infections in patients with rheumatoid arthritis especially in the first 6 months of treatment: updated results from the British Society for Rheumatology Biologics Register with special emph. Rheumatology (Oxford). 2011;50:124–31. doi:10.1093/rheumatology/keq242.

40. Galloway JB, Mercer LK, Moseley A, et al. Risk of skin and soft tissue infections (including shingles) in patients exposed to anti-tumour necrosis factor therapy: results from the British Society for Rheumatology Biologics Register. Ann Rheum Dis. 2013;72:229–34. doi:10.1136/annrheumdis-2011-201108.

41. Mercer LK, Lunt M, Low ALS, et al. Risk of solid cancer in patients exposed to anti-tumour necrosis factor therapy: results from the British Society for Rheumatology Biologics Register for Rheumatoid Arthritis. Ann Rheum Dis. 2014. doi:10.1136/annrheumdis-2013-204851.

42. Semble AL, Davis SA, Feldman SR. Safety and tolerability of tumor necrosis factor-α inhibitors in psoriasis: a narrative review. Am J Clin Dermatol. 2014;15:37–43. doi:10.1007/s40257-013-0053-5.

43. Collamer AN, Battafarano DF. Psoriatic skin lesions induced by tumor necrosis factor antagonist therapy: clinical features and possible immunopathogenesis. Semin Arthritis Rheum. 2010;40:233–40. doi:10.1016/j.semarthrit.2010.04.003.

44. Joyau C, Veyrac G, Dixneuf V, Jolliet P. Anti-tumour necrosis factor alpha therapy and increased risk of de novo psoriasis: is it really a paradoxical side effect? Clin Exp Rheumatol. 2012;30:700–6.

45. Nguyen K, Vleugels RA, Velez NF, et al. Psoriasiform reactions to anti-tumor necrosis factor α therapy. J Clin Rheumatol. 2013;19:377–81. doi:10.1097/RHU.0b013e3182a702e8.

46. Włodarczyk M, Sobolewska A, Wójcik B, et al. Correlations between skin lesions induced by anti-tumor necrosis factor-α and selected cytokines in Crohn's disease patients. World J Gastroenterol. 2014;20:7019–26. doi:10.3748/wjg.v20.i22.7019.

47. Ryan C, Leonardi CL, Krueger JG, et al. Association between biologic therapies for chronic plaque psoriasis and cardiovascular events: a meta-analysis of randomized controlled trials. JAMA. 2011;306:864–71. doi:10.1001/jama.2011.1211.

48. Gottlieb AB, Kalb RE, Langley RG, et al. Safety observations in 12095 patients with psoriasis enrolled in an international registry (PSOLAR): experience with infliximab and other systemic and biologic therapies. J Drugs Dermatol. 2014;13:1441–8.

49. Puel A, Cypowyj S, Bustamante J, et al. Chronic mucocutaneous candidiasis in humans with inborn errors of interleukin-17 immunity. Science. 2011;332:65–8. doi:10.1126/science.1200439.

50. Hueber W, Sands BE, Lewitzky S, et al. Secukinumab, a human anti-IL-17A monoclonal antibody, for moderate to severe Crohn's disease: unexpected results of a randomised, double-blind placebo-controlled trial. Gut. 2012;61:1693–700. doi:10.1136/gutjnl-2011-301668.

51. Lebwohl M, Yeilding N, Szapary P, et al. Impact of weight on the efficacy and safety of ustekinumab in patients with moderate to severe psoriasis: rationale for dosing recommendations. J Am Acad Dermatol. 2010;63:571–9. doi:10.1016/j.jaad.2009.11.012.

52. Lecluse LLA, Driessen RJB, Spuls PI, et al. Extent and clinical consequences of antibody formation against adalimumab in patients with plaque psoriasis. Arch Dermatol. 2010;146:127–32. doi:10.1001/archdermatol.2009.347.

53. Roubille C, Richer V, Starnino T, et al. The effects of tumour necrosis factor inhibitors, methotrexate, non-steroidal anti-inflammatory drugs and corticosteroids on cardiovascular events in rheumatoid arthritis, psoriasis and psoriatic arthritis: a systematic review and meta-analysis. Ann Rheum Dis. 2015;74:480–9. doi:10.1136/annrheumdis-2014-206624.

54. Solomon DH, Massarotti E, Garg R, et al. Association between disease-modifying antirheumatic drugs and diabetes risk in patients with rheumatoid arthritis and psoriasis. JAMA. 2011;305:2525–31. doi:10.1001/jama.2011.878.

55. Wu JJ, Poon K-YT, Channual JC, Shen AY-J. Association between tumor necrosis factor inhibitor therapy and myocardial infarction risk in patients with psoriasis. Arch Dermatol. 2012;148:1244–50. doi:10.1001/archdermatol.2012.2502.

56. Fleming P, Roubille C, Richer V, et al. Effect of biologics on depressive symptoms in patients with psoriasis: a systematic review. J Eur Acad Dermatol Venereol. 2014. doi:10.1111/jdv.12909.

57. Tyring S, Gottlieb A, Papp K, et al. Etanercept and clinical outcomes, fatigue, and depression in psoriasis: double-blind placebo-controlled randomised phase III trial. Lancet. 2006;367:29–35. doi:10.1016/S0140-6736(05)67763-X.

58. Mrowietz U, Chouela EN, Mallbris L, et al. Pruritus and quality of life in moderate-to-severe plaque psoriasis: post hoc explorative analysis from the PRISTINE study. J Eur Acad Dermatol Venereol. 2014. doi:10.1111/jdv.12761.

59. Revicki DA, Willian MK, Menter A, et al. Impact of adalimumab treatment on patient-reported outcomes: results from a Phase III clinical trial in patients with moderate to severe plaque psoriasis. J Dermatolog Treat. 2007;18:341–50. doi:10.1080/09546630701646172.

60. Motaparthi K, Stanisic V, Van Voorhees AS, et al. From the Medical Board of the National Psoriasis Foundation: recommendations for screening for hepatitis B infection prior to initiating anti-tumor necrosis factor-alfa inhibitors or other immunosuppressive agents in patients with psoriasis. J Am Acad Dermatol. 2014;70:178–86. doi:10.1016/j.jaad.2013.08.049.

61. Lebwohl M, Bagel J, Gelfand JM, et al. From the Medical Board of the National Psoriasis Foundation: monitoring and vaccinations in patients treated with biologics for psoriasis. J Am Acad Dermatol. 2008;58:94–105. doi:10.1016/j.jaad.2007.08.030.

62. Carter JD, Ladhani A, Ricca LR, et al. A safety assessment of tumor necrosis factor antagonists during pregnancy: a review of the food and drug administration database. J Rheumatol. 2009;36:635–41. doi:10.3899/jrheum.080545.

63. Crijns HJMJ, Jentink J, Garne E, et al. The distribution of congenital anomalies within the VACTERL association among tumor necrosis factor antagonist-exposed pregnancies is similar to the general population. J Rheumatol. 2011;38:1871–4. doi:10.3899/jrheum.101316.

64. Verstappen SMM, King Y, Watson KD, et al. Anti-TNF therapies and pregnancy: outcome of 130 pregnancies in the British Society for Rheumatology Biologics Register. Ann Rheum Dis. 2011;70:823–6. doi:10.1136/ard.2010.140822.

65. Scarpa R, Manguso F, D'Arienzo A, et al. Microscopic inflammatory changes in colon of patients with both active psoriasis and psoriatic arthritis without bowel symptoms. J Rheumatol. 2000;27:1241–6.

66. Mahadevan U, Wolf DC, Dubinsky M, et al. Placental transfer of anti-tumor necrosis factor agents in

pregnant patients with inflammatory bowel disease. Clin Gastroenterol Hepatol. 2013;11:286–92; quiz e24. doi:10.1016/j.cgh.2012.11.011.

67. Nielsen OH, Loftus EV, Jess T. Safety of TNF-α inhibitors during IBD pregnancy: a systematic review. BMC Med. 2013;11:174. doi:10.1186/1741-7015-11-174.

68. Cheent K, Nolan J, Shariq S, et al. Case report: fatal case of disseminated BCG infection in an infant born to a mother taking Infliximab for Crohn's disease. J Crohns Colitis. 2010;4:603–5. doi:10.1016/j.crohns.2010.05.001.

69. Pompili M, Biolato M, Miele L, Grieco A. Tumor necrosis factor-α inhibitors and chronic hepatitis C: a comprehensive literature review. World J Gastroenterol. 2013;19:7867–73. doi:10.3748/wjg.v19.i44.7867.

70. Davies R, Dixon WG, Watson KD, et al. Influence of anti-TNF patient warning regarding avoidance of high risk foods on rates of listeria and salmonella infections in the UK. Ann Rheum Dis. 2012;72:461–2. doi:10.1136/annrheumdis-2012-202228.

Biologic Therapy of Psoriatic Arthritis

29

Philip J. Mease

Abstract

Biologic medications, therapeutic proteins which inhibit or modulate pro-inflammatory immune cells and cytokines, have significantly altered our ability to effectively treat psoriatic arthritis (PsA). The first widely used biologics have been those targeting TNFα. Five agents, etanercept, infliximab, adalimumab, golimumab and certolizumab have shown significant benefit in all clinical domains of PsA including arthritis, enthesitis, dactylitis, spondylitis, skin and nail disease, as well as inhibiting progressive joint destruction, improving function and quality of life. Although the anti-TNFs have been significantly beneficial for the majority of patients, some may not respond and other may lose efficacy over time. Thus, it has been important to develop new medicines which target other key cytokines and immunologic pathways. Ustekinumab inhibits both IL12 and IL23 and thus is felt to work in both the TH1 and TH7 pathways of inflammation. This agent has been approved for the treatment of PsA. An emerging group of therapies, the IL17 inhibitors, have demonstrated significant effectiveness in psoriasis and also in musculoskeletal manifestations of PsA. Other medicines in development include the co-stimulatory blockade agent, abatacept and an emerging group of therapies which inhibit IL23. As modulators of immune cell function, these agents have the potential to increase risk for infection, as well as other side effects. These must be discussed with the patient and considered when determining overall risk benefit regarding their use. Treatment strategies such as treating PsA early in disease course to reduce damage risk, treating-to-target and tight control, use of background methotrexate to reduce immunogenicity, and various cost-saving strategies are all being tested with biologic medicines for PsA.

P.J. Mease, MD
Department of Rheumatology,
Swedish Medical Center,
601 Broadway, Suite 600, Seattle, WA 98122, USA
e-mail: pmease@philipmease.com

© Springer International Publishing Switzerland 2016
A. Adebajo et al. (eds.), *Psoriatic Arthritis and Psoriasis: Pathology and Clinical Aspects*,
DOI 10.1007/978-3-319-19530-8_29

Keywords

Psoriatic arthritis • Psoriasis • Biologics • TNF inhibition • IL12-23 inhibition • IL17 inhibition • IL23 inhibition

Introduction

Biologic therapy refers to use of parenterally administered (subcutaneous or intravenous) complex proteins which are biologically manufactured in mammalian or yeast cell lines, and typically function by binding to inflammatory cytokines or cell receptor sites to diminish immunologic cell function that is pro-inflammatory. Many biologics mimic human immunoglobulin structure. It is possible that antibodies may develop in the human recipient against the foreign protein which may diminish therapeutic effectiveness. This issue has been diminished by the creation of humanized or fully human therapeutic proteins, or by the concomitant use of medications such as methotrexate, which may reduce antibody formation. Prior to the introduction of biologic therapy for rheumatic diseases such as rheumatoid arthritis (RA) in the late 1990s, therapy of psoriatic arthritis (PsA) consisted primarily of synthetic medicinals such as methotrexate, sulfasalazine, and non-steroidal anti-inflammatory medications, along with adjunctive approaches including physical and occupational therapy [1, 2]. Although partially effective, these medicines were not typically able to achieve low disease activity or remission states and often were not well tolerated. The first biologic therapies to be studied and approved for the treatment of PsA were the TNFα inhibitors [1, 2]. These agents have literally revolutionized our ability to effectively treat all of the clinical manifestations of PsA, including arthritis, enthesitis, dactylitis, spondylitis, skin and nail disease as well as associated inflammatory bowel disease and uveitis. PsA treatment recommendations developed by international groups such as the Group for Research and Assessment of Psoriasis and Psoriatic Arthritis (GRAPPA) and the European League Against Rheumatism (EULAR) recommend the use of biologic agents for patients with moderate to severe disease [3, 4]. Sustained remission or low disease activity state is now achievable with these agents. With time, however, effectiveness may diminish and be lost, necessitating cycling between TNFα inhibitors or to agents with a different mechanism of action.

TNF Inhibition

TNFα was one of the first pro-inflammatory cytokines to be implicated in the pathogenesis of numerous inflammatory/autoimmune diseases. It is produced by several types of immune cells and activates a number of key effector cells involved in tissue inflammation and destruction in psoriasis and PsA including lymphocytes, macrophages, chondroctyes, osteoclasts, and keratinoctyes. There are now five agents which inhibit TNFα including etanercept, infliximab, adalimumab, golimumab and certolizumab (Fig. 29.1). These were first demonstrated to be effective in the treatment of rheumatoid arthritis, and subsequently have also shown effectiveness in PsA and ankylosing spondylitis (AS) [1, 2, 5]. Etanercept, infliximab and adalimumab are approved for the treatment of psoriasis and all five have demonstrated effectiveness in psoriasis. All except for etanercept are classified as monoclonal antibodies and have demonstrated effectiveness in inflammatory bowel disease, whereas etanercept has not. It also appears that these agents are effective in treating the associated condition, uveitis, although the data has been variably collected, including demonstration of fewer flares of uveitis than expected while these agents are used, especially the monoclonal antibody constructs. The effects of the individual agents in PsA are reviewed in the following section and American College of Rheumatology (ACR) 20/50/70 responses are summarized in Table 29.1 [1, 2, 5].

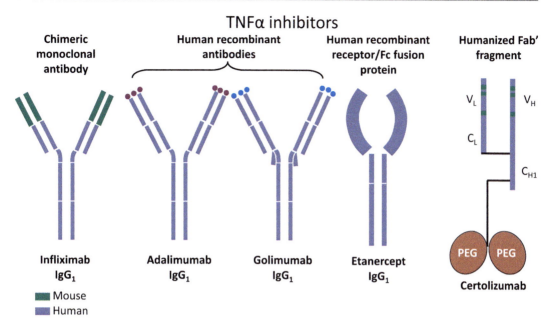

Fig. 29.1 TNFα inhibitors (Courtesy of Philip J. Mease, MD)

Table 29.1 Anti-TNF therapies in PsA: ACR responses

Trial	n	ACR 20 %		ACR 50 %		ACR 70 %	
		Rx	P	Rx	P	Rx	P
Adalimumab[a] [6]	315	58	14	36	4	20	1
Certolizumab[a] [7]	409	58	24	36	11	25	3
Etanercept[a] [8]	205	59	15	38	4	11	0
Golimumab[b] [9]	405	52	8	32	3.5	18	0.9
Antoni ref infliximab[b] [10]	200	58	11	36	3	15	1

[a]12 weeks
[b]14 weeks

Etanercept

Etanercept is a soluble receptor antibody administered subcutaneously 50 mg per week. Its efficacy in PsA was first demonstrated in an investigator-initiated trial of 60 patients [11], later confirmed in a phase 3 trial in 205 patients [8] (Table 29.1). Dosing in PsA is 50 mg subcutaneously weekly. This was the first anti-TNFα agent to be approved for PsA and was the first of this class to demonstrate ability to inhibit progressive joint damage as measured by serial radiographs of hands and feet [8]. Ability to improve enthesitis and dactylitis with this agent was demonstrated in the PRESTA study [12], in which the 50 mg weekly regimen was compared to 50 mg twice weekly for 12 weeks followed by 50 mg weekly in patients with moderate-to-severe arthritis and severe skin disease. The latter regimen is the approved regimen for this agent in psoriasis. Improvement of musculoskeletal domains (arthritis, enthesitis and dactylitis) was similar between these two dosage regimens. However, it was noted that skin manifestations of psoriasis were more effectively treated in the initial higher dose arm of the study. Etanercept can be administered with or without background methotrexate and durability of effectiveness does not appear to be affected by background methotrexate use, implying lesser tendency to immunogenicity [13].

Infliximab

Infliximab, an intravenously administered anti-TNFα agent, demonstrated effectiveness in a 200 patient study using 5 mg/kg every 2 months after a loading dose regimen [10]. As with other anti-TNFα agents, the multiple clinical domains of PsA improve significantly, including inhibition of structural damage (Table 29.1). This agent has a murine component, and may generate more immunogenicity with subsequent neutralization of effect over time. Thus, although it can be administered without background methotrexate, its efficacy may be more enduringly sustained if methotrexate is used concomitantly (Nor-DMARD study).

Adalimumab

Adalimumab is a fully human subcutaneously-administered anti-TNFα antibody given at a dose of 40 mg every other week. Its efficacy in PsA was established in the ADEPT trial of 313 patients [6] (Table 29.1). Sustained effectiveness has been demonstrated in various PsA clinical domains, including inhibition of structural damage and patient-reported outcomes of function, quality of life, and fatigue, as have other anti-TNFα agents [14]. Durability of effectiveness has been demonstrated with or without background methotrexate (NOR-DMARD).

Golimumab

Golimumab is an anti-TNFα antibody with a prolonged half-life, allowing for monthly subcutaneous administration, approved for PsA, in 50 mg dose based on a 405 patient study [9]. It is also available in intravenous formulation, although that is only approved for RA. Effectiveness in all clinical domains of PsA as well as long term efficacy through 5 years [9, 15], (Table 29.1).

Certolizumab

Certolizumab is a unique antibody composed of the Fab portion of an immunoglobulin molecule attached to two polyethylene glycol moieties to prolong half-life. It is administered subcutaneously at a dose of 200 mg every 2 weeks or 400 mg every 4 weeks. At 12 and 24 weeks In the RAPID-PsA trial, 405 patients were evaluated with both doses vs. placebo, showing statistically significant benefit in ACR responses (Table 29.1), as well as significant improvement in DAS28, HAQ-DI, enthesitis, dactylitis, skin and nail measures, inhibition of radiologic damage progression, as well as improvement in SF-36 and work productivity measures [7]. Uniquely in this study, 20 % of patients had been previously exposed to anti- TNFα therapy and similar degrees of response were seen in this group compared to anti- TNFα-naïve patients. Safety results were similar to other agents of this class.

Safety of TNFi

Detailed safety review of the TNFi class of medications is beyond the scope of this chapter, but a few key points can be described. As immuno-modulatory medications, an increased risk for infection, including serious infections, can be observed. In addition to bacterial infections, this can include opportunistic infections such as tuberculosis, invasive fungal infections such as histoplasmosis and coccidiodomycosis, and listeria and legionella. Other more rare potential side effects include risk for lymphoma and non-melanoma skin cancer, autoimmune reactions such as drug-induced lupus, psoriasis, or multiple sclerosis, hypersensitivity reactions, skin reactions, congestive heart failure, and hematologic aplasias. TNFi safety has been recently reviewed across disease indications in the context of one of the TNFi agents, adalimumab [16].

Co-stimulatory Blockade Modulating T Lymphocyte Function

Abatacept

Abatacept is a co-stimulatory blockade agent which inhibits T cell activation through second signal inhibition. Specifically it is a combination of the Fc portion of an immunoglobulin molecule and CTLA4, a natural inhibitor of the CD80-86 second signal molecule on an immune cell surface [15]. Abatacept is approved for rheumatoid arthritis. A phase 2 study of 170 PsA patients, using various doses of its intravenous formulation, demonstrated significant improvement of ACR20 response [17]. Magnetic resonance imaging (MRI) study of hands or feet at 24 weeks demonstrated improved synovitis, erosion, and osteitis scores. Skin psoriasis responses were modest. This agent is now in phase 3 development in its subcutaneous form in PsA. As with other immunomodulatory medications, abatacept can increase risk for infection.

IL-6 Inhibition

Like TNFα, IL-6 is a pleiotropic pro-inflammatory cytokine which has a significant role in RA and has been shown to be elevated in psoriasis skin lesions and PsA synovium [18]. Tocilizumab is an IL-6 receptor blocker approved for RA. There have been mixed results from case reports about its efficacy in PsA [19].

Clazakizumab

Clazakizumab is a direct IL-6 inhibitor that has shown efficacy in RA [20]. This agent was studied in a phase 2 dose ranging trial with 165 PsA patients, 70 % of whom were on background MTX [21]. ACR20 response was observed in 29/46/52/39 % of patients in the placebo/25 mg/100 mg/200 mg monthly groups at the Week 16 primary endpoint, which was statistically significant in the 100 mg group. PASI 75 responses were observed in 12/15/17/5 % of placebo/25 mg/100 mg/200 mg groups. Improvements in enthesitis and dactylitis were most noted in the 100 mg group. The safety profile was that expected for an IL-6 inhibiting agent. Thus, this trial did show an effect in musculoskeletal inflammation domains, supporting the concept that IL-6 inhibition may be helpful for this set of domains, but minimal effect for treatment of psoriasis lesions. The trial also

lacked a true dose effect given the underperformance of the 200 mg group, due partly to use of non-responder imputation analysis and a greater number of adverse effects and droputs in the higher dose group. As with other immunomodulatory agents, IL-6 inhibitors can increase risk for infection. Other potential side effects include elevation of liver enzymes, cholesterol, neutropenia and thrombocytopenia, intestinal perforation, and administration reactions.

B Lymphocyte Inhibition

Rituximab, a B lymphocyte ablating agent, has been approved for the treatment of RA and vasculitis. In RA, B lymphocytes play a prominent role and subsets of RA patients have significant B cell aggregation in synovial tissue, denoting a more severe phenotype. Although some B cell aggregation has been noted in PsA synovium [22], in general B cells are not considered to be important players in psoriasis or PsA pathogenesis. Small series of patients have been treated with rituximab [23, 24] and in general, although modest efficacy in arthritis has been demonstrated in such open label use, not enough efficacy has been demonstrated in joints or psoriasis skin lesions to lead to conduct of placebo-controlled studies of this agent in PsA. Side effects can include increased risk for infection as well as hypersensitivity/infusion reactions.

Targeting the TH17 Cell Axis in PsA

The cytokine interleukin 17A (IL-17A) was discovered in 1993 [25]. Since then, a family of related cytokines, IL-17A-F has been characterized, which led to the discovery, in 2005, of a distinct form of T cells, TH17, distinguished by their ability to produce a distinct repertoire of cytokines, including IL-17 s, IL-21, and IL-22 and not interferon-γ(IFN γ) or interleukin-4, which are reflective of TH1 and TH2 lineage cells [26–28] (Fig. 29.2). Since then, there has been a large amount of discovery about the functional and immunological significance of this T cell lineage, including front-line antimicrobial

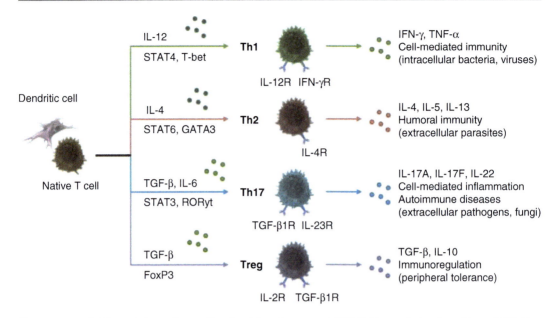

Fig. 29.2 T cell differentiation pathways (Reprinted from Leung et al. [29]. With permission from Nature Publishing Group)

defense via the innate immune response as well as the its pro-inflammatory role in several different immunological diseases such as psoriasis, the spondyloarthritides, including psoriatic arthritis (PsA) and axial spondyloarthritis, inflammatory bowel disease (IBD), and rheumatoid arthritis (RA).

TH17 cell differentiation is induced by IL-1β plus IL-23, and possibly TGF β in the presence of inflammatory cytokines such as IL-6, IL-21, and IL-23 [26]. Human TH17 cells produce IL17A through IL17F, IL22, IL26 and the chemokine CCL20. IL17A is more potent than IL17F, IL17E (also known as IL25) is involved in TH2 responses, and IL17B, C and D are less well characterized in terms of their biological significance [26]. In the quiescent state, IL17A and F are primarily observed in spleen and small intestine lamina propria cells. In inflammatory states, activated T cells, particularly TH17 cells are the main producers of both, but also CD8+, NK T cells, γ δ T cells, mast cells, neutrophils, myeloid and type 3 innate lymphoid cells may be sources [28]. The receptor is broadly expressed in the immune cell pathway and includes cells of the endothelium, epithelium, fibroblasts, keratinocytes, osteoblasts, monocytes, and macrophages

[28]. In a pioneering murine study, Sherlock and Cua found that injection of IL23 encased in minicircles preferentially gravitated to enthesial insertion sites and the aortic root where a local inflammatory reaction occurred involving a unique group of T cells which were CD3+CD-CD8-ROR-γt+IL23R+ [30]. The enthesitis inflammatory response was primarily driven by IL17 produced by these cells whereas IL22 expression activated STAT3-dependent osteoblast-mediated bone remodeling. Lories and McInnes have subsequently proposed the model that in humans, a variety of factors such as microbial antigens, alterations in the gut microbiome, the HLA-B27 unfolded protein response, biomechanical stress, and other factors may lead to expression of IL23 [31] (Fig. 29.3). IL23 then incites differentiation and activation of specific populations of T cells, including TH17 cells, which in turn produce cytokines such as IL17 and IL22 with IL17 driving an inflammatory response which may result in such consequences as bone erosion, in addition to clinical features such as inflammation in synovium and skin, whereas IL22 may, among other inflammatory activities, lead to osteoproliferation as is seen in the periostitis and ankylosis of PsA and ankylosis of

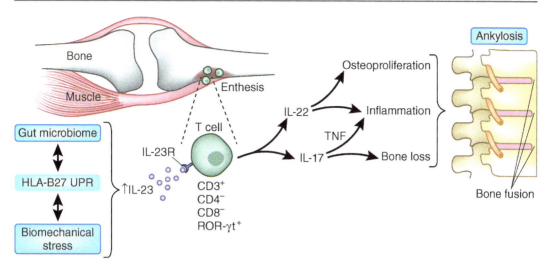

Fig. 29.3 IL-23 and resident T-cells promote enthesitis and osteoproliferation (Reprinted from Lories and McInnes [31]. With permission from Nature Publishing Group)

ankylosing spondylitis (AS). Such a model could help explain the fact that both osteolysis and osteoproliferation, seemingly opposite processes, are both seen in parallel in the SpA conditions. This model also posits a greater role for the innate immune system relative to the adaptive immune system, distinct from some other autoimmune diseases such as RA.

Numerous studies have shown that IL23, IL17, and IL22 are richly expressed in the psoriatic skin lesions and the synovium of PsA patients and participate in the pathophysiological aspects of these diseases including hyperproliferation of keratinocytes and promotion of synovitis [28, 32–35]. Inhibition of key cytokines in this pathway, including IL23 and IL17 results in clinical improvement in diseases such as psoriasis and the spondyloarthritides, as will be discussed in the following sections.

IL-12-23 Inhibitors

Ustekinumab

Ustekinumab is a fully human monoclonal IgG1 antibody which binds to the common p40 subunit of IL12 and IL23, thus inhibiting their activity and presumably, the T cell pathways which they influence, TH1 and TH17 respectively.

Ustekinumab is now approved by the FDA for the treatment of psoriasis and PsA in a weight based regimen: 45 mg for patients less than 100 kg and 90 mg for those that are greater. The drug is administered subcutaneously at baseline, 4 weeks, then every 12 weeks thereafter.

Ustekinumab was assessed in 2 phase 3 trials in psoriasis. In the first study, 766 patients treated with 45, 90 mg, or placebo achieved PASI 75 responses of 67.1, 66.4, and 3.1 % respectively at the primary endpoint of 12 weeks [36]. In the second study, PASI 75 responses in the 1230 subjects were 66.7, 75.7, and 3.7 % in the 45 mg, 90 mg, and placebo arms respectively [37]. Other key measures of response, including nail disease and quality of life also showed significant improvement. No major serious side effect issues emerged in these trials.

Ustekinumab was assessed in 2 phase 3 trials in PsA. In PSUMMIT 1, 615 patients who had inadequate response to methotrexate were randomized to receive 45 or 90 mg of ustekinumab vs placebo [38]. Ustekinumab was given at week 0, 4, and every 12 weeks thereafter subcutaneously. At the primary endpoint, week 24, 42.4 and 49.5 % of the 45 and 90 mg treated patients achieved ACR 20 response compared to 22.8 % of placebo-treated patients, statistically significant. Other key measures of enthesitis, dactylitis, skin and nail disease, function, and quality of life also improved. Similar rates of adverse events were noted between the groups and there were no opportunistic infections or major cardiovascular events. PSUMMIT 2 was similar in design but allowed two thirds of its subject population to have previously been treated with anti-TNF agents [39]. ACR20 response was observed in 43.7, 43.8 and 20.2 % of the 45 mg, 90 mg, and placebo treated patients in the overall population, and 36.7, 34.5, and 14.5 % of the anti-TNF-experienced population. In a separate report in which radiographic data from the two trials was pooled, inhibition of structural damage was observed, although this benefit was driven by the methotrexate inadequate response population from PSUMMIT 1 rather than the subjects from PSUMMIT 2 who had been previously exposed to anti-TNF therapy [40].

It is anticipated that development of this drug for the treatment of AS/axial spondyloarthritis will occur based on promising results from an open label trial in ankylosing spondylitis [41]. There is no published data for ustekinumab in rheumatoid arthritis.

IL-17 Inhibitors

Three IL17 inhibitors are in development and/or are approved for the treatment of psoriasis, psoriatic arthritis, and axial spondyloarthritis/ankylosing spondylitis, as well as other conditions, secukinumab, ixekizumab and brodalumab.

Secukinumab

Secukinumab is a human monoclonal IgG1k antibody that targets IL-17A, which has recently gained FDA approval for psoriasis. Two phase 3 52-week trials, ERASURE (Efficacy of Response and Safety of Two Fixed Secukinumab Regimens in Psoriasis) and FIXTURE (Full Year Investigative Examination of Secukinumab vs. Etanercept Using Two Dosing Regimens to Determine Efficacy in Psoriasis). In ERASURE, 738 patients and in FIXTURE, 1306 patients were randomized to subcutaneous secukinumab at doses of 300 mg or 150 mg administered once

weekly for 5 weeks then every 4 weeks thereafter, vs. placebo [42]. In the ERASURE study, PASI 75 was met at week 12 by 81.6 %, 71.6 % and 4.5 % with 300 mg, 150 mg and placebo respectively. PASI 90 was met by 59.2 %, 39.1 %, and 1.2 % respectively. In the FIXTURE study, PASI 75 was met by 77.1 %, 67.0 %, 44 %, and 4.9 % with 300 and 150 mg of secukinumab, etanercept 50 mg twice weekly, and placebo respectively. PASI 90 was met by 54.2 %, 41.9 %, 20.7 %, and 1.5 % respectively. All responses statistically separated from placebo. Improvements in nail disease, itch, and quality of life were also significant. Serious adverse events were infrequent and similar in frequency across all groups. There were no deaths. Rates of infections were similar across all three treatment arms, including etanercept, and were numerically greater than in the placebo arm. Candida infections, of specific interest because of the potential for IL-17 inhibition to increase the rate of these infections, occurred in a mild to moderate form in 4.7 % of the 300 mg, 2.35 of the 150 mg Secukinumab groups, and 1.2 % in the etanercept group, half of which were considered severe in the FIXTURE study. Grade 3 neutropenia occurred in 9 patients (1.0 %) in all Secukinumab groups and none in the etanercept or placebo groups. Rates for these adverse events were similar between the two studies.

Two phase 3 trials in PsA have recently been reported [43, 44]. FUTURE 1 enrolled 606 patients who were randomized to an IV loading dose of secukinumab, 10 mg/kg at baseline, week 2 and 4 and then either 150 mg or 75 mg every 4 weeks from week 8 vs. placebo. Thirty percent had received prior anti-TNF therapy and 60 % were on concomitant MTX, randomized equally. At 24 weeks, the 150 mg dose arm demonstrated 50.0 %, 34.7 %, and 18.8 % ACR 20/50/70 responses whilst the 75 mg arm demonstrated 50.5 %, 30.7 %, and 16.8 % responses and placebo arm 17.3 %, 7.4 %, and 2.0 % responses respectively. Key secondary measures of enthesitis, dactylitis, skin disease, radiographic evidence of inhibition of x-ray progression, function and quality of life all separated statistically from placebo in the treatment arms compared to placebo.

FUTURE 2 [45] enrolled 397 patients to receive subcutaneous Secukinumab 300 mg, 150 mg, 75 mg and placebo at weeks 1, 2, 3, 4 and every 4 weeks thereafter. Thirty-five percent had received previous anti-TNF therapy. ACR, enthesitis, dactylitis, skin, function, and quality of life responses were similar to those seen in FUTURE 1. However, analysis of the TNF inadequate response subgroup did demonstrate lower responses in the 75 and 150 mg groups as compared to the 300 mg group. Overall serious adverse events were few and similar in frequency between the treatment and placebo arms through week 16 in both studies. In FUTURE 1, overall infection rate was slightly greater in the secukinumab arm than placebo; there were no opportunistic infections, including TB.

Two phase 3 trials in AS have been recently reported as well. In MEASURE 1, 371 patients with AS were randomized to receive secukinumab 75, 150 mg subcutaneously every 4 weeks after a 10 mg/kg weekly × 4 loading dose or placebo. At 16 weeks, the ASAS20 responses were 59.7, 60.8, and 28.7 % respectively [46]. In MEASURE 2, subjects received either 75 mg or 150 mg secukinumab subcutaneously weekly X 4 followed by this dose every 4 weeks or placebo. ASAS20 responses were 41.1, 61.1 and 28.4 % respectively [47]. Other key measures, such as ASAS40, ASAS partial remission, and function measures also improved. No new safety issues emerged.

Interestingly, results with secukinumab in RA have not been as robust. In a phase 2 trial in 237 RA patients with an inadequate response to methotrexate, subjects receiving 25, 75, 150, and 300 mg of secukinumab demonstrated 36.0–53.7 % ACR 20 response vs. 34 % in the placebo group; no dose arm statistically separated from placebo [9]. On the other hand, it was noted that the continuous measure, DAS28, did show statistical separation as did hs-CRP reduction.

Ixekizumab

Another IL-17A inhibitor, ixekizumab, is in development for psoriasis and PsA. In a phase 2 study of 142 subjects with psoriasis, at 12 weeks, PASI 75 response in those treated with 25, 75, or 150 mg of ixekizumab at weeks 0, 2, 4, 8 and 12 was 76.7 %, 82.8 %, and 82.1 % respectively compared to 7.7 % in the placebo arm [48]. A 10 mg dose arm did not achieve statistical significance. In the highest two dose groups, 150 mg and 75 mg, PASI 100 response was noted in 39.3 % and 37.3 % respectively. Separation from placebo was seen as early as 1 week. No new safety issues were noted as compared to the secukinumab data, thus this agent appears to have overall similar good effect in psoriasis.

A phase 3 trial program in PsA is being conducted and results are pending.

Ixekizumab has been studied in a phase 2 study in RA [49]. In this trial, 260 biologic naïve and 188 patients with inadequate response to anti-TNF therapy were studied. Subcutaneous doses of 3, 10, 30, 80 and 180 mg of ixekizumab vs placebo were studied in the former group and 80 or 180 mg vs placebo in the latter group. At week 12 in the biologics naive group, ACR 20 responses of 45, 43, 70, 51, and 54 % in the 5 different drug doses vs placebo response of 35 %. Of these, only the 30 mg response seen in 70 % achieved statistical significance. In the anti-TNF inadequate response group, ACR 20 response of 40 and 39 % were seen vs placebo response of 23 %. These values were statistically significant. As was seen in the secukinumab RA study, significant response was seen in DAS28 improvement and CRP reduction, thus supporting the concept that there was some treatment effect of the agent even though a true dose response was not seen and most doses failed to achieve statistically significant ACR 20 response. No new safety signals were seen. It is not clear whether further development of this agent or secukinumab will occur in RA.

Brodalumab

Brodalumab is a fully human monoclonal antibody which blocks the IL17A receptor. Since this receptor joins with other IL-17R subunits to form the receptor complex for IL17A through IL17-F, it has the capability to broadly block IL17 signaling. As in the trials of the direct IL17A inhibitors, brodalumab has demonstrated significant efficacy in psoriasis. Effectiveness in psoriasis studies was similar to that seen with secukinumab, described above [50].

A phase 2 study in 168 PsA patients has been conducted with brodalumab [51]. At the pre-specified 12 week primary endpoint, ACR20 response was experienced by 37 and 39 % of 140 and 280 mg treated subjects vs 18 % in the placebo group, statistically superior for both treatment arms. As these same patients continued into open label use of brodalumab on these same doses, ACR20 responses were observed in 51 and 64 % respectively of the 140 and 280 mg treated patients. As a result of this observation, the primary endpoint in the phase 3 program will be extended beyond 12 weeks, as it appeared that in multiple clinical domains, responses were still increasing at that point in time. During the open label extension, 2 events of Grade 2 neutropenia occurred.

At the time of writing of this chapter, the brodalumab development program has been put on hold. Rare instances of suicidal ideation and suicide were noted, primarily in the psoriasis program. It is unknown whether this was related to a biological effect of the drug or background patient-related factors or both. Development hold was instituted because of the anticipated regulatory restrictions for its clinical use.

The IL17 inhibitors will not be studied in IBD. Pilot work suggests that there is no benefit for this disease and there could possibly be a signal of potential flare of IBD with IL17 inhibition, which is a caution.

IL23 Inhibitors

As previously discussed, IL23 is a key cytokine involved in the differentiation and proliferation of TH17 cells, thus acting upstream from IL17 expression and potentially capable of inhibiting the production of several different types of cytokines from TH17 cells and other immune cells, including both IL17 and IL22. Two IL23 inhibitors have reported preliminary results in the treatment of psoriasis and there is contemplation of their development in PsA and axial spondyloarthritis.

Guselkumab

Guselkumab is a human monoclonal antibody directed against the p19 subunit of IL23. In a phase 1 single ascending dose study, patient response was evaluated at 12 weeks after single doses of 10, 30, 100, or 300 mg of guselkumab [52]. PASI75 responses were demonstrated in 50, 60, 60 and 100 % respectively compared with 0 % in the placebo group. Adverse effect frequency was similar between the treatment and placebo groups.

Tildrakizumab

Tildrakizumab is a humanized IgG1/x antibody targeting the p19 subunit of IL23. A phase 2 study was reported at the American Academy of Dermatology in 2013. In 355 patients at 12 weeks, PASI75 response was reported in 33, 64, 66, and 74 % of patients receiving 5, 25, 100 and 200 mg of tildrakizumab vs 2 % of patients receiving placebo. A low rate of adverse effect was noted [53, 54].

Therapeutic Strategies with Biologic Therapy

Early Treatment

In an open label trial of MTX vs. MTX + infliximab, in early PsA patients not yet exposed to MTX, the RESPOND trial, significant better ACR and PASI responses were noted in the combination group [55]. A more substantial controlled trial is now initiating which will compare clinical and radiographic outcomes in early PsA patients being blindly randomized to MTX alone, anti-TNFα biologic alone, and combination of the two. This should give us a better understanding of the potential value of early intervention, as more substantial data on MTX and biologic monotherapy vs. combination therapy.

Avoidance of Immunogenicity

Because biologic agents are therapeutic proteins with varying degrees of "foreignness" to the human body, it is theoretically possible that antibodies to the therapeutic protein may be formed and have a potential effect of neutralizing or diminishing therapeutic efficacy. This has generally been seen most frequently with the chimeric antibody, infliximab, and with lesser frequencies with the human or humanized antibody constructs. Some observational registries have demonstrated decreased durability of use of anti-TNFα agent, presumably partly due to diminished efficacy with time, when used in monotherapy format vs. combination with MTX. An at least partial explanation of this observation is that MTX can function to diminish immunogenicity, which may be contributing to loss of efficacy in the monotherapy situation. This has most clearly been observed with infliximab and least with etanercept, of the three agents most studied in these registries, infliximab, adalimumab, and etanercept [13, 56]. Consideration should be given to use of MTX for this purpose.

Treating to Target

An evolving paradigm of rheumatoid arthritis treatment is that a combination of "tight control" and "treat-to-target" strategies (seeing patients frequently and trying to achieve a quantitative target of low disease activity or remission) yields better long-run disease control and clinical, functional, and radiologic outcomes [57, 58]. Although it has been assumed that a similar beneficial outcome would be seen in PsA [59], this had not been studied formally until the recent TICOPA trial [60]. When such a strategy was used in PsA, comparing a tight control arm aiming for Minimal Disease Activity (MDA) criteria [61], there were indeed significantly improved ACR and PASI response outcomes in the tight control vs. standard care arms [60]. However, it should be noted that there were more serious adverse events and greater financial costs due to greater combination and biologic therapy use in the tight control group.

Cost

Biologic therapy is expensive due to complex manufacturing processes and the cost of develop-

ment. In the future, forces which may bring cost down and make these agents affordable for more people globally include competition, as more products become available, and the introduction of "biosimilar" agents which closely mimic the pharmacokinetic properties of the innovator compound and which have been shown in clinical trials to yield results similar to the original innovator trials. Although rules of regulatory agencies are still evolving, it appears that if a biosimilar agent is effective in a disease such as rheumatoid arthritis, then it will be approved, with some possible exceptions, for other indications for which the innovator is approved, including psoriatic arthritis.

Conclusion

The treatment of PsA has been revolutionized in the last decade and a half by the introduction and use of biologic medications, therapeutic proteins which inhibit and modulate the effects of pro-inflammatory immune cells and cytokines. During this time, agents which inhibit the key cytokine TNFα have become widely utilized and consistently demonstrated to improve all clinical domains of PsA including arthritis, enthesitis, dactylitis, spondylitis, skin and nail disease, inhibit progressive joint damage as assessed by radiographs, and improve function, quality of life and fatigue. Serious side effects can occur, particularly infections, so for each patient a careful risk-benefit evaluation should occur to assure that use of the medicine makes sense in light of potential risk. In a minority of patients, the medicine may have no effect or yield side effects that do not allow continuation of use, and in a greater number, loss of efficacy occurs gradually with time. The latter may partly be due to immunogenicity, for which one therapeutic strategy is to use concomitant methotrexate. Whatever the reason, we need to cycle between agents – either to another anti-TNFα agent or to an emerging suite of biologics with a different mode of action, for example the IL12/23 inhibitor, ustekinumab. More recently, the IL17 inhibitors have shown significant promise in PsA in clinical trials.

Although they are not yet approved for use in PsA, it is anticipated that such approvals will be forthcoming and one agent, Secukinumab, is approved for the treatment of psoriasis. As our understanding of the pathophysiology of PsA increases, it is clear that new targets of treatment have been and will be identified for which new biologic treatment approaches will be developed, tested, and if successful and relatively safe, may be added to the therapeutic armamentarium for PsA.

References

1. Mease PJ, Armstrong AW. Managing patients with psoriatic disease: the diagnosis and pharmacologic treatment of psoriatic arthritis in patients with psoriasis. Drugs. 2014;74(4):423–41.
2. Acosta Felquer ML, Coates LC, Soriano ER, et al. Drug therapies for peripheral joint disease in psoriatic arthritis: a systematic review. J Rheumatol. 2014;41(11):2277–85.
3. Ritchlin CT, Kavanaugh A, Mease PJ, et al. Treatment recommendations for psoriatic arthritis. Ann Rheum Dis. 2009;68(9):1387–94.
4. Gossec L, Smolen JS, Gaujoux-Viala C, et al. European League Against Rheumatism recommendations for the management of psoriatic arthritis with pharmacological therapies. Ann Rheum Dis. 2012;71(1):4–12.
5. Mease P. Psoriatic arthritis and spondyloarthritis assessment and management update. Curr Opin Rheumatol. 2013;25(3):287–96.
6. Mease PJ, Gladman DD, Ritchlin CT, et al. Adalimumab for the treatment of patients with moderately to severely active psoriatic arthritis: results of a double-blind, randomized, placebo-controlled trial. Arthritis Rheum. 2005;52(10):3279–89.
7. Mease PJ, Fleischmann R, Deodhar AA, et al. Effect of certolizumab pegol on signs and symptoms in patients with psoriatic arthritis: 24-week results of a Phase 3 double-blind randomised placebo-controlled study (RAPID-PsA). Ann Rheum Dis. 2014;73(1):48–55.
8. Mease PJ, Kivitz AJ, Burch FX, et al. Etanercept treatment of psoriatic arthritis: safety, efficacy, and effect on disease progression. Arthritis Rheum. 2004;50(7):2264–72.
9. Kavanaugh A, McInnes I, Mease P, et al. Golimumab, a new human tumor necrosis factor alpha antibody, administered every four weeks as a subcutaneous injection in psoriatic arthritis: twenty-four-week efficacy and safety results of a randomized, placebo-controlled study. Arthritis Rheum. 2009;60(4):976–86.
10. Antoni C, Krueger GG, de Vlam K, et al. Infliximab improves signs and symptoms of psoriatic arthritis: results of the IMPACT 2 trial. Ann Rheum Dis. 2005;64(8):1150–7.
11. Mease PJ, Goffe BS, Metz J, et al. Etanercept in the treatment of psoriatic arthritis and psoriasis: a randomised trial. Lancet. 2000;356(9227):385–90.
12. Sterry W, Ortonne JP, Kirkham B, et al. Comparison of two etanercept regimens for treatment of psoriasis and psoriatic arthritis: PRESTA randomised double blind multicentre trial. BMJ. 2010;340:c147.
13. Fagerli KM, Lie E, van der Heijde D, et al. The role of methotrexate co-medication in TNF-inhibitor treatment in patients with psoriatic arthritis: results from 440 patients included in the NOR-DMARD study. Ann Rheum Dis. 2014;73(1):132–7.
14. Mease PJ, Ory P, Sharp JT, et al. Adalimumab for long-term treatment of psoriatic arthritis: two-year data from the Adalimumab Effectiveness in Psoriatic Arthritis Trial (ADEPT). Ann Rheum Dis. 2009;68(5):702–9.
15. Kavanaugh A, van der Heijde D, Beutler A, et al. Patients with psoriatic arthritis who achieve minimal disease activity in response to golimumab therapy demonstrate less radiographic progression: results through 5 years of the randomized, placebo-controlled, GO-REVEAL study. Arthritis Care Res. 2015.
16. Burmester GR, Panaccione R, Gordon KB, et al. Adalimumab: long-term safety in 23,458 patients from global clinical trials in rheumatoid arthritis, juvenile idiopathic arthritis, ankylosing spondylitis, psoriatic arthritis, psoriasis and Crohn's disease. Ann Rheum Dis. 2013;72(4):517–24.
17. Mease P, Genovese MC, Gladstein G, et al. Abatacept in the treatment of patients with psoriatic arthritis: results of a six-month, multicenter, randomized, double-blind, placebo-controlled, phase II trial. Arthritis Rheum. 2011;63(4):939–48.
18. Fonseca JE, Santos MJ, Canhao H, et al. Interleukin-6 as a key player in systemic inflammation and joint destruction. Autoimmun Rev. 2009;8(7):538–42.
19. Costa L, Caso F, Cantarini L, et al. Efficacy of tocilizumab in a patient with refractory psoriatic arthritis. Clin Rheumatol. 2014;33(9):1355–7.
20. Mease P, Strand V, Shalamberidze L, et al. A phase II, double-blind, randomised, placebo-controlled study of BMS945429 (ALD518) in patients with rheumatoid arthritis with an inadequate response to methotrexate. Ann Rheum Dis. 2012;71(7):1183–9.
21. Mease PJ, Gottlieb A, Berman A, et al. A phase IIb, randomized, double-blind, placebo-controlled, dose-ranging, multicenter study to evaluate the efficacy and safety of clazakizumab, an anti-IL-6 monoclonal antibody, in adults with active psoriatic arthritis. Arthritis Rheum. 2014;66(S10, abstract 952).
22. Celis R, Planell N, Fernandez-Sueiro JL, et al. Synovial cytokine expression in psoriatic arthritis and associations with lymphoid neogenesis and clinical features. Arthritis Res Ther. 2012;14(2):R93.
23. Mease PJ. Is there a role for rituximab in the treatment of spondyloarthritis and psoriatic arthritis? J Rheumatol. 2012;39(12):2235–7.

24. Mease P, Kavanaugh A, Genovese M, et al. Rituximab in psoriatic arthritis provides modest clinical improvement and reduces expression of inflammatory biomarkers in skin lesions. Arthritis Rheum. 2010;62(Suppl 10):S818.
25. Rouvier E, Luciani MF, Mattei MG, et al. CTLA-8, cloned from an activated T cell, bearing AU-rich messenger RNA instability sequences, and homologous to a herpesvirus saimiri gene. J Immunol. 1993;150(12):5445–56.
26. van den Berg WB, McInnes IB. Th17 cells and IL-17 a – focus on immunopathogenesis and immunotherapeutics. Semin Arthritis Rheum. 2013;43(2):158–70.
27. Miossec P, Korn T, Kuchroo VK. Interleukin-17 and type 17 helper T cells. N Engl J Med. 2009;361(9):888–98.
28. Frleta M, Siebert S, McInnes IB. The interleukin-17 pathway in psoriasis and psoriatic arthritis: disease pathogenesis and possibilities of treatment. Curr Rheumatol Rep. 2014;16(4):414.
29. Leung S, Liu X, Fang L, et al. The cytokine milieu in the interplay of pathogenic Th1/Th17 cells and regulatory T cells in autoimmune disease. Cell Mol Immunol. 2010;7(3):182–9.
30. Sherlock JP, Joyce-Shaikh B, Turner SP, et al. IL-23 induces spondyloarthropathy by acting on ROR-gammat + CD3 + CD4-CD8- entheseal resident T cells. Nat Med. 2012;18(7):1069–76.
31. Lories RJ, McInnes IB. Primed for inflammation: enthesis-resident T cells. Nat Med. 2012;18(7):1018–9.
32. Nestle FO, Kaplan DH, Barker J. Psoriasis. N Engl J Med. 2009;361(5):496–509.
33. Raychaudhuri SP. Role of IL-17 in psoriasis and psoriatic arthritis. Clin Rev Allergy Immunol. 2013;44(2):183–93.
34. Jandus C, Bioley G, Rivals JP, et al. Increased numbers of circulating polyfunctional Th17 memory cells in patients with seronegative spondylarthritides. Arthritis Rheum. 2008;58(8):2307–17.
35. Suzuki E, Mellins ED, Gershwin ME, et al. The IL-23/IL-17 axis in psoriatic arthritis. Autoimmun Rev. 2014;13(4–5):496–502.
36. Leonardi CL, Kimball AB, Papp KA, et al. Efficacy and safety of ustekinumab, a human interleukin-12/23 monoclonal antibody, in patients with psoriasis: 76-week results from a randomised, double-blind, placebo-controlled trial (PHOENIX 1). Lancet. 2008;371(9625):1665–74.
37. Papp KA, Langley RG, Lebwohl M, et al. Efficacy and safety of ustekinumab, a human interleukin-12/23 monoclonal antibody, in patients with psoriasis: 52-week results from a randomised, double-blind, placebo-controlled trial (PHOENIX 2). Lancet. 2008;371(9625):1675–84.
38. McInnes IB, Kavanaugh A, Gottlieb AB, et al. Efficacy and safety of ustekinumab in patients with active psoriatic arthritis: 1 year results of the phase 3, multicentre, double-blind, placebo-controlled PSUMMIT 1 trial. Lancet. 2013;382(9894):780–9.
39. Ritchlin C, Rahman P, Kavanaugh A, et al. Efficacy and safety of the anti-IL-12/23 p40 monoclonal antibody, ustekinumab, in patients with active psoriatic arthritis despite conventional non-biological and biological anti-tumour necrosis factor therapy: 6-month and 1-year results of the phase 3, multicentre, double-blind, placebo-controlled, randomised PSUMMIT 2 trial. Ann Rheum Dis. 2014;73(6):990–9.
40. Kavanaugh A, Ritchlin C, Rahman P, et al. Ustekinumab, an anti-IL-12/23 p40 monoclonal antibody, inhibits radiographic progression in patients with active psoriatic arthritis: results of an integrated analysis of radiographic data from the phase 3, multicentre, randomised, double-blind, placebo-controlled PSUMMIT-1 and PSUMMIT-2 trials. Ann Rheum Dis. 2014;73(6):1000–6.
41. Podubbnyy D, Callhoff J, Listing J, et al. Ustekinumab for the treatment of patients with active ankylosing spondylitis: results of a 28-week, prospective, open-label, proof-of-concept study (TOPAS). Arthritis Rheum. 2013;65(10 Suppl):S766.
42. Langley RG, Elewski BE, Lebwohl M, et al. Secukinumab in plaque psoriasis – results of two phase 3 trials. N Engl J Med. 2014;371(4):326–38.
43. Mease P, McInnes I, Kirkham B, et al. Secukinumab, a human anti–interleukin-17A monoclonal antibody, improves active psoriatic arthritis and inhibits radiographic progression: efficacy and safety data from a phase 3 randomized, multicenter, double-blind, placebo-controlled study. Arthritis Rheum. 2014;66(S10):S423.
44. van der Heijde D, Landewe R, Mease P, et al. Secukinumab, a monoclonal antibody to interleukin-17A, provides significant and sustained inhibition of joint structural damage in active psoriatic arthritis regardless of prior TNF inhibitors or concomitant methotrexate: a phase 3 randomized, double-blind, placebo-cotrolled sudy. Arthritis Rheum. 2014;66(S10):S424.
45. McInnes I, Mease P, Kirkham B, et al. Secukinumab, a human anti-interleukin-17A monoclonal antibody, improves active psoriatic arthritis: 24-week efficacy and safety data from a phase 3 randomized, multicenter, double-blind, placebo-controlled study using subcutaneous dosing. Arthritis Rheum. 2014;66(S10).
46. Baeten D, Braun J, Baraliakos X, et al. Secukinumab, a monoclonal antibody to interleukin-17A, significantly improves signs and symptoms of active ankylosing spondylitis: results of a 52-week phase 3 randomized placebo-controlled trial with intravenous loading and subcutaneous maintenance dosing. Arthritis Rheum. 2014;66(S10):S360.
47. Sieper J, Braun J, Baraliakos X, et al. Secukinumab, a monoclonal antibody to interleukin-17A, significantly improves signs and symptoms of active ankylosing spondylitis: results of a phase 3, randomized, placebo-controlled trial with subcutaneous loading and maintenance dosing. Arthritis Rheum. 2014;66(Suppl 10):S232.
48. Leonardi C, Matheson R, Zachariae C, et al. Anti-interleukin-17 monoclonal antibody ixekizumab

in chronic plaque psoriasis. N Engl J Med. 2012;366(13):1190–9.

49. Genovese MC, Greenwald M, Cho CS, et al. A phase II randomized study of subcutaneous ixekizumab, an anti-interleukin-17 monoclonal antibody, in rheumatoid arthritis patients who were naive to biologic agents or had an inadequate response to tumor necrosis factor inhibitors. Arthritis Rheum. 2014;66(7):1693–704.

50. Papp K, Leonardi C, Menter A, et al. Safety and efficacy of brodalumab for psoriasis after 120 weeks of treatment. J Am Acad Dermatol. 2014;71:1183–90.

51. Mease PJ, Genovese MC, Greenwald MW, et al. Brodalumab, an anti-IL17RA monoclonal antibody, in psoriatic arthritis. N Engl J Med. 2014;370(24):2295–306.

52. Sofen H, Smith S, Matheson RT, et al. Guselkumab (an IL-23-specific mAb) demonstrates clinical and molecular response in patients with moderate-to-severe psoriasis. J Allergy Clin Immunol. 2014;133(4):1032–40.

53. Tausend W, Downing C, Tyring S. Systematic review of interleukin-12, interleukin-17, and interleukin-23 pathway inhibitors for the treatment of moderate-to-severe chronic plaque psoriasis: ustekinumab, briakinumab, tildrakizumab, guselkumab, secukinumab, ixekizumab, and brodalumab. J Cutan Med Surg. 2014;18(3):156–69.

54. Leonardi CL, Gordon KB. New and emerging therapies in psoriasis. Semin Cutan Med Surg. 2014;33(2 Suppl 2):S37–41.

55. Baranauskaite A, Raffayova H, Kungurov NV, et al. Infliximab plus methotrexate is superior to metho-

trexate alone in the treatment of psoriatic arthritis in methotrexate-naive patients: the RESPOND study. Ann Rheum Dis. 2012;71(4):541–8.

56. Mease P, Collier D, Karki N, et al. Persistence and predictors of biologic TNFi therapy among biologic naïve psoriatic arthritis patients in a US registry. Arthritis Rheum. 2014;66(Suppl 10):abs 1853.

57. Smolen JS, Steiner G. Therapeutic strategies for rheumatoid arthritis. Nat Rev Drug Discov. 2003;2(6):473–88.

58. Smolen J, Breedveld F, Burmester G, et al. Extended report: treating rheumatoid arthritis to target: 2014 update of the recommendations of an international task force. Ann Rheum Dis. 2015 [Epub 12 May 2015].

59. Smolen JS, Braun J, Dougados M, et al. Treating spondyloarthritis, including ankylosing spondylitis and psoriatic arthritis, to target: recommendations of an international task force. Ann Rheum Dis. 2014;73(1):6–16.

60. Coates L, Moberley A, McParland L, et al. Results of a randomised, controlled trial comparing tight control of early psoriatic arthritis (TICOPA) with standard care: tight control improves outcome. Arthritis Rheum. 2013;65(Supp 10):814.

61. Coates LC, Fransen J, Helliwell PS. Defining minimal disease activity in psoriatic arthritis: a proposed objective target for treatment. Ann Rheum Dis. 2009;69(1):48–53.

62. Patel DD, Lee DM, Kolbinger F, et al. Effect of IL-17A blockade with secukinumab in autoimmune diseases. Ann Rheum Dis. 2013;72 Suppl 2:ii116–23.

Index

© Springer International Publishing Switzerland 2016
A. Adebajo et al. (eds.), *Psoriatic Arthritis and Psoriasis: Pathology and Clinical Aspects*,
DOI 10.1007/978-3-319-19530-8